LIFE
IN THE
BALANCE

《   》

Mickey S. Eisenberg, M.D., Ph.D.

LIFE
IN THE
BALANCE

« »

Emergency Medicine
and the
Quest to Reverse
Sudden Death

OXFORD UNIVERSITY PRESS
New York   Oxford
1997

Oxford University Press

Oxford   New York
Athens   Auckland   Bangkok   Bogotá   Bombay
Buenos Aires   Calcutta   Cape Town   Dar es Salaam
Delhi   Florence   Hong Kong   Istanbul   Karachi
Kuala Lumpur   Madras   Madrid   Melbourne
Mexico City   Nairobi   Paris   Singapore
Taipei   Tokyo   Toronto

and associated companies in
Berlin   Ibadan

Copyright © 1997 by Mickey S. Eisenberg

Published by Oxford University Press, Inc.,
198 Madison Avenue, New York, New York 10016

Oxford is a registered trademark of Oxford University Press

Library of Congress Cataloging-in-Publication Data
Eisenberg, Mickey S.
Life in the balance : emergency medicine
and the quest to reverse sudden death /
Mickey S. Eisenberg.
p. cm.   Includes bibliographical references and index.
ISBN 0-19-510179-0
1. Resuscitation—Popular works.
2. Sudden death—Popular works. I. Title.
RC87.9.E37 1997   615.8'043—dc20   96-36114

1 3 5 7 9 8 6 4 2

Printed in the United States of America
on acid-free paper

In memory of my parents
Mrs E. and Louie

CONTENTS

《 》

PREFACE

« »

The scream of a siren cuts through the air as you walk down the street. You look up to see an ambulance racing through traffic, on its way to an emergency. Somewhere, a man or woman has suffered a heart attack, or drowned, or in some other fashion swept past the edge of death.

A hundred years ago, that person would have almost certainly died. Today, he or she stands a fair to excellent chance of being brought back to life. *You* stand a fair to excellent chance of being brought back to life. For it could be you lying on the living room floor, or hanging from the power pole, or rescued from the ocean breakers. It could be you who has suffered sudden death. It could be you on whom the paramedics swiftly work, striving with all their might and technology, to pull you back over the line marking the boundary between the quick and the dead.

Humanity's journey from the inevitability of irreversible sudden death to the nearly routine ability to reverse the process of death has been a winding path, indeed. It begins with a grief-stricken mother who brings her lifeless child to a prophet and continues with, among others, a physician to gladiators, two London doctors who offered medals to good Samaritans, a Danish masseur, a Baltimore fire chief, smooth-talking medical quacks, and a crusty cardiologist. This improbable but true story also includes magnets, bellows, rectal tobacco smoke, frog legs, executed criminals, a miner overcome by fumes, the French Revolution, bells attached to coffins, "reanimation chairs," fresh corpses, polio epidemics, a long car ride from Kansas City to Baltimore, paralyzed subjects, electrocuted linemen, a serendipitous dog experiment, and a one-story hospital in Belfast.

Life in the Balance: Emergency Medicine and the Quest to Reverse Sudden Death is the story of that journey. For the first time in the million-plus years of our existence, we have the ability to reverse sudden death. It happens every day, in thousands of cities and towns around the world. It may be happening even as you read these words.

Successful cardiac resuscitation requires both the will and the way. The will is the human belief and desire that resuscitation is possible and should be attempted. The way is the physical means to resuscitate someone successfully. In 1600 neither the will nor the way existed. By 1760 the will was emerging from centuries of quiescence—but the way, the technology, was unknown. For 200 years, from about 1760 to 1960, various pioneers struggled with the knowledge available, but not until 1960 did the individual pieces come together and the means to achieve resuscitation become reality.

In *Life in the Balance* I have tried to keep jargon and medical usage to a minimum; though some terms are unavoidable, they are all defined. The book also includes a glossary of medical terms. In telling this history I may have drawn connections that perhaps never existed. Any faults of distortion or oversimplification are, of course, mine. It is also difficult to separate the perception of someone in the present from that of preceding generations. How exactly did prior generations view death? Was resuscitation a fantasy or something conceivable to them? When was death viewed as reversible?

In ancient times reversal of death required divine intervention. Today, it requires rapid CPR and defibrillation. How this came to be, and the individuals who brought it about, is the story of this book.

Seattle, Washington   M. S. E.
October 1996

ACKNOWLEDGMENTS

« »

I am indebted to many individuals who so willingly gave of their time and energy; without their assistance *Life in the Balance* would not be what it is today.

First, I wish to thank "John and June Colven" who allowed me to describe John's sudden death and resuscitation. My interviews with them proved to be a moving experience—they are determined to lead the fullest lives possible and refuse to let John's sudden death turn them into emotional cripples. I wish them many more fulfilling and enjoyable years.

Second, I salute the paramedics, emergency medical technicians, and emergency dispatchers who saved John's life. They did a perfect job, and I know the fulfillment they feel. In addition, I would like to acknowledge the dedication and professionalism of the emergency medical technicians, paramedics, and emergency dispatchers not only in Seattle and King County, Washington, but throughout the world. They face an exceedingly difficult job. Their professional lives consist of 90 percent routine responsibilities punctuated with moments of adrenalin-fueled high stress. The sorrow of unsuccessful resuscitation is balanced by the joy of snatching life from the jaws of premature death. They stare mortality in the face, and appreciate life's preciousness.

I am especially grateful to the people who agreed to be interviewed for this book, and who freely shared their recollections. They include: Ellen Adams, Pyramid Films, Santa Monica, California; David Allen, paramedic, Seattle Medic-1; Greg Brace, paramedic, Seattle Medic-1; John Chadbourn, M.D., St Vincent's Hospital, New York; Leonard Cobb, M.D., University of Washington, Seattle; Richard Crampton, M.D., University of Virginia, Charlottesville, Virginia; Michael Criley, M.D., UCLA, Los Angeles, California; James Elam, M.D. (who died in 1995), Valpairiso, Indiana; John Geddes, M.D., University of Manitoba, Winnipeg; Archer Gordon, M.D., Ph.D. (who died in 1994), Los Angeles, California; Claude Haggard, Medford, Oregon, James Jude, M.D., University of Florida; Jack Howard, Seattle, Washington; K. Garth Huston, Jr., M.D., Del Mar, California; Guy Knickerbocker, Ph.D., Emergency Care Research Institute, Plymouth Meeting, Pennsylvania; Costas Lambrew, M.D., Maine Medical Center; Richard Lewis, M.D., Ohio State University, Columbus, Ohio; Bernard Lown, M.D., Brigham and Women's Hospital, Brookline, Massachusetts; Martin McMahon, Baltimore, Maryland; Eugene Nagel, M.D., Winter Haven, Florida; Frank Pantridge, M.D., Belfast, Northern Ireland; Leonard Rose, M.D., Portland, Oregon; Peter Safar, M.D., University of Pittsburg; Felix Steichen, M.D., New York City; Henry Thomas III, M.D., Will Rogers Pulmonary Research Labs, White Plains, New Jersey; Dan Yerkovich, Physio-Control Corporation, Redmond, Washington; Paul Zoll, M.D., Boston, Massachusetts.

Several colleagues at the University of Washington created opportunities and welcomed me into the world of emergency medicine and emergency medical services. In particular I wish to thank Gil Omenn, M.D., Ph.D., Robert Petersdorf, M.D., Loren Winterscheid, M.D., Ph.D., Philip Fialkow, M.D., Ph.D., Paul Ramsey, M.D., Leonard Cobb, M.D. and Michael Copass, M.D.

Many others gave assistance of various kinds. Albert Jonson, Ph.D., James Whorton, Ph.D., Keith Benson, Ph.D., and Jon Bridgman, Ph.D., all of the University of Washington, were immensely helpful in offering an overview and suggestions on where to begin. Tom Hearne, Ph.D., King County Emergency Medical Services Division, Seattle, shared insights into the history of resuscitation. Dick Dickenson, Royal Humane Society, London, loaned me valuable original source material from the eighteenth century. Martha Fulton and Sheryl Stiefel, Museum of History & Industry, Seattle shared material from their collection of medical devices. Nancy Caroline, M.D., Metulla, Israel, gave me many insights into key individuals from the sixties. Pat Evans, London, helped me track down a painting and her husband, Tom Evans, M.D., shared some interesting references. Walter La-Strange, Bellevue Hospital, New York, provided photos of early ambulances from Bellevue Hospital. Robert Niskanen of Physio-Control Corporation, Redmond, Washington, and Carl Morgan of Heartstream Corporation, Seattle, gave me physics lessons in joules. James Green, R.N., San Francisco Department of Public Health, Paramedic Division, supplied information about emergency medical services in San Francisco during the late 1960s. Susan Lucius, American Heart Association, Dallas, Texas, provided original source material on Heart Association CPR committee meetings during the 1960s. W. Douglas Weaver, M.D., University of Washington, taught me subtleties of cardiac physiology and defibrillation. My colleague Richard Cummins, M.D., kindly interviewed Paul Zoll and Guy Knickerbocker on my behalf, and offered many helpful perspectives on the history of resuscitation. Tore Laerdal, Stavanger, Norway, offered valuable insights into the topic of resuscitation and, most important, served as an unwavering friend who constantly encouraged me in this undertaking.

Elizabeth Ihrig, Bakken Library and Museum, Minneapolis, Minnesota, provided invaluable aid in finding original seventeenth- through twentieth-century manuscripts and material. Her colleague Albert Kufeld, Ph.D., willingly explained how the electrical devices in their fine collection worked. I also appreciate the tireless efforts of many librarians at the University of Washington, especially those at the Health Sciences Library. Robin Maberry was particularly helpful in tracking down obscure references.

For secretarial and research assistance I am grateful to Judy Prentice and Gussie Litwer of the University of Washington. Susan Damon, of the King County Emergency Medical Services Division, assisted in writing the Glossary. Shelly Dixon, also of the Emergency Medical Services Division, transcribed many interviews. Marsha Donaldson, of the University of Washington, helped solve some perplexing word-processing problems. Rowena Lee, Stacey Levine, and Sherry Smith, also of the University of Washington, along with my son David Eisenberg, spent countless hours organizing and obtaining copyright permissions for the illustrations. My daughter, Devora Eisenberg, as well as my other son, Daniel Eisenberg, assisted with typing and bibliographic work. Peggy McKinley helped reproduce illustrations with clarity and attention to detail. I also happily acknowledge a study grant from the Bakken Library and Museum of Electricity in Life, as well as the University of Washington for its ongoing support and encouragement of this project.

Over the last eighteen years my associates at the Emergency Medical Services Division of the Seattle-King County Department of Health have taught me what I know about emegency medical services and have opened doors of opportunity. I am grateful for their support and friendship. My sincere thanks to Health Department directors Larry Bergner, M.D., Bud Nicola, M.D., Jess Tapp, M.D., David Lurie, and Alonzo Plough, Ph.D.; Division Managers Del Tilton, Dick Landis, Jill Marsden, Judy Pierce, and Steve Call; research associates, Tom Hearne, Ph.D., Linda Becker, Deborah Berger, Barbara Blake, Sheri Schaeffer, Linda Culley, Jill Clark, Judy Graves, Elena Andresen, Rosalie Wendt, Jessica Schubach, Susan Damon, Richard Cummins, M.D., Hendrika Meischke, Ph.D., and Mary Ho, M.D.; medical directors Christy Horton, M.D. and Jack Murray, M.D.; biostaticians Alfred Hallstrom, Ph.D., Paul Litwin, M.S., Mary Pat Larsen, M.S., Dan Henwood, and Eric Duhlberg, Ph.D.; paramedics Ed Stuhlman, and Bill Marsh; EMT trainer Tom Torell (who died in 1990) and Douglas Austin; program coordinator Linda Culley; and data coordinator Jill Clark.

I am especially grateful for the hundreds of hours my brother, Melvin Eisenberg, and his wife, Rosalie Eisenberg, spent scouring antique shops in Michigan, Connecticut, Illinois, Indiana, Ohio, and Nevada for historic medical electrical devices. Mike Riggins, at the University of Washington Scientific Instruments Department, used his wizardry to put them all in working order. I learned a great deal examining these machines and experiencing firsthand what the electric therapies felt like. I can categorically state that the violet ray hair attachment does not cure thinning hair, but it sure is a hair-raising experience. I was tempted to try all the attachments, but there is a limit to my curiosity.

My agent, Joshua Bilmes, never lost faith in this project and I thank him for his perseverance. Joan Bossert, editor at Oxford University Press, was immensely helpful. Considering that I accepted virtually all of her suggestions, I'd say she was batting almost 1000. Rosemary Wellner assisted with the final editing. Her green pencil curbed my literary excesses and I thank her for a fine job.

My wife, Jeanne, was a constant source of support. As I slavishly hunched over the computer keyboard, her tolerance and unflagging encouragement only confirmed why we have been the closest of friends for twenty-eight years.

I am profoundly grateful to Joel Davis who helped me throughout the writing of the book. He was a consultant, editor, guide, and mentor. An accomplished scientific writer himself, Joel wrote the first drafts of most of the profiles. He also edited and improved the entire text. I can't say whether the book would have been published without his help, but I can say it would have been a lot less readable.

Last, the historian David Lindberg in his preface to *The Beginnings of Western Science,* expresses my sentiments exactly: "If this list is remarkable for its length, I can only explain that I needed all the help I could get."

PROLOGUE

《 》

Everything just went black. I didn't see any light
at the end of a tunnel, and there certainly weren't any angels singing.
—John Colven

APRIL 1991

《　》

On April 6, 1991, at 12:50 P.M., John Colven died.[1] Twenty minutes later, he was brought back to life. A miracle? Perhaps—but a "miracle" with a long history, and one that happens every day in cities and towns around the world. It is the miracle of modern-day resuscitation.

For John Colven and June, his wife of forty years, it was simply a miracle that gave them back their life together.

John had no premonition that anything unusual was about to happen that early April afternoon. He and June had lived for many years in the same affluent community south of Seattle, bordering a golf course where he enjoyed playing eighteen holes with his friends. He was in reasonably good health, still active and vigorous, though he had infrequent attacks of chest pains and was suffering from diabetes. And his smoking didn't help—John knew he should stop, but every time he tried it was too uncomfortable. It wasn't worth trying anymore.

Each person has two "electrical circuit boxes," one near the top of the heart and one in its center, both helping the heart to keep a steady beat. Normally the circuit boxes work silently and efficiently, signaling the heart to pump tens of millions of times a year (about thirty-one million beats per year, at a rate of sixty beats per minute). In John Colven's heart the circuit boxes were about to short out. John had been having mild chest pain—mostly when he overexerted himself—and his doctor had placed him on two drugs, Norpace and Procardia, to help with the problem. It seemed to be working—at least enough so that the doctor discontinued the Norpace.

For the last several days John had felt mildly fatigued. It was nothing specific; maybe a virus, he reasoned. He had always been physically active, and worked for years in the construction industry. He enjoyed using his body, loved golf, and enjoyed traveling with June. The enjoyment had been wearing off for some time, though; Colven could feel his body slowing down. He was only sixty-two.

John himself says today, "I'm like most other people. I still feel I'm going to live forever, even though I know intellectually that's not true." That day, however, John Colven's lifeline came close to permanently breaking.

John and June had purchased a painting during their last visit to Hawaii. On the morning of April 6, John Colven went to a local picture framing store to pick up the newly framed artwork. He came home and hung the painting. Feeling very tired, he decided to go to the bedroom and take a nap. All these things he did on the day he died. He knows he did, because his wife and friends have told him so. But John still has no recollection of them. In fact, he can remember nothing of his life from four hours before his cardiac arrest until three days after he was taken to the hospital.

Shortly before noon, June went to see how her husband was doing. She was only mildly concerned about his lack of energy. After all, what's so out of the ordinary about a little tiredness?

When June entered the room John was lying facedown on the bed. As she later recalled: "He rose up and made this horrible noise. It was just as though he was really trying to get a tremendous breath, and it caught in his throat. And then he just went—flat." To her, John's breath sounded like the worst snore she had ever heard. It seemed almost demonic.

John's desperate attempt to breathe lasted only one or two seconds. Then it was over. He recalls no feeling of pain (of course; he can remember nothing of those hours or days). He didn't clutch his hands to his chest in some histrionic movie-scenario action. He simply tried to grab one breath, could not, and collapsed back onto the bed.

John Colven had suffered cardiac arrest. His heart's electrical system had short circuited and his heart was unable to pump any blood to his body or brain. His attempt at breathing was not a normal respiration—it was the respiration triggered by a brain not receiving any oxygen. His rate of breathing had suddenly gone from a normal rate of about fifteen per minute to less than four. When the brain is deprived of oxygen, this "agonal" or death-like respiration will stop within two to three minutes. Brain death—final death—soon follows.

June Colven knew at once that something terrible had happened. She suspected the worst—but the worst, as she would later recall, "was simply not an acceptable alternative for me. Absolutely not."

"John!" she screamed. "John! Don't you do this to me!" Almost instinctively, she wrestled his large inert body over onto its back, leaned over him, placed her mouth on his—and breathed out. "His mouth was clenched so tight, so tight," she remembers. "I just literally yanked his mouth open." Completely untrained in the medical technique of cardiopulmonary resuscitation (CPR, as it is popularly known by its initials), she still knew enough from TV shows casually seen and educational broadcasts barely overheard to do the right thing at the right time.

Then she did the second right thing at the right time. "I gave him one quick breath," June recalled, "and at the same time I reached for the phone."

She dialed 911.

"It was very quick, the time that it happened and the time I got to the telephone. They were in close proximity, and there wasn't any time to think about it," June said. "It was very obvious that this was something that John was not going to come out of—you know, where I could sit him up and say, 'Well! Don't you ever do anything like that again!' He was gone."

When John Colven had collapsed, his heart went from a normal beat of about eighty per minute to a rhythm known as ventricular fibrillation, or VF as it is commonly called. In ventricular fibrillation the heart begins to quiver uncontrollably. Blood pressure drops to zero; the pulse in the body disappears; within five seconds the person becomes unconscious. Because the heart is ineffectually quivering, no blood supply gets to the body's organs and brain.

At the moment of ventricular fibrillation a person is clinically dead. Consciousness, pulse, blood pressure, bodily response—all stop. The person appears dead, but there is a fleeting potential for reversal. If the body is deprived of blood flow and oxygen for more than about five minutes, there is no possibility of restoring pulse or blood pressure. In Colven's case, if nothing more had happened—if no efforts had been made to revive him—his state of clinical death would have become biological death within five minutes. The chance of resuscitating him would have been lost forever.

June Colven dialed 911 from the bedroom phone, and in so doing trig-gered a complex and highly effective emergency medical response. It was 12:52 P.M.: only two minutes had passed since John had taken his horrifying agonal breath. After only three rings a specially trained 911 dispatcher answered, "Fire department emergency."

The first words out of June's mouth in reply were her address. Normally calm and melodious of voice, she now sounded nearly panic-stricken. But again she did the right thing.

"What is the problem?" asked the dispatcher, his voice calm, soothing, but commanding instant respect and response.

"Please!" June sobbed, "I need an ambulance. I think my husband's had a heart attack."

"Is he conscious?"

"No!" Sobbing. "No!"

"OK, where is he right now?"

"Yes. He just breathed—he can breathe, my God!"

"Ma'am, ma'am," the dispatcher interrupted, trying to get her back on track. The information he was gathering was absolutely vital to saving John Colven's life, and he needed it now.

June cried, "He's not dead!"

"Ma'am, the aid car is coming now." The dispatcher had sent Aid Unit 33, staffed with three firefighters, from the Federal Way Fire Station and Medic Unit 8, carrying two paramedics, from its headquarters at Auburn General Hospital, eight miles from the Colvens. This all happened unheard by June. The dispatcher pushed several buttons on his console and entered numeric codes designating which units to send. He was following standard proce-dures. Determine the address—always get the address first—then the nature of the problem. If it's a minor problem, dispatch the closest aid unit. In this case Aid Unit 33 was only a mile from the Colvens' home. If it's a major problem, send both the aid unit and the medic unit simultaneously. Sending both allows the aid unit's trained personnel to arrive quickly and begin emer-gency treatment. The medic unit, literally a mobile emergency department, arrives several minutes later to take over and provide definitive care. It's not possible to have a medic unit on every street corner, but this system is the next best thing.

"OK," said June, calming down a bit.

The dispatcher asked, "Can you tell me if he's breathing normally?"

"No, he's not."

"Do you know how to do C——"

She interrupted the dispatcher, screaming, "He just took a deep breath but he's not doing anything!" John Colven had taken another agonal breath. His body was fighting desperately to live—to get a little oxygen to its brain—anything—a few more instants of anything at all.

"Ma'am, ma'am, do you know how to do CPR? I can give you instructions," said the dispatcher.

June replied, "I'm going to try."

"Do you need help?" the dispatcher asked again, trying to get as much clarity on the situation as possible. "I can give you instructions."

"Please! Please!" cried June, talking over him.

"Do you need instructions?"

"Yes, please."

The dispatcher then "walked" June through the steps leading to CPR. First, June got the phone next to the bed where John lay and turned him over so he was faceup. She could not get him onto the floor, which would have given her a solid and unyielding surface on which to work. That wasn't essential, though, since he was now at least faceup on the bed. The dispatcher quickly moved her to the next step. Following his instructions, she stripped John's shirt off his chest, knelt by his side, pinched his nose with one hand and with the other lifted John's chin so his head bent back.

"OK," said the dispatcher. "Completely cover his mouth with yours and force two deep breaths of air into his lungs, just like you're blowing up a big balloon."

"I'm listening. I'm listening."

"OK, you do that—get the two breaths in. OK?"

"OK."

"OK. Now, remember, flat on his back, strip the chest, pinch the nose. OK."

June gave her husband two big breaths of air as the dispatcher waited at the other end. First, the breaths: now, the chest.

"Now, I want you to put the heel of your hand—ma'am?" he stopped to check that June was at the phone.

"Yes."

"Put the heel of your hand on the center of his chest, right between the nipples."

"Yes."

"Put the other hand on top of that hand—"

"Yes"

"Push down firmly on the heels—"

"Yes!"

"—one and a half to two inches. Do that fifteen times, and count for me. One . . . two . . . three . . . "

"three" June pushed and counted.

"Four"

"Four"

"Five"

"Five"

"Six"

"Six—Oh, come on, honey," June begged, "breathe!"

The count-up continued, the dispatcher and the wife counting from one to fifteen, the wife's breathing getting heavier and more labored as she pushed down on her husband's chest, counting up and pressing down, pushing as if her life depended on it, as if his life depended on it. "Fourteen."

"Fourteen"

"Fifteen"

"Fifteen"

"OK, I want you—ma'am?" said the dispatcher. "Ma'am, we're going to give him two more breaths now." June gave her husband two more breaths, counting "One" and "Two" after each one. "Now we're going for fifteen compressions," he continued. "OK. Fifteen compressions, now. One . . . "

"One"

"Two"

"Two"

They moved through the count-up again. At "fifteen" June suddenly heard someone at the door. "I think they're here," she cried to the dispatcher. "Oh my God, they're here!" June dropped the phone on the floor and ran to the front door.

It was 12:54 P.M. Incredibly, only two minutes had passed since June had dialed 911, four minutes since John Colven had collapsed clinically dead on his bed. The aid unit quickly pulled up in front of the manicured lawn of Colvens' well-kept one-story home. The three firefighters, all trained as emergency medical technicians (EMTs)—Mark McNally, Jerry Nevin, and Robert Wallace—grabbed their equipment and trotted to the front door. McNally was carrying a machine called a defibrillator, designed to provide an electrical shock that would restart the heart. Nevin brought a ventilation kit consisting of bags and mouthpieces to open an airway and provide a person with life-sustaining oxygen. In one hand Wallace carried an all-purpose aid kit with bandages, splints, and other paraphernalia; in the other he held a green metal cylinder of compressed oxygen.

June let them in and quickly led them to the bedroom. She picked up the phone.

"They're here!" she cried, relief pouring from her voice.

"Ma'am," the dispatcher said, "stay on the phone for just a minute. Ask them if they've got CPR." The dispatcher wanted to confirm that John had indeed suffered cardiac arrest. If so, he would pass this information on to the paramedics in Medic 8; perhaps they would drive a little faster knowing this was "the real McCoy" and not a false alarm.

"Do you have CPR?" June asked the EMTs as she held the phone to her ear.

"Are they doing what you were doing?" the dispatcher asked.

"Yes, but not right now. They're setting up for it."

"OK," he replied. "That's fine. Tell them they have another medic unit coming."

"Thank you!" said June. "Thank you so much!"

The three EMTs quickly moved John from the bed to the floor, and continued the CPR June had begun just minutes before. They started a small tape recorder to make a record of everything they did and said. The EMTs were trained to verbally describe what they were doing while they did it. Later, the medical director of the EMT-defibrillation program, Dr. Richard Cummins, would review the recording and evaluate their performance. McNally pulled some cables from a small pouch connected to the defibrillator and attached the machine to John.

"We have a sixty-two-year-old male. We had telephone CPR in progress when we got here," said McNally to no one in particular.

"He does have a heart condition," June interrupted.

"Does he?" said Jerry Nevin.

"OK, we're hooking up the Lifepak, white to right," said McNally. "Boy, we've got a lot of hairy chest here. And red to ribs. Go ahead." The Lifepak McNally mentioned was the defibrillator. The reference to white and red had to do with the color of the cables, which needed to be attached to different areas of John Colven's chest. Meanwhile, Jerry Nevin continued to do CPR.

"OK, we're going to analyze," McNally said to Nevin. "Stop CPR."

The machine they were using was an automatic external defibrillator. Once attached to a person's chest, it could automatically interpret the heart's rhythm. Such "smart" defibrillators, developed in the 1980s, are now standard equipment in many fire department aid units. The patient could not be touched or jiggled before or during the analysis because it would throw off the machine's interpretation. If the rhythm was ventricular fibrillation, the machine would advise the operator to deliver a shock. It took about six seconds to analyze the heartbeat and another five to charge up for the shock.

The machine advised a shock to John Colven's heart. McNally ordered his partners to stand clear—a safety measure to prevent anyone touching John from getting shocked by the electrical charge. He pressed the shock button and called out (for the tape), "Shock delivered."

It was about 12:57 P.M., just seven minutes since John Colven had died. "Reanalyzing; stand clear," McNally said. The machine analyzed the heart's reaction to the shock. Nothing. Colven was still in ventricular fibrillation. McNally ordered a second shock.

John Colven's heart began beating normally again. Another emergency medical technician was "breathing" for John. He had a bag over John's mouth and a tube down his throat to keep his tongue from getting in the way. The oxygen bottle was attached to the bag, delivering 100 percent oxygen. The technician compressed the bag fifteen times per minute. Once more, oxygenated blood began moving through Colven's body, replenishing his organs and brain.

"Do we have a pulse?" McNally asked. "I've got a pretty good rhythm here."

"Yeah, we do," said Nevin, "a real weak one."

"OK, well keep up with the respirations."

"Oh, come on," said June to her still-unconscious husband. "Don't do this to me!"

Less than a minute later, it happened again: John Colven's heart went into ventricular fibrillation. McNally pressed the "analyze" button and the machine advised a third shock. "Stand clear," he ordered. "We're gonna go ahead—OK, I am clear. Everybody's clear." He pushed the shock button. "Shock delivered. OK, reanalyze—don't touch the patient." It was not enough. They delivered a fourth shock. Again Colven's heart jumped back into normal rhythm. Again his organs and brain were flooded with oxygenated blood. The EMTs noted that John now had a strong pulse rate and blood pressure, both good signs.

Medic Unit 8 arrived at the Colven home at 1:03 P.M., nine minutes after June Colven's call. It was staffed by two paramedics, Tony Scoccolo and Doug Weigand. Like all paramedics, they were highly trained in emergency medicine. In order to be certified they had completed a one-year course in emergency management with special training in how to treat sudden cardiac death.

Paramedics can give definitive care at the scene of critical emergencies. Like EMTs, they carry defibrillators,[2] but because of their advanced training paramedics can administer emergency medications and intravenous fluids and insert endotracheal tubes into the trachea for advanced airway control. They can be likened to a hospital emergency room on wheels. Paramedics reached national attention through their portrayal in *Emergency!*—the dramatic and successful TV series of the 1970s. *Emergency!* showed paramedics in constant radio contact with an emergency room doctor. The show was accurate in that respect for its time. Today, however, standing orders issued by the program's medical director authorize paramedics to provide immediate care at the scene without requiring radio contact with a hospital emergency room. Once they have established a strong pulse and blood pressure, the paramedics contact the local hospital for further instructions and approval from the emergency physician.

John and June Colven were fortunate to live in King County, Washington. Fifteen medic units are scattered throughout that county, with an average response time of just ten minutes. Because there are many more of them—more than a hundred throughout the entire county—the local fire department aid units can arrive at an emergency scene more quickly than the medic units. The aid units have an average response time of five minutes. The result is a "tiered" or layered emergency response system. The first tier is the aid unit staffed with firefighters trained as emergency medical technicians. The second is the medic unit with the paramedics. The third tier is the hospital emergency room. But below the first tier is the most important part of the system: people like June Colven, who either know CPR themselves or can follow a 911 dispatcher's instructions—and do it well enough the first time to bring a person back from the dead.

McNally quickly briefed Scoccolo and Weigand on the status of their patient. As he did, the two paramedics went into action. First, they attached electrodes from their defibrillator to John Colven's chest. McNally reported, "After the second shock we got a rhythm, and then he went back to VF."

Scoccolo nodded acknowledgment, then said, "Set up an IV for Doug. We need to get some lidocaine on board." The instruction was to put an intravenous tube into John's arm and give him lidocaine, a drug that helps keep the heart's rhythm stable and prevents it from slipping back into ventricular fibrillation. "I want you to turn the lidocaine drip open to a drop every two seconds," Weigland advised one of the EMTs.

Then, "He's in VF—start CPR," he ordered. John Colven's heart had once again reverted to the chaotic tremors of ventricular fibrillation. One of the EMTs began CPR and Weigland prepared to shock John's heart yet again. He did a final check before he simultaneously pressed the red button on each paddle—"everybody clear"—and the shock was delivered.

"Shocking back into supraventricular rhythm," Weigand announced. "It's seems pretty regular." The regular nature of the pulse was a very good sign and meant that the heart was able to beat normally on its own, so long as the fibrillation didn't return.

Someone else called out, "He's breathing on his own, about twenty a minute."

"We have the lidocaine drip going. We want to give him another 100 of lido. Okay let's go ahead and intubate now." By "intubate," Weigland was instructing his partner to put a tube down John Colven's trachea. This would not only help him breathe easier, but would also keep material in his stomach from possibly getting up into his throat and lungs."

"Now he's going about ninety; he looks like a sinus rhythm." Sinus rhythm is the normal human heartbeat. The ninety stands for ninety beats per minute. Colven was alive again, with his heart once more sending blood to his brain and body.

The paramedics and EMTs spent a few extra minutes checking Colven over, making sure he was getting enough air, sufficient lidocaine, and had a strong heart rhythm. They took his blood pressure, checked for other possible injuries he might have suffered, and prepared to administer some additional medications. While Scoccolo did a final check and stabilization prior to departure for the hospital, Weigland began the inevitable paperwork. Every time EMTs and paramedics respond to an emergency call, they must complete a detailed incident report form. Sometimes the forms describe resuscitations in which the last entry shows zero blood pressure and a flat line on the ECG followed by a cryptic "DC efforts," meaning discontinue efforts of resuscitation. But this time the outcome was strong vital signs with an excellent prognosis; it would be a pleasure to compete the form.

"OK, Tony," said Weigland at last, "get ready to move him." John Colven was about to take his third trip of the day. The first had been to a frame shop. This one would be to the hospital. Between the journeys by car and ambulance, he had made yet another.

To death and back.

O, that I could but call these dead to life!
—William Shakespeare, *King Henry VI*

JUNE 1778

《 》

John Colven is fortunate to live where and when he does. Four key factors made his journey to death and back possible:

- His wife performed artificial respiration that oxygenated his blood.
- Artificial circulation brought the blood to his brain and heart.
- Defibrillation restored a normal heart rhythm.
- A system of emergency services moved quickly enough so that the first three happened before death became irreversible.

It is an easy system to activate; merely dial three numbers on the telephone. Yet behind this simple act lies decades and centuries of effort.

Resuscitation in times past was founded on intuitive—but erroneous—principles. Some of those historical techniques bear a striking resemblance to today's methods. Yet those early "correct" methods were jumbled together with a hodgepodge of competing and often incorrect measures. For resuscitation to succeed, the proper techniques must be applied quickly—literally within minutes. That kind of swift response was not possible until the mid-1960s. In the past, people simply did not understand the physiology of death.

What, then, *was* sudden death like 200 years ago? How would the rescue effort and techniques of resuscitation differ from those of today? What were the chances of returning to life? Here's a look at how it used to be, based on an actual event from the records of the Royal Humane Society in London.[1]

The Humane Society was established in 1774 to promote resuscitation, or reanimation as it was then called, of victims of drowning or other accidents. The Humane Society was the eighteenth-century equivalent of today's emergency medical services. Heart disease as a cause of sudden death was considered rare in the 1700s. Most sudden, unexpected death was accidental, and drowning was by far the most common accident.

The date is June 1778, just two years after John Hancock put his pen to the Declaration of Independence. The location is the banks of the River Stour, at the small country village of Chilham near Canterbury, England. It is late morning and the maid servant, Mary Macintyre, is carrying her employer's one-year-old son for a stroll along the river. ("Mary" is a made-up name. The account, written by a Dr. Mantill, does not disclose the maid's identity— patient confidentially is an age-old tradition.) Mary is employed by Thomas Thompson, the town's miller. What begins as an idyllic walk will inexplicably end in a double drowning. The circumstances are somewhat obscure—all the account states is that "It was at least fifteen minutes before she was missed; how long she had been in the water from that time is uncertain, but by the water being clear and still about the place, it was conjectured she had not struggled or disturbed it for near the above period."

Today, two centuries after this real-life event, the questions beguile us: How could both the maid and the baby be in the water? Was this really an accident? Perhaps Mary slipped on a rock, striking her head as she fell, with heavy clothing weighing down both her and the child. Or perhaps Mary was despondent. Did her low station in life and the lack of future prospects plunge her into despair? Was she pregnant with an unwanted child—her employer's? Such a situation was hardly uncommon. Perhaps Mary was working under intolerable conditions, and her rage got the better of her. Was the double drowning a botched murder—an attempt to kill the child of her employer and call it an accidental drowning? The account remains silent, though there is enough doubt for the circumstances to be justly called a "supposed" accident.

Once Mary and the baby were found and the alarm sounded, it took fifteen minutes to pull them from the water. The rescuers carried them to the miller's house, and another twenty minutes elapsed before Dr. Mantill could be summoned. By now nearly an hour had probably passed since the two had fallen into the water and drowned. Both Mary and the Thompson baby were described as "totally dead." Until the doctor arrived, no one attempted to revive the victims. This is not surprising, since it is unlikely that anyone had ever even heard of the Royal Humane Society—much less read any of its recommendations for reanimation.

Not so Dr. Mantill—he was aware of the Society's "Methods of Treatment of Drowned Persons," which outlined resuscitative measures. Generating heat was the first step recommended by the Humane Society. A variety of methods were used at the time, including rubbing wool or flannel (preferably warmed), warmed rock salt or ashes, or heated brandy over the body. It was also recommended practice to place the victim in a warmed bath or cover the body with heated sand, stones, or grains. And it was suggested that "if the body be of no great bulk," a naked person lie next to victim and change position frequently. Applying friction or heat was both intuitive as well as supported by countless observations made of near-drowning victims. In a near drowning, the victim is cold when pulled from the water, and as breath returns the body begins to warm. Of course, this is a classic example

FIGURE I.   *1787 engraving of a young man being taken out of a river, apparently dead, in sight of his distressed parents; by Robert Pollard (1755–1838) after Robert Smirke (1752–1845). (Courtesy of Wellcome Institute Library, London)*

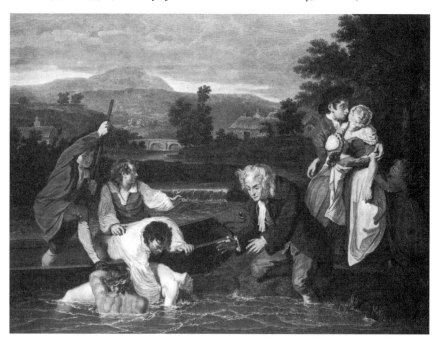

of confusing cause with effect. The breathing causes the warmth to return to the body, but to the untutored it appears as though the return of heat makes the breath become visible. In actuality, the breath and pulse are often initially imperceptible.

Dr. Mantill followed the first recommended step. He ordered the baby undressed and placed before a large fire, and Mary carried upstairs, undressed, and put in bed. He directed a bystander to use friction to warm the baby's skin. The bystander rubbed his hand quickly back and forth over the baby's body. The doctor next asked that flannel and warmed clothing also be rubbed over the baby's skin for additional warmth. Dr. Mantill then ordered that warm wood ashes from the hearth be rubbed on Mary's body. He also asked for warmed rock salt to be placed on her abdomen, arms, and legs.

By this time Dr. Mantill's father, a surgeon, had also been summoned to help with the resuscitation. On the advice of his father, Dr. Mantill proceeded to blow into the baby's mouth. Although the exact technique is not described, one can only assume that the nose was pinched closed and sufficient air exhaled into the mouth to cause the baby's chest to rise—concrete evidence that mouth-to-mouth artificial breathing was a lifesaving technique used in the eighteenth century. As we will later see, this method eventually fell out of favor—only to be rediscovered in 1954.

The two doctors also held "volatile spirits" (a liquid form of smelling salts) under the baby's nose and rubbed some of the fluid to the baby's temples. These administrations achieved the intended results. The Humane Society record notes: "Soon we had the pleasure, and the mother the inexpressible joy, of perceiving he showed some small signs of life, which increased, and continued still more visible." The child survived, and in a few days was well, "likely to become a useful, if not a valuable member of society," as the records somewhat tactfully phrase it. The possibility of poor neurologic outcomes following resuscitation was presumably appreciated in 1778.

The obviously successful reanimation spurred the doctors and bystanders to greater efforts on Mary's behalf. Activity centered around providing stimulants to the lifeless body. The rationale for stimulation stemmed from the prevailing belief in the "vital principle" of life—an inclusive term referring to the activity of the brain and nervous system. Even if circulation or respiration ceased, the vital principle existed for a period of time, and had the potential, if accompanied by proper stimulation, of restoring life. Belief in this vital principle came about in part from experiments with the newly discovered energy called electricity. Long after an animal died, electricity could still evoke a muscular contraction. With enough stimulation, reanimation itself might occur. Today we know that oxygenated blood is essential for life, including a properly functioning nervous system, so restoring circulation should have the highest priority. But 200 years ago scientists and doctors had the sequence backward. They recommended stimulating the nervous system first, which they believed would restart breathing and circulation. To some extent their reasoning was correct; at least they had noted the close relationship of circulation to the proper functioning of the brain and nerves. They erred, however, in assuming that the vital principle lasted for a considerable period. At the time of Mary's attempted resuscitation it was thought that the vital principle could remain alive for up to several hours. In reality, the vital functions of the nervous system can last only about four minutes before permanent damage occurs.

Dr. Mantill first held volatile smelling salts under Mary's nose and rubbed the potent smelling liquid on her temples. Because of the temples' proximity to the brain, many scientists believed it was a nearly direct route to stimulating the nervous system. The technique did not work. Mantill next tried a more potent stimulant—tobacco smoke in the rectum. This approach required a bit of setting up, but most of the apparatus was readily at hand. Mantill grabbed a bellows from the fireplace and placed a tube from his bag on the nozzle end. He then asked for tobacco smoke (a pipe was quickly offered) to be vigorously puffed into the tube, filling up the bellows. Next he inserted the tube in Mary's rectum and compressed the bellows, expelling the smoke directly into her large intestine. Tobacco smoke is a potent stimulant and Mantill knew from his scientific reading that this technique was reported to be both safe and effective. But again, it was to no avail.

Since the mouth-to-mouth breathing for the baby seemed to have helped, the doctor decided to try it on Mary. In eighteenth-century England, the practice of placing one's mouth on the mouth of a lifeless adult was considered particularly repugnant. Mantill instead inserted a tube into one nostril and, closing the other as well as his mouth, proceeded to blow into the tube. Most of the air entered Mary's stomach, and as he saw the abdomen begin to protrude, Mantill decided the effort was counterproductive. Mary was faceup, and her tongue and soft tissues at the back of her throat had fallen backward, blocking her airway. The only place for the air to go was down the esophagus into the stomach, something not understood in those days.

Dr. Mantill would likely have read the first report of the Humane Society in 1774, in which electricity was used to stimulate life back into a drowning victim four hours after every other measure had failed. Unfortunately, Mantill did not have the proper equipment to generate electricity, or almost certainly he would have tried using it.

As a last resort, Mantill removed a scalpel from his bag and made an incision directly over Mary's jugular vein. Bleeding was recommended for drowning in order "to relieve congestion, which almost constantly occurs in the veins of the head, and is probably a frequent cause of the death of drowned persons." Not surprisingly, considering the lack of circulation, only a small ooze of blood emerged. Mantill took this as a bad sign, and, after conferring with his father, decided to stop the reanimation attempt. Over two hours had passed since Mary was recovered from the water.

Why did the baby live, and not the maid? It is impossible to know, given the paucity of details about the length of submersion. Perhaps the baby may have floated on the surface for a while. A more likely explanation involves the ability of a baby's brain to better tolerate lack of oxygen compared to an adult brain. Within four minutes of submersion, Mary had suffered irreversible brain damage. The baby may have been able to survive up to ten minutes without oxygen. In addition, the water temperature could have been low enough to slow the brain's metabolism, protecting it from irreparable damage for another several minutes. Because the baby's brain was so small, it would have cooled very quickly—certainly more rapidly than Mary's adult-sized brain.

Did the techniques of 1778 really save the Thompson baby? Based on what we know today about resuscitation, it's doubtful. More probably, the baby had a very weak pulse and shallow respirations, too imperceptible for either the bystanders or the two doctors to notice, but enough to sustain life. The heating techniques undoubtedly helped, but little else did. Even the mouth-to-mouth breathing, which we know today is an essential component of CPR, was delivered far too late to be meaningful.

At the same time, it's easy to see why the Humane Society's rules and methods had so many believers. All it would take is one or two "saves" to reinforce such totally unsubstantiated practices as bleeding and tobacco stimulation. The supposed logical connection between tobacco smoke in the rectum and reanimation certainly would have seemed unassailable then. In fact, it was a false connection, as were most of the other "logical" and "totally proven" resuscitation techniques of that era. We humans have brains that are built to detect patterns, to find connections. Most of the time, our "connec-

tion finders" work quite well. The downside is that we often perceive patterns or connections where none exist.

The attempt to resuscitate Mary did not succeed, but two aspects of that
attempt are rather remarkable. The first and most important is that it even
took place. As we will see, the quest to reverse sudden death has not been a
constant in human history. Second, many of the components of modern
resuscitation were already being advocated more than two centuries ago. In
particular, the methods of mouth-to-mouth respiration and electric shocks to
the chest were almost identical to today's techniques. But without consistent
success, these techniques quickly fell into obscurity. A multitude of competing—and usually unsuccessful—recommendations took their place. Medicine in the eighteenth century was empirically based. Techniques that seemed
to work received support from the medical community. What didn't got
dumped. And because effect and cause were often confused, wheat got
thrown out at least as often as chaff. Sadly, some valuable techniques were
lost. It would be 200 years before several courageous and stubborn men
rediscovered them.

Part I

THE QUEST

《 》

If I'd known I was going to live this long, I'd have taken better care of myself.
—Eubie Blake

THE MOMENT OF DEATH

《　》

The Sudden Death of John Colven

John Colven's death was sudden and totally unexpected—one moment active and animated, the next moment stilled and flaccid, with the silence broken only by his deathlike rattle. Regrettably, sudden death occurs thousands of times per day in the United States. It happens in homes, at work, in malls, and on freeways. It can take place during the most mundane of activities—raking leaves, washing dishes, watching a video. Why does it occur? Is there any way to prevent it?

Sudden death is caused by underlying heart (or cardiac) disease; therefore it is often referred to as sudden cardiac death.[1] The event can be defined as the sudden and complete loss of circulation in a person not expected to die at that time. Since it is unexpected, most sudden deaths occur outside hospitals. What's more, sudden death is truly sudden, though the collapse may often be preceded by minutes or sometimes an hour or two of heart symptoms such as chest pain.

Heart disease is the leading cause of death in industrialized countries. This simple statement belies both the true magnitude of the problem as well as its emotional impact. In the United States, heart disease accounts for almost one million deaths per year, twice as many as all cancers, ten times as many as all accidents, and forty times as many as AIDS. To put it another way, if the deaths from heart disease could be reduced by only 5 percent, there would be almost twice as many lives saved as currently die from AIDS in one year. The economic cost is staggering, estimated at $125 billion per year. If heart disease magically disappeared tomorrow, the savings could double the amount the nation spends on education. This figure of $125 billion is a cold economic statistic—It can't possibly begin to indicate the disease's emotional impact.

Sudden cardiac death usually strikes men in their early sixties, and women in their seventies. This age difference reflects the earlier onset of heart disease in men than in women. But it is not uncommon for the disease to strike people in their forties or fifties. They are not only vigorous, active, productive members of society, they are husbands, wives, parents, and grandparents.

The only good piece of news in these otherwise grim figures is that heart disease has decreased 35 percent in the last decade. The probable reasons include improvements in life style (less smoking, more exercise, low-cholesterol and low-fat diets), and better health care and medications.[2] Despite this reduction, heart disease is still our leading killer.

John Colven had heart disease before his sudden death, but his disease was mild and well controlled with medications. We often think of the heart, which essentially is a specialized muscle, as a pump, but actually it is four pumps. Two, the right and left ventricles, are the large pumps that supply blood to the body and lungs. The other two, the right and left atria, are much smaller pumps that serve as antechambers for propelling the blood into the ventricles. The heart muscle is supplied with nutrient and oxygen-containing blood by heart arteries (coronary arteries). Even though the heart chambers are constantly bathed in blood, the muscle requires its own internal supply of blood. In addition to the blood supply through the coronary arteries, the heart has an electrical system that signals it to contract rhythmically and repeatedly.

The most common form of heart disease, and what Colven had, is a partial blockage caused by a buildup of fat in the coronary arteries. This is known as *atherosclerosis*, the medical term for fat deposits in the lining of the artery wall. The heart muscle does not receive enough nutrients and oxygen, and it responds with pain. The pain is not unlike a muscle cramp. When it occurs in the heart muscle, it is known as angina. "Angina" means "gripping," which is the sensation described by people feeling this type of pain.

A more serious form of heart disease is a complete blockage of the coronary artery. Such a blockage destroys the portion of the heart muscle down-stream from it. The medical term for this is *myocardial infarction*. A myocardial infarction (MI) is not necessarily fatal. If only a small part of the heart is damaged, the person can go on to lead a normal life. If a large portion of the heart is destroyed (more than 40 percent of the muscle), death is inevitable.

A common expression often used to describe heart disease is "heart attack." This is an imprecise term and often refers to a spectrum of disease ranging from angina to sudden death. Nevertheless, it is very descriptive and clearly tells what is happening—namely, a person feels as if attacked because the heart suddenly fails or becomes damaged.

Colven had several episodes of angina, but his heart suffered no permanent damage. He was leading a normal life and enjoying his retirement. While he complained of fatigue and went to lie down, he said nothing to his wife about chest pain. John cannot recall the moments before his sudden death, so it is not completely clear whether he experienced any pain. From other patients with sudden death who are resuscitated, we learn that approximately half experience symptoms, usually chest pain, even if only for a few minutes or seconds. The other half have no symptoms whatsoever. Presumably, the group with symptoms is having a partial or complete blockage of a coronary artery, thus leading to chest pain. The other group is experiencing primary ventricular fibrillation. Perhaps this group is also experiencing partial blockage, but without symptoms, a condition known as silent angina.

During a previous checkup Colven's doctor had noticed some irregular heartbeats. An electrocardiogram showed extra beats, called premature ventricular contractions. John was only vaguely aware of this irregular heart rate and sometimes felt his heart skip a beat or experienced a fluttering sensation in his chest for a second or two. John passed it off as being insignificant, but his doctor was not as unconcerned. He realized that these premature contractions are dangerous in someone with underlying heart disease and therefore placed John on a medication to help control those premature beats. Because the extra beats happen randomly (in John's case, six to ten times per minute) they can occur at a vulnerable time in the cardiac cycle and trigger ventricular fibrillation (VF). These premature beats are somewhat like tiny lit matches thrown into a room with a glass of gasoline sitting on the floor. If one match happens to land in just the right spot, the room will catch on fire. Similarly, if the extra beat occurs at just the right split second, it will trigger fibrillation. These premature contractions are very common and millions of people have them. They are dangerous, however, only in individuals with underlying heart disease. The diseased heart is apparently more sensitive to the effects of the extra beats.

John reported no aura or out-of-body experience. As he put it, "The lights went out." Death itself was not painful. The many out-of-body experiences described by patients are probably associated with near-death situations completely different from Colven's sudden death. In a near-death experience the brain is not receiving enough blood and dreamlike visions can occur. In sudden death the brain receives no blood and no dreamlike states are possible.

Colven's heart progressed from a normal beating heart rhythm to a fatal rhythm, literally in an instant. The heart's electrical signaling system went haywire. It was like an orchestra, in revolt against the rhythmic beat of the conductor's baton, suddenly deciding to play random and cacophonous notes. The heart changed from a powerful pump into a seething mass of fibers feebly quivering. If you could observe the heart at the moment of ventricular fibrillation, you would see it appear to wiggle chaotically. Some have described it as a bag of worms undulating. At the instant of fibrillation, the heart pumps no blood, so the pulse is lost and blood pressure falls to zero.[3] The goal of a defibrillatory shock is to jolt the heart into a momentary standstill. In other words, the electric current causes all the heart's muscle cells to contract at the same instant in response to the electricity. All these cells will discharge simultaneously and thereby become synchronized. This eliminates the chaotic pattern of contractions so that all the cells have the chance to march together again in an orderly fashion.

Colven's heart went into VF with no warning, other than mild fatigue. Such an event would be called primary VF—in other words, there was no identifiable precipitating event. Primary VF accounts for approximately half of all sudden cardiac deaths. The remaining 50 percent result from myocardial infarction or angina. In a myocarcial infarction there is damage to the heart muscle cells that causes leakage of irritating enzymes; this in turn can trigger VF. During angina, a portion of the heart muscle is inadequately supplied with oxygen and nutrients. For reasons poorly understood, this lack of oxygen may set off an episode of VF.

When John's heart went into fibrillation, events happened fast and Death's stopwatch began counting down. At this point he was, by definition, clinically dead. In other words, he was totally unresponsive to external stimuli. There was no evidence of life, no consciousness, no reaction to stimuli, no movement. He became a mass of dying cells. In approximately four to five minutes, his state of clinical death would begin to turn to biologic death. By fifteen minutes, biologic death would be complete.

This "window of opportunity" to reverse clinical death is brief and with each passing minute the likelihood of resuscitation diminishes. When John's heart fibrillated, his heart stopped pumping blood and thus blood circulation ceased. With the onset of fibrillation, John lost consciousness. If June had attempted to take a pulse, she would have found none. Every cell in John's body was suddenly deprived of oxygen and nutrients carried by the bloodstream. In addition, the blood could no longer carry off waste from the cells and toxic substances began to build up. Each cell is like a tiny furnace. It requires fuel (oxygen, sugar, and other nutrients) and removal of its combustion products (acids, carbon dioxide). Complex biochemical processes continually occur in normal cells. During stress or periods of no oxygen, a different set of biochemical reactions takes place. Certain organs of the body are more sensitive than others to loss of oxygen. The brain is by far the most sensitive.

If the brain is deprived of oxygen, unconsciousness occurs within seconds. All the oxygen stores in the brain are used up within ten to fifteen seconds. Normally, atoms of sodium, potassium, and calcium travel back and forth across cell membranes. This constant movement maintains the proper chemical balance between the outside and inside of the cell. With depletion of oxygen, this reciprocal pumping of atoms ceases. Calcium begins to accumulate within the cell because it cannot be pumped outside. Chemical chain reactions start that break down the genetic material within the cell's nucleus. Once this happens, the cells are irreparably damaged since the genetic code, which serves to regulate all activity including repair and reproduction, is destroyed. A by-product of all this damage is the production of acid within the cell that then enters the bloodstream. Normally, the blood contains the proper balance of acids and bases. Too much acid or too much base is fatal, and only a narrow range of balance is compatible with life. This acid reaches a plateau within ten to fifteen minutes. The sugar within the brain cells (known as glucose) is depleted within five minutes. Glucose is almost as critical as oxygen since sugar serves to fuel all the chemical reactions within the cell. Without glucose there is no potential for brain recovery. Once the glucose is depleted, an acceleration of destructive and irreversible processes begins. If there is restoration of circulation after just ten minutes of total cardiac arrest, there will probably be irreversible brain damage. The longer the interval without CPR, the greater the damage.

When the heart goes into the fatal rhythm of fibrillation, time-dependent critical events begin to occur within its muscle cells. The events in the heart are only slightly less time- critical than those in the brain. Initially the fibrillation is very coarse. There is still energy in the individual heart muscle cells to contract, even though these contractions are occurring in a totally chaotic and unorganized fashion (and thus pumping no blood). The heart muscle is itself supplied with blood from the coronary arteries at the base of the aorta. With fibrillation the forward flow of blood within the coronary arteries ceases. As the heart remains in fibrillation, the oxygen, glucose, and other nutrients are consumed without being replenished. The strength of each cell's contractions weakens. Within fifteen minutes the contractions disappear completely.

The heart is now in a state called asystole, which means "no motion." At this time the heart is completely dead with no chance of resuscitation. If John Colven had an electrocardiogram monitor attached to him at the moment of collapse, the pattern on the monitor screen would go from an organized normal rhythm to the chaotic ventricular fibrillation. If June did not do CPR, the fibrillation pattern on the monitor would become smaller and smaller, until at about fifteen minutes when there would be only a straight line, or asystole. The potential of the heart to convert from fibrillation to a normal rhythm is directly related to the duration of fibrillation. As the fibrillation becomes weaker and weaker, the chances of converting to a normal rhythm become very small.

CPR delays the onset of irreversible damage in the brain and heart by keeping a flow of oxygenated blood circulating throughout the vital organs.[4] This flow is far from normal and probably achieves only ten to thirty percent of normal circulation. However, this trickle of oxygenated blood entering the carotid arteries and reaching the brain and the coronary arteries is better than nothing. It's enough to slow the dying processes within the cells, particularly the sensitive brain cells. By itself, CPR cannot defibrillate a heart that is fibrillating. This requires an electric shock delivered by a defibrillator. But CPR can buy time until the defibrillator arrives.

Within one minute of John Colven's sudden collapse and the onset of fibrillation, June began CPR. Her efforts allowed both John's brain and heart to receive oxygenated blood. When the EMTs arrived several minutes later, John's heart was still in a coarse pattern of ventricular fibrillation. Had June not performed CPR, the heart would have been more difficult or even impossible to convert to a normal rhythm. More important, had she not done CPR John might have been resuscitated but with brain damage. Her actions, along with the assistance of the emergency dispatcher, kept John's brain alive.

Why Does Sudden Death Happen?

What causes the heart to fibrillate? Why do only some episodes of angina and infarction lead to fibrillation? Unfortunately, no straightforward answers exist for these straightforward questions. Determining them is the greatest challenge facing cardiology today. The lack of definitive answers does not preclude speculation and many possible reasons have been put forth. Theories about why the electrical disturbance occurs range from irritation in the heart muscle to the influence of emotions and stress.

Can Sudden Death Be Prevented?

Could Colven's sudden death have been prevented? Since the exact trigger of sudden death is not known, it's impossible to design a specific prevention. But since sudden death is associated with heart disease, it follows that if heart disease can be eliminated, so too can sudden death. Regrettably, heart disease cannot be prevented, at least with our current understanding. Exercise, proper diet, control of high blood pressure, and, perhaps most important, quitting smoking can help delay or retard heart disease, but we do not know how to prevent it.

This is not to belittle the benefit of reducing risk factors. For example, a smoker has a 50 percent increase in likelihood of heart disease compared to a nonsmoker. A smoker who has high cholesterol has a 300 percent likelihood of heart disease compared to a nonsmoker without high cholesterol. And if the person also has high blood pressure, the risk of heart disease goes up almost 400 percent compared to someone without these three risk factors.

No one can peer into a crystal ball to determine how death will come. Yet this obvious reality should not lead to fatalism. I have heard so many patients and friends respond to advice about heart disease with, "Well, something's got to kill me." I find such reasoning silly, though I try to keep my moralistic comments to myself. Sure, something is going to kill all of us, but why play Russian roulette?

It all comes down to risk factors and probabilities. Reduce—better yet, eliminate—risks and you delay or even prevent heart disease. Some risks cannot be changed—genetic inheritance, for example. Some can be changed only with concerted effort by many people—legislation to prohibit smoking in public places, for example. But some can be changed through personal choice. A person decides whether or not to exercise, to eat low-cholesterol and low-fat foods, to take medications for high blood pressure, to smoke. Smoking is, in my mind, the top of the personal risk pile, but admittedly more problematic since its addictive property complicates the element of choice. Virtually all smokers want to stop smoking. (All three of my children started smoking as teenagers—the power of peer pressure is impressive—and only one has been able to quit.) I think in a hundred years historians will look back on our era and marvel at the addictive poisons we tolerated in our society.

The limitations in knowledge and inability to prevent heart disease in no way detract from the remarkable accomplishment of resuscitation. Colven's resuscitation and countless others may truly be called a miracle. Death, the eternal and dreamless sleep, was not permanent. Life was restored—a feat consigned to the gods or fantasy in previous generations. True, it wasn't the ultimate miracle of immortality itself—death is, after all, still inevitable. But its premature visitation, though allowed to cross the threshold of mortality, could now unceremoniously be ushered back. Sudden and untimely death was reversed.

The fear of some divine and supreme powers keeps men in obedience.
—Robert Burton (1577–1640)

THE FIRST
RESUSCITATION

« »

Death is part of my job. I work in a university hospital emergency room and I have trained paramedics and accompanied them on resuscitations. Admittedly this gives me a rather skewed view. I don't see the quiet, ideally peaceful, and painless deaths that conclude a terminal disease. These happen in hospital rooms, nursing homes, or private residences. Hospice nurses have a different image of death. Mine is of a person wearing street clothes, whose pockets and purses are filled with keys, coins, credit cards, and photos of loved ones, who only a few minutes ago was fully animated and is now silent and still. I see sudden death and my image is that of someone walking on a glacier snow bridge that suddenly breaks, plunging the person into a bottomless crevasse. The person is too startled to even shout for help. And my job, like that of countless other emergency personnel, is to throw a lifeline in time to reach the falling victim and while there is still enough "life" or energy to catch and hold onto that line. It's the suddenness I have such a hard time accepting.

John Colven made the journey to death and back. Two hundred years earlier, Mary Macintyre didn't. The resuscitations were completely different, yet each was motivated by an unwillingness to accept premature and sudden death. How we reached that motivation and how we achieved the skill to succeed is a story peopled by some remarkable individuals.

Yet the quest to reverse sudden death is not a struggle against death itself.

Instead, it is a struggle against death that rudely arrives unannounced. It is one thing to accept death in a body wasted with the ravages of disease; it is quite another to accept death in a seemingly healthy person. Sudden death in the eighteenth century was mostly the result of accidents. Today's epidemic of heart disease was unknown 200 years ago. For one thing, people usually did not live long enough to develop heart disease. For another, heart disease may have been less frequent because of diet, exercise, lack of smoking, or other factors.

The most unacceptable type of sudden death is that in which the body appears normal. Mutilating accidents, however horrific, can at least be understood as an irreversible process. But in drowning or suffocation there is no disfigurement or distortion of the body, making death appear all the more unfair. Today, drownings and suffocations are an uncommon cause of accidental death—motor vehicle accidents and urban violence head the list. However, accidental deaths pale in frequency to death from heart disease, a far more stealthy killer.

As we have seen with the death of John Colven, it frequently arrives totally unannounced. There are few causes of death that occur so unexpectedly, and certainly none so common. (Perhaps the only other condition that can cause death in a matter of seconds is rupture of a cerebral aneurysm, a burst vessel in the brain—a relatively infrequent event.) The affront of ventricular fibrillation is that the body and even the heart itself can look completely normal. The only defect is a small disruption in the electrical signal to the heart. It's like a million dollar piece of machinery failing because of a defective twenty-cent fuse. Ventricular fibrillation is the quintessential sudden death—occurring in the community, often with no warning, striking in the prime of life.

When was the first successful resuscitation? Did it begin in biblical times? During the eighteenth-century Enlightenment? Or with the first human defibrillation in 1947? Or with the rediscovery of chest compression in 1959? What about the establishment of the world's first mobile coronary care unit in 1966—was that the start of modern resuscitation?

We could choose each of these dates—and for that matter, many others. And yet no single date is really accurate. The selection of a specific date or event implies an epochal event that led directly to modern practice. It just didn't happen that way. For one thing, many different discoveries had to occur, since resuscitation involves complex procedures. Each discovery had its own timeline and a unique history.

The very act of reversing death has a history clouded in obscure begin-nings. Technology—procedures and devices—must make the intervention possible, but the culture itself must question deaths's final sentence and want to bring its victims back to life. Moreover, the causes of sudden death have changed. Sudden death in the premodern era meant death from accidents such as drowning, smoke inhalation, or trauma. Today sudden death is usu-ally the result of ventricular fibrillation caused by heart disease. The history I unfold here will tell of the discoveries and devices, the cultures that came to believe that death was reversible, and the event of death itself. The begin-nings of such a history, alas, lie far in the past, out of our reach.[1]

Sudden Death and Resuscitation in Ancient Times

Imagine what must have gone through the prehistoric man's mind as he encountered death. He saw life—its vivacity, glistening eyes, coherent thought, moist lips, warm skin, and all its other hallmarks—suddenly turned to a cold, inanimate corpse. Did prehistoric man cry in pain? Did he shake the body and rail at the mysterious forces in the universe? Did he attempt to breathe into the body? Did he attempt to warm it? Did he accept death's irre-versibility?

The breath of life is an ancient image. In Genesis, the graphic account of God breathing the breath of life into Adam could properly be called the first "suscitation." The etymology for suscitation is *suscitare*, Latin for "to stir up, arouse, excite."

The first written account of a resuscitation is that of Elijah the Prophet. The story in the Hebrew Bible tells of an anguished mother who brings her lifeless child to Elijah, but the incident itself is related in Kings I: "And the son of the woman, the mistress of the house, became ill; and his illness was so severe that there was no breath left in him." Unwilling to accept her son's death, the grief-stricken mother carried her lifeless child to Elijah who had been staying in her home. The prophet placed her son on his own bed and prayed to the Lord. Then he stretched himself on the child three times, and crying out, "O Lord my God, let this child's life return to his body." The account continues: "And the Lord hearkened to the voice of Elijah, and the soul of the child came into him again, and he revived." To Elijah and onlook-ers, it was clear that the prophet brought the child back to life with the assis-tance of God. It is not clear what action is meant by the phrase "stretched

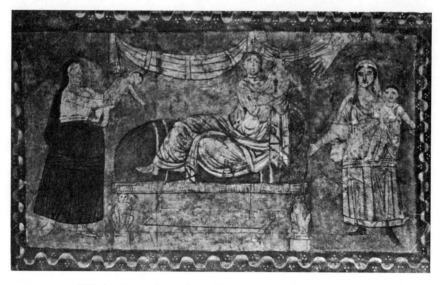

FIGURE 2.   Elijah. *Fresco from Dura Europas, synagogue in ancient Syria. On the left panel the mother is shown in mourning clothes carrying her child to Elijah and begging for help. Elijah, with the assistance of God (as depicted here with God's hand reaching down), brings the child back to life. On the far right the grateful mother has taken her child back in her arms and is no longer dressed in mourning clothes. (Courtesy of Yale University Press)*

himself on the child." Was this a form of chest compression or an attempt to stimulate respiration? Was it a means for Elijah to invoke God's intervention, perhaps like a priestly benediction? Or was the action allegorical and its meaning lost through the ages?

A fascinating and even more detailed account of a resuscitation is related in Kings II and involves Elisha the Prophet, a disciple of Elijah. According to the biblical account, an elderly Shunamite woman was rewarded with a son for her kindness and hospitality to Elisha. One day, the child suffered from a severe headache and collapsed, dying several hours later after being carried to his home. Not accepting her son's death, the mother quickly rode to a neighboring village, where she found Elisha and reproached him for allowing her a child only to have the child die. Elisha dispatched his servant to be with the boy, having given his staff to his servant with instructions as to the manner in which it was to be placed on the boy's face. Elisha and the mother soon followed the servant.

When they arrived the servant informed them, "The boy has not awakened." Elisha entered the house and saw the boy laid out on his bed. He first prayed to the Lord and then "placed himself over the child. He put his mouth on his mouth, his eyes on his eyes, and his hands on his hands, as he bent over him. And the body of the child became warm. He stepped down, walked once up and down the room, then mounted and bent over him. Thereupon, the boy sneezed seven times, and the boy opened his eyes." Some authorities speculate that the weight of Elisha caused chest compression and Elisha's beard tickled the child's nose and caused subsequent sneezing. Perhaps this is the origin of "God Bless You" in answer to a sneeze.[2] The wooden staff was not a powerful enough talisman to reverse death. In this case, the prophet and his belief in the active intervention of God succeeded.

In Biblical Israel it is doubtful that the Hebrews would have accepted the notion that anyone other than God could intervene in critical illness and death. Whatever the real message of Elijah and Elisha may be, these early accounts are revealing in that resuscitation required divine intervention, either directly with the hand of God or through his prophets. Mere mortals cannot resuscitate someone.[3]

In the first chapter we witnessed the real-life resuscitation of John Colven.

FIGURE 3. Elisha Raising the Son of the Shunamite. *Painting by Lord Frederick Leighton. (Courtesy of Kensington and Chelsea Libraries)*

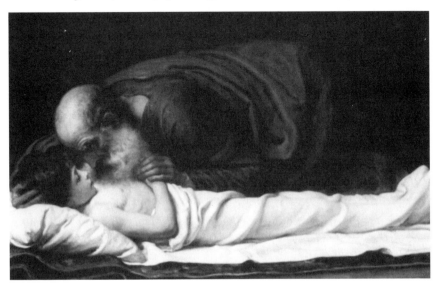

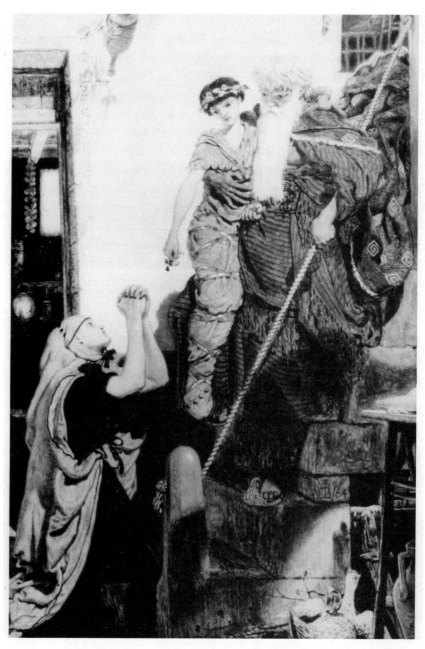

FIGURE 4.   Elijah Descending the Ladder. *Ford Madox Brown, 1864. Elijah is carrying a revived child to his joyous mother. The child is partially shrouded in grave clothes that resemble Egyptian funereal dressing rather than Israeli custom. (Courtesy of Birmingham Museum and Art Gallery)*

He escaped from death's clutches through the timely intervention of his wife, the assistance of trained medical personnel, and the availablity of some high-tech equipment. But if the Colvens had lived 3000 years ago in Biblical Israel, John's fate would have been considerably different. First of all, John—or Jacob ben Isaac in the Hebrew form—would not have died from heart disease. Atherosclerosis was unrecognized then—in fact, the disease probably didn't even exist. Perhaps diet factors, such as more grains and less red meat, or the people's life style (no smoking, fewer sedentary activities, perhaps less stress) meant the near-total absence of heart disease. Also, the average life expectancy in biblical times was probably under twenty-five years. Few lived long enough to develop atherosclerosis.

Three thousand years ago the most common causes of death were accidents and infections. Though some types of infections, such as meningitis or bubonic plague, could kill someone in twenty-four hours or less, signs of illness and infection were always present. The only sudden and totally unexpected forms of death were accidents and fights, including wars.

The real John Colven experienced sudden death from heart disease. Let's assume that sudden death overtook Jacob ben Isaac of 1000 B.C.E. One likely cause of such a death was drowning. Perhaps Jacob (John) is a fisherman on the Sea of Galilee. An oar strikes him and he falls insensate into the water just offshore from Tiberius. By the time his crew retrieves him and hauls him onto shore twenty minutes have elapsed. There are no signs of life. Someone runs to tell his wife Sarah (the name June didn't exist then). His boatmates stand by his lifeless body. Perhaps one shakes him or turns him on his belly. Sarah arrives and cries out, "Dear God, what have you done?" and flings herself onto his body. The bystanders feel pity, and his friends sorrow. But all believe that Yahweh, in some unknowable and mysterious way, has taken Jacob's life. Though they might fervently wish it, no one would even think that such an event could be reversed. Jacob ben Isaac is dead, and he will not return to life. The vigorous effort made on behalf of Mary Macintyre in 1778 would not be seen for centuries.

*The Heart of all creatures is the foundation of their life, the Prince
of all their parts, the sun of their microcosm, that on which all growth depends
and from whence all strength and vigour flows.*
—William Harvey, 1628

BUILDING
THE FOUNDATION

« »

Three millennia lie between the divine resuscitations in biblical Israel and the CPR and defibrillation of John Colven. So much had yet to be understood—anatomy, circulation, physiology, electricity—before sudden death could be reversed. The first steps begin in ancient Roman times.

Galen: The First Physician

Galen (129–210+ C.E.), the ancient physician, was a Greek living much of his life in Rome whose writings influenced medicine for the next 1300 years. Galen wrote several hundred distinct works (the ones that survive fill twenty-two volumes[1]), and their sheer magnitude undoubtedly contributed to the Roman emperor Marcus Aurelius's calling him the "first of physicians and philosophers."[2]

Galen was born in Pergamon, a city in Asia Minor (now western Turkey), then part of the Roman Empire. He was a bright child, and by age fourteen had mastered the classic teachings in philosophy and mathematics. After his father's death Galen left Pergamon to study with medical teachers and learn the skills of a doctor. Medical schools as we know them today did not exist during Galen's time—those who would be physicians studied and apprenticed with mentors, older and experienced practitioners of medicine.

At the age of twenty-eight, Galen returned to his home and was appointed physician to the gladiators. Human vivisection was taboo, so physicians learned anatomy on living patients. The moral prohibition against human dissection was probably a result of veneration of the dead as well as magical beliefs about the corpse.[3] Thus, much of Galen's experience in human anatomy was gained through tending the wounds of mauled and mutilated men, the victims of war and combat. However, Galen does describe an occasional corpse washed up on the shores of the river with muscles and bones visible. He writes of these events with the glee of a child receiving an unexpected present. After three years he left for Rome and eventually became a special physician to the emperor and other high officials.

Until the sixteenth century, Galen was considered the final authority on all matters related to health and disease. His experiments, conducted mostly on pigs and monkeys, constituted a fund of anatomical and physiological knowledge. It was a fund with limited assets, though. Galen had been hindered in his appreciation of respiratory and cardiac function. He wrote

FIGURE 5. *Galen tending to the wounds of a gladiator in the amphitheater at Pergammon. Based on an original painting by Jan Verhas, 1870. (Reproduced from Figuier L,* Vies des Savants Illustres, Vol. I, *Librairie Hachette, Paris)*

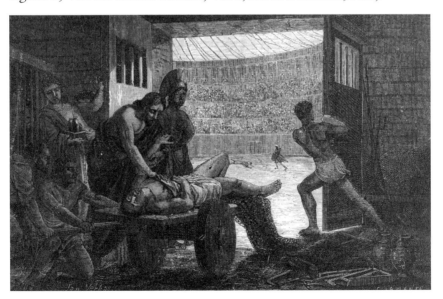

about the difficulty of studying respirations, since thoracotomy inevitably led to the collapse of the lung and the animal's ultimate death: "For which this perforation (of the pleural membrane) the whole process of respiration is destroyed, while if it be not perforated you cannot see within the thorax at all."[4]

Throughout the Middle Ages, there could be no appeal from the "truth of Galen." One must, of course, judge Galen in the context of second-century knowledge. His systematic acquisition of anatomical information and his strong belief in the ethical practice of medicine were quite remarkable. However, Galen was wrong in many of his writings and those errors remained unchallenged for many centuries, thus inhibiting the development of medical science.

To begin to comprehend Galen's view of the human body, we must set aside rational Western scientific belief and enter a world in which magic and spirit were prominent. Galen believed in a vital spirit, which dwelled in all animate objects and was drawn into the body through the lungs. This vital spirit, called "pneuma," is not exactly air. Rather, it is "spirit air," which travels from the lung into the left side of the heart where it is mixed with blood, warmed by the innate heat of the heart, and then transported via the arteries throughout the body.[5]

According to Galen, the three principal organs—the heart, liver, and brain—each had an innate ability to modify the pneuma. Blood was synthesized from food in the liver and then transported to the body through the veins. It traveled from the right side of the heart to the left side. Galen speculated that pores existed in the heart's septum to allow this right-to-left journey. There was no circulation of blood, only ebb and flow—veins to carry nutrients and arteries to carry pneuma. In reality, there are no pores in the heart and blood travels from the right to left side only through the lungs. In order to explain thinking, feeling, and movement, Galen postulated that the brain acted on the blood to create psychic pneuma that then traveled down hollow nerves.

In the final analysis, it wasn't Galen's erroneous anatomy that prevented progress in resuscitation. His physiology dogmatically required a belief in vital spirits and the "furnace of life," an innate heat that animates the body. Galen taught that this innate heat was produced in the furnace of the heart. It was turned on at birth and extinguished at death, never to be lit again.[6] This strongly held belief, passed on through centuries, is one reason why no one thought that death could be reversed.

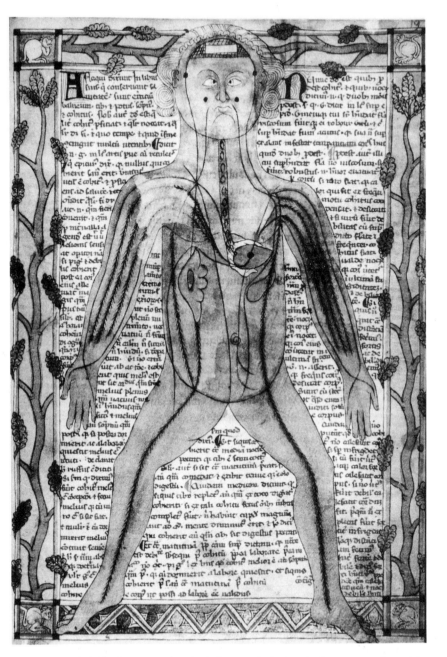

FIGURE 6. *Medical manuscript depicting Galen's circulation system, late thir-teenth century. (Courtesy of Bodleian Library, Oxford)*

Resuscitation in Rome, 200 C.E.

Suppose our real-life couple from Seattle, John and June Colven, lived in Rome around 200 C.E., the year of Galen's death. Galen's theories were well known and widely adhered to by physicians of the time. Life expectancy was now about thirty years, though members of the ruling class often survived into their sixties. As in biblical times, the most common causes of death remained infectious diseases and accidents. Infant mortality was very high, but if one made it past infancy, one had a reasonable chance of living into adulthood. What happens to John if he becomes a victim of sudden accidental or violent death? Are his chances of resuscitation any better than when he lived in Israel around 1000 B.C.E.?

John Colvin—let us make his name Colvinius—is a member of the Senate. A protracted debate about financing defenses in southern Gaul lasts late into the evening. As Colvinius returns to the home where he lives with his wife Aurelia, he is mugged and strangled. His purple striped senatorial robe is torn away. From his limp body thieves roughly strip a gold pendant, a signet ring, and two rings set with precious stones.

A Praetorian guard hears the last few grunts of struggle, sounds an alarm, and rushes to the scene—but too late. The gathering crowd, some carrying lanterns, watch as the body is loaded sideways onto a horse and taken to Colvinius's home. A physician is called, yet he does little but offer advice on the preparation of the body. He has seen at once that Colvinius is not breathing, not taking in pneuma. Without pneuma, the fire of life cannot be sustained. In fact, a quick examination makes it clear that the furnace has already cooled considerably. The physician has no reason to doubt Galen's teachings, and there is no possibility of reactivating Colvinius's vital spirit. Aurelia weeps and wails, and asks the gods why this has happened. The physician shakes his head in sympathy.

The only exception to this slavish adherence to Galen's belief involved attempted resuscitation of newborns. Occasional accounts of midwives using artificial respiration to turn on the "furnace of life" have survived. These attempts over the centuries lacked any physiological understanding. Consider the advice of Bagellardus to midwives in 1472: "If she find it [the newborn] warm, not black, she should blow into its mouth, if it has no respiration." So far so good, but then he adds this final piece of wisdom, "or into the anus."[7]

The Dark Ages

Science did not make great strides until the fifteenth century. The first stir-
rings of modern scientific inquiry occurred during the Renaissance and
reached fruition in the eighteenth-century Enlightenment. The period from
the fall of ancient Rome until the first flowering of the Renaissance was a
millennium characterized by superstition and magic. Historians date the
beginnings of Rome's final decline to about 400 C.E. At about that time
some 40,000 Visigoths, Huns, and freed Roman slaves crossed the Alps and
entered Italy. Ten years later they sacked Rome. The long period known popularly as the Dark Ages began. The term, by the way, was not invented by
modern historians, but by those living in the Renaissance. The name is apt,
given the lack of progress and learning. The Dark Ages (roughly 400 to 1000
C.E.) flowed seamlessly into the Middle Ages (roughly 1000 to 1400 C.E.).

In his book *A World Lit Only by Fire*, William Manchester paints a
depressing picture of life during these years. Famines and plagues periodically decimated the population. During its recurring visits the Black Death
(bubonic plague) would often destroy half a community's people. There was
virtually no commerce or trade. No roads were built, and even after a thousand years of neglect, the ancient Roman roads were still the best in Europe.
Those foolish enough to travel faced the likelihood of being robbed,
abducted, or murdered. Few murderers were caught and abduction for ran-
som was a common means of livelihood for unemployed knights. According
to Manchester, the peril was so ever present that "people huddled closely
together in communal homes. They married fellow villagers and were so
insular that local dialects were often incomprehensible to men living only a
few miles apart." Except for cathedrals, there were virtually no stone build-
ings erected throughout the continent. One has an image that is less a civilization and more small clusters of isolated villagers living in constant fear
and superstition.[8]

What is remarkable during this long period is the unchanging constancy
of the centuries. A village farmer in central Europe in the year 600 lived a life
almost identical to that of one in the year 1200. Daily survival was a timeless
blur of passing seasons. The succession of popes, kings, and emperors had no
effect on the masses. Wars and natural disasters were part of the fabric of
existence; they were not events to be marked. It was not a time of intellectual
achievement. Manchester writes, "Saint Bernard of Clairvaux (1090–1153),

the most influential Christian of his time, bore a deep distrust of the intellect and declared that the pursuit of knowledge, unless sanctified by a holy mission, was a pagan act and therefore vile." Innovation and progress were inconceivable and could only invite suspicion of witchcraft. And the only good witch was a burnt witch.

Equally unchanging throughout these centuries was the view of the human body. Thomas Moore in his book *Care of the Soul* describes these different perceptions. In the Middle Ages the human body was a manifestation of the soul—body and soul were interwoven. The concept of soul was more than religious soul; it was part of the very essence of life and one's character.[9] Given such a view, it is understandable that death should be regarded as an irreversible process. When the body dies, the soul departs to enter either the religious cosmos or the spirit of the world. The heart contains the soul. So when the heart stops beating, the soul must vanish. To someone in the Middle Ages this was simply fact. The modern view, by contrast, is mechanistic. The body is an efficient machine. The heart is merely a muscle and its function simply to pump blood. If one tends to the machine and cares for it, it can function smoothly for many decades. If something goes wrong, it can be cured with a chemical to correct the error, or fixed with a new part. And when the machine stops, it can be restarted. The soul has no influence or bearing on this modern view.[9]

The Renaissance

The first stirring of the Renaissance appeared in the 1400s. It is of course impossible to determine the precise year of the onset of such a sweeping renewal of Western civilization. Certain events heralded its beginning, however. Prior to the fall of Constantinople to the Turks in 1453, scholars and merchants transferred many ancient Greek manuscripts to Rome. The "rediscovery" of these classics by Western Europeans led to a rebirth of interest in the ancient arts and humanities. "Renaissance" means "renewal," and it refers to this rediscovery. In 1458 Gutenberg developed movable type and used it to print the Bible. Within twenty-five years, presses existed in every major city in Europe. And by the end of the century edited books of Aristotle's writings appeared in Italy. By 1515 the works of all the Hellenic giants were available. The great artists—Leonardo, Rabelais, Botticelli, Perugino, Ghirlandajo, Raphael, Michelangelo, Cellini, Crivelli, Signorelli, and Titian—all lived and worked in the late 1400s. The first schools that might be called universities had appeared in England (Oxford and Cambridge), France (Paris), and Italy (Bologna) in the twelfth century. By the end of the fifteenth century, however, colleges and universities as we would eventually know them had been established throughout Europe.

Historians consider the Polish astronomer Nicolaus Copernicus (1473–1543) the first great Renaissance scientist. He literally changed our view of the cosmos from an Aristotelian geocentric view with the earth as the center to a heliocentric one revolving around the sun. Though emblazoned forever in the science hall of fame for his theory of the universe, it was really Copernicus's method of study that revolutionized science. He was the first to insist that science and its hypotheses be based on realities, not fictions. His predecessors manufactured convenient hypotheses, irrespective of truth, in order to save hallowed beliefs. Copernicus rejected this easy approach; for him there was only one truth and the goal of science was to discover it.[10]

Vesalius and the "Truth of Galen"

For medicine, the previously inviolable "truth of Galen" finally began to crumble under the weight of the work of the Renaissance's two great anatomists, Andreas Vesalius and William Harvey. In 1543 Andreas Vesalius (1514–1564), at the age of twenty-eight, wrote *De Humani Corporis Fabrica* (*The Structure of the Human Body*),[11] a remarkable treatise on human anatomy. With its publication, he began to overthrow the ancient Galenic superstitions that had held firm for centuries.

Vesalius's ability to refute the statements of Galen was largely the result of his work on cadavers. The judge of the Padua criminal court became interested in Vesalius's early research and in 1539 made the bodies of executed criminals available to the young scientist. Apparently he even delayed executions to suit Vesalius's convenience. Vesalius heretically declared that human anatomy could only be learned from dissection and observation of the body. The prevailing wisdom was that anatomy was taught just from texts, mainly those of Galen.

Vesalius's writings contain a description of the first known attempt to resuscitate the stilled hearts of pigs and dogs. He used tracheostomies, tracheal intubation, and bellows to intermittently expand the lungs, attempting to simulate natural respirations. The medical historian A. Barrington Baker observes that such a remarkable achievement is understated almost to the point of disguise and speculates that Vesalius feared the wrath of the Church and thus drew little attention to his experiments. The Church surely would not have taken kindly to such meddling in God's province.[12]

Vesalius finally broke the stranglehold Galen held on medical belief and practice. Of course, there was still much to discover. For example, though Vesalius doubted that blood traveled from the right side of the heart to the left through pores in the septum, he was unwilling to repudiate the ancient Greek's belief about blood flow or its manufacture in the liver.[13]

A story, probably apocryphal, is told about Vesalius who, while conducting an autopsy on the body of a woman, found that when he opened the rib cage her heart was still beating. Rather than face the Inquisition, Vesalius left for a pilgrimage to the Holy Land. The known facts are that he did visit the Holy Land with the approval of the king. On his return journey, however, a storm caused a forced landing on a Greek island, where he subsequently died.[14]

William Harvey and Circulation

Seventy-five years later, the English physician William Harvey continued in the tradition of Vesalius and was the first to definitively describe the circulatory system. It was a time of great intellectual ferment during the Renaissance, and Harvey contributed mightily. Not only did he demonstrate the true nature of the heart's function and the circulation of blood, along with William Gilbert, whose investigations of the magnet helped create contemporary physics, Harvey laid the foundations for scientific experimental research as we know it today.

William Harvey, said his contemporaneous biographer John Aubrey, was a small man with "a little eie, round, very black, full of spirit." He was born on April 1, 1578, in the town of Folkestone, just a few miles southeast of Dover, the oldest of nine children. All his brothers were successful in either business or at the royal court, and his father, Thomas Harvey, was a well-to-do businessman who later became Folkestone's mayor. Little is known of Harvey's childhood before the age of ten, but from 1588 to 1593 he was a student at the King's School at Canterbury Cathedral. When he was sixteen, Harvey began attending Gonville and Caius College at Cambridge University. Caius specialized in educating doctors, so it is reasonable to assume that

Harvey's interest in the subject was well developed by then. He received his B.A. in 1597 but continued his studies at Caius. However, he missed much of his last year (1598–99) because of illness, possibly malaria. Yet Harvey was determined to complete his studies and decided to do them at the best medical school in Europe—the University of Padua in Italy. There he studied with the famous anatomist Hieronymous Fabricius (1537–1619).

Harvey was one of the best and brightest students in Fabricius's class. He returned to England in 1602 with his doctor's degree, fully trained by the standards of his time with clinical experience gained at the hospitals in Padua. By late 1604 he had passed a series of examinations given by the College of Physicians in London and began practicing as a fully licensed physician.

Not long after he married Elizabeth Browne, the daughter of Lancelot Browne, the physician to King James I. Little is known about Harvey's family life except that he had no children. In 1609, possibly through the help of his father-in-law or the efforts of his brother John (who worked in the King's household), the King recommended Harvey for an appointment at St. Bartholomew's Hospital, where he soon became head physician. He received an annual salary of twenty-five pounds, and held his position for the next thirty-four years. He eventually developed a thriving private practice as well. One of his patients was Sir Francis Bacon.

The spark that led to his discovery about circulation of the blood was the result of long and careful observation. Harvey believed in direct observation instead of relying on others' writings or philosophizing: "I do not profess either to learn or to teach anatomy from books or from the maxims of philosophers, but from dissections and from the fabric of Nature herself." What Harvey observed were valves located inside the large veins. These valves were placed to give "free passage to blood towards the heart, but opposed the passage of the venal blood the contrary way." As Harvey reasoned, the valves pointing toward the heart were not placed without design. The only logical conclusion is that they were there to facilitate the one-way flow of blood—through the veins to the heart and from the heart through the arteries.

William Harvey was good at his profession, and his peers recognized his ability. By 1615 he was a fellow of the Royal College of Physicians and the same year the Royal Society gave Harvey the lifetime post of Lumleian Lecturer. In his first series of lectures, delivered in 1616, he described the circulation of blood and concluded, "It is proved by the structure of the heart that the blood is continuously transferred through the lungs into the aorta. . . . It is proved by the ligature that there is a passage of blood from the arteries to the veins. It is therefore demonstrated that the continuous movement of the blood in a circle is brought about by the beat of the heart."[15]

For the next twelve years Harvey carried out even more experiments to prove his theories on blood circulation. They went well and, by 1628, he published his epochal work on blood circulation, *Exercitatio Anatomica de Motu Cordis et Sanguinis in Animalibus* (*An Anatomical Disputation Concerning the Movement of the Heart and Blood in Living Creatures*).[16] *De Motu Cordis*, as it is commonly known, was only seventy-two pages long, with two dedications, an introduction, and seventeen brief chapters. But in that short work, Harvey wrought a revolution in medicine and biology.

In his later years, Harvey liked to be in the dark, believing that it helped him think better, and he had caves constructed under his home. The violent change in power wrought by the Civil War had left Harvey a political "undesirable." He often had to live at one or another of his brothers' homes outside London. However, his skill as a doctor and his shrewd investments following his brothers' financial advice had made William Harvey a wealthy man. In 1652 he gave his fellow physicians a new library, which contained his own extensive collection of books and presumably some of his surviving manuscripts. (Sadly, the library burned to the ground in the Great Fire of 1666, along with all of Harvey's books.)

By now William Harvey was old and ill, suffering from kidney stones and gout. One morning he awoke partly paralyzed and unable to speak. He died shortly thereafter, on June 3, 1657.[17]

Anne Green and Resuscitation

Obtaining humans for dissection was a challenging problem for Harvey and other scientists. Up until then, the sanctity of the human body and the belief in its resurrection prevented any dissection or advances in anatomy. This problem was partially solved in England in 1636 by a section of the great charter of Charles I to the University of Oxford. This charter allowed an anatomy reader to demand, for the purpose of anatomical dissection, the body of any person executed within twenty-one miles of Oxford. This exception to the rule led to one of the earliest known instances of human resuscitation. Anne Green was a maid employed by Sir Thomas Read. She was twenty-two years old and described as "of middle stature, strong, fleshy, and

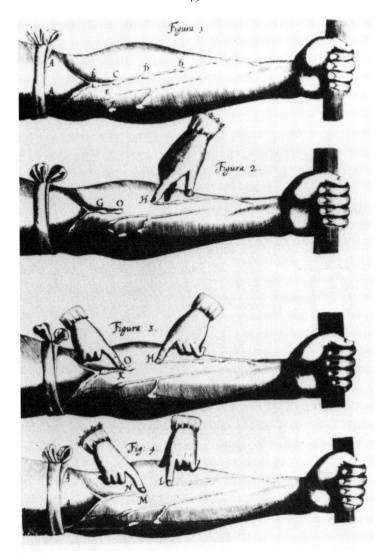

FIGURE 7. *Drawing of arm veins from Harvey's* De Motu Cordis *(1628) demonstrating circulation and directional flow of blood. (Courtesy of National Library of Medicine, Bethesda, Maryland)*

of an indifferent good feature." She was seduced by Read's grandchild and became pregnant, but early in her third trimester delivered a premature, still-born boy. Green concealed the infant's body, and when it was discovered she was suspected of murder. She was condemned to death and on December 14, 1650, was hanged at Cattle yard in Oxford. She hung for half an hour; during that time some of her friends hung "with all their weight upon her legs, sometimes lifting her up, and then pulling her down again with a sudden jerk, thereby the sooner to dispatch her out of her pain." Finally, the under-sheriff required them to desist lest they break the rope. When everyone thought she was dead, they lowered her body, put it in a coffin, and carried it to the private house of Dr. William Petty, the reader in anatomy.

Much to his surprise, when Petty opened the coffin, he observed that Anne Green took a breath and heard a rattle in her throat. Thoughts of dissection were abandoned and efforts to revive her began. Petty poured cordials into her throat, tickled it with a feather, applied heating plasters to her chest, and used other heating plasters as an enema. He eventually revived her, and the story ends happily. Anne Green later married, bore three children, and lived for fifteen years after her resuscitation. Her father, either an inveterate opportunist or a shrewd businessman, charged admission for the curious to come see the person snatched from the coffin.[18]

The resuscitation of Anne Green was a unique event. Although the

FIGURE 8. *Execution and resuscitation of Anne Green. Part of the resuscitation involved placing Anne Green in a warm bed next to a woman. (Courtesy of Bodleian Library, Oxford)*

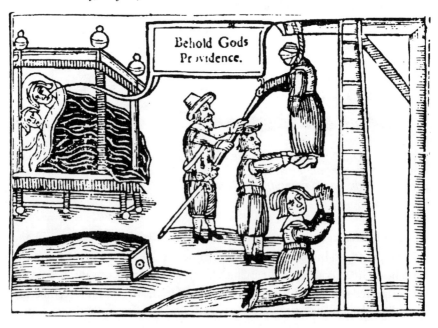

Renaissance witnessed an awakening of intellectual activity, the artists, writers, and thinkers of that period were not rebellious. Most accepted the orthodoxy of the Christian Church and worked within the assumptions of religious belief. Writers, painters, and architects used and unquestioningly accepted religious themes. Not surprisingly, there are virtually no recorded attempts at resuscitation during the Renaissance. Such efforts would be almost unthinkable since no rational scientific basis existed for such an act. For resuscitation to become an accepted procedure, and for death to be considered reversible, two historical developments were required. One was the secularization of society—the all-pervasive grip of orthodox religion on everyday life had to diminish. The other was the infiltration of science and the scientific method into intellectual thought.

Prior to and well into the Renaissance the strength of Christianity was unshakable. Orthodox belief held that individual spiritual judgment took place at death, followed by salvation or eternal damnation. And death is the will of God. An example of the conflict between secular and theological forces occurred in 1669 in Uppsala, Sweden. The mayor's ten-year-old daughter was being buried, but as the casket lid was being lowered the town's chief physician noted signs of life. He wanted to try to revive the dead child but was reviled by a professor of theology who proclaimed how bad it would be to bother a dead body. Though nothing was done, the child awoke spontaneously and lived, if accounts can be believed, to age ninety-two.[19]

The concept of judgment at death, of course, is not unique to Christianity. Judaism has numerous references in prayers and writings to the fate that awaits us all. Similar themes appear in the great holy books of Hinduism, Buddhism, and other religions. But more important than references to death as the final chapter is the belief that God has total power over our fate and somehow "knows" when the time of reckoning will come. For example, much of the liturgy during Rosh Hashanah and Yom Kippur revolves around God's closing the Book of Life at the end of the religious service. At that moment one's fate is sealed for the coming year. Not everything is totally predetermined; prayer and repentance during these religious days of atonement can help ensure a good "fate" for the coming year. Similarly, Ecclesiastes speaks of the acceptance of a proper time for everything, "a time for being born and a time for dying."

The secularization of society accelerated with the Reformation during the sixteenth century. Reformers challenged the power of Rome and created a plethora of alternative religious doctrines. While it is true that some of the more fundamental Protestant sects believed in predestination, others taught just the opposite. Skepticism about the old teachings became the rule. No longer was it believed that only a select few would be saved from eternal damnation; now anyone could be. People were the masters of their fate. The new religious ethic was "God helps those who help themselves." One can't help supposing that the same concept diffused into the science of medicine: "Anyone could and should be saved." Such beliefs provided the cultural substrate for Anne Greene's resuscitation in 1650.

Scientific thought did not of course permeate human consciousness overnight. Old ways of thinking and the power of religion only reluctantly gave way. In 1720 Edward Jenner's smallpox vaccine was opposed on religious grounds. This ambivalence, which lasted even into the late nineteenth century, is well typified in this passage from *Middlemarch*, published in 1871 by George Eliot:

> "this Doctor Lydgate," who was capable of performing the most astonishing cures, and rescuing people altogether given up by other practitioners. But the balance had been turned against Lydgate by two members, who for some private reasons held that this power of resuscitating persons as good as dead was an equivocal recommendation, and might interfere with providential favors. In the course of the year, however, there had been a change in the public sentiment.[20]

The rise of secularism and science allowed the first attempts at resuscitation. A belief in resuscitation emerged from centuries of pre-Enlightenment thinking, but the will to achieve it was not solidly established until it was fixed in the human consciousness of the eighteenth century.

Part II

THE BREATH
OF LIFE

《 》

Thou takest away their breath, they die, and return to dust.
—Psalms 104, 29

THE SEARCH FOR ARTIFICIAL RESPIRATION

《 　 》

With the Enlightenment, the search for the best means of resuscitation began in earnest. It was, of course, impossible at the time to know that success would require tools and means not yet invented. The crucial factor is that sudden and unexpected death was no longer passively accepted. Enlightenment scientists[1] and physicians started their quest attempting to emulate the most basic and fundamental property of life—breath itself.

The first account of mouth-to-mouth resuscitation appeared in 1744—though it actually occurred in 1732. A Scottish surgeon named William Tossach wrote that he was called to a patient who had been overcome by "nauseous steam arising from coals set on fire in the pit." The patient was laid on his back, "his skin was cold, there was not the least pulse in either heart or arteries and not the least breathing could be observed." Tossach described his actions: "I applied my mouth close to his and blowed my breath as strong as I could, but having neglected to stop all his nostrils, all the air came out of them, wherefore taking hold of them with one hand . . . I blew again my breath as strong as I could, raising his chest fully with it and immediately I felt six or seven beats of the heart." From that point conventional therapy was used—bleeding an arm vein, rubbing the skin, and applying smelling salts to the nose and lips. The story has a happy ending. "In an hour or more he came pretty well back to his senses and could take drink," Tossach noted, "but knew nothing of all that had happened. . . . Within an hour, he walked home." After several days the man returned to his job. Tossach modestly concluded his account, "I must submit to better Judges to determine whether the experiment I design to relate was the mean of saving the man's life on whom it was tried; it is at least very simple, and absolutely safe, and therefore can at least be no harm, if there is not an advantage in acquainting the publick of it."[2]

In 1745 John Fothergill, a leading London physician, happened to read Tossach's account. He thought it deserved a wider audience and decided to report the resuscitation to the Philosophical Society. Fothergill acknowledges the case as the first instance of successful mouth-to-mouth ventilation. Clearly impressed, he advised using mouth-to-mouth respiration on all cases of drowning and suffocation whenever possible. "The blast of a man's mouth" was simple, inexpensive, harmless, and could be administered by unskilled bystanders directly at the scene. According to Fothergill, mouth-to-mouth ventilation "may possibly do *great good*, but cannot do harm." It was preferred over bellows, a common fireplace implement, for the following reasons: "(1) as the bellows may not be at hand; (2) as the lungs of one man may bear, without injury, as great a force as those of another man can exert, which by the bellows cannot always be determined; (3) the warmth and moisture of the breath would be more likely to promote the circulation than the chilling air forced out of a pair of bellows."[3] Fothergill inquired in a later writing, "In what cases, and under what circumstances there may be a prospect of applying this, and other similar methods, with success?" He answers his own question, "The diseases in which they may be of use, are those called sudden deaths from an invisible cause, apoplexies, fits of various kinds . . . and many other disorders, wherein persons in a moment sink down and expire."[4]

In addition to his suggestions about artificial respiration, Fothergill deserves mention for his description of angina and sudden death. In 1776 he wrote a case report in a London medical journal of a sixty-three-year-old man with symptoms of angina after exertion who "fell down and expired immediately." The autopsy revealed findings consistent with atherosclerotic heart disease, though not recognized as such.[5] At the time of the Declaration of Independence there were only a few case reports of angina and very little anatomical understanding of the disease that would become so pandemic. The immediate death of Fothergill's patient was most likely caused by ventricular fibrillation, a condition that would not be defined for another 100 years.

Fothergill's belief that mouth-to-mouth ventilation was superior to the use of bellows was supported by other physicians. William Buchan, a London physician, provides a remarkable description of how to perform mouth-to-mouth respiration: "To renew the breathing a strong person may blow his own breath into the patient's mouth with all the force he can, holding his nostrils at the same time. When it can be perceived by the rising of the chest or belly that the lungs are filled with air, the persons ought to desist from blowing, and should press the breast and belly so as to expel the air again; and this operation may be repeated for some time, alternately inflating and depressing the lungs so as to imitate natural respiration." Buchan recommended the use of bellows only if mouth-to-mouth respiration was unsuccessful.

Buchan's recommendations were published in a textbook, popular in England and the United States, entitled *Domestic Medicine or the Family Physician*.[6] Its early editions made no mention of how to resuscitate victims of drowning but by the eighth edition, published in 1784, such advice was included. Clearly, Buchan's text reflected the influence of English Rescue Societies that came into existence after 1774.

Fothergill's belief in mouth-to-mouth resuscitation was entirely consistent with a mechanistic view of the body. He reflects the Enlightenment notion of viewing the universe and the body as a harmonious mechanism whose inner workings have only to be understood. He writes, "It does not seem absurd, to compare the animal machine to a clock . . . without some impulse communicated to the pendulum, the whole continues motionless. . . . Inflating the lungs, and by this means communicating motion to the heart, like giving the first vibration to a pendulum, may possibly, in many cases, enable this something to resume the government of the fabric."[7]

Fothergill also recommended rolling the drowning victim on a barrel before trying mouth-to-mouth. The facedown position allows water to drain. As the victim is rolled back over the barrel, the abdomen and chest are compressed, leading to exhalation and, as the victim is rolled forward, pressure is removed, allowing inhalation. Barrels were readily available on ships and in seaports, thus placing the rescue device in close proximity to the drowning victim. Though easy to perform, the barrel roll was not effective.

Variations on the barrel roll as well as the inversion methods in which the victim was placed upside down were apparently universal. Woodcuts from

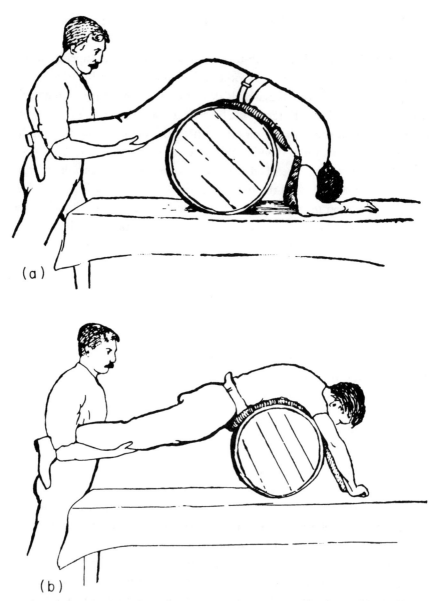

FIGURE 9. *The barrel-roll method of artificial respiration. Top figure depicts initiation of inspiration and bottom figure shows expiration. (Courtesy of The Lancet)*

Japan depict these procedures. Perhaps the intuitive nature of this method accounted for its widespread use.

Amsterdam Rescue Society

Organized efforts to deal with sudden drowning were carried out by rescue societies, which sprang up in most European capitals as well as in New York, Philadelphia, and Boston. In August 1767, the first society, the Society for the Recovery of Drowned Persons, was formed by a few wealthy and benevolent gentlemen in Amsterdam. They were "struck with the variety of instances in which persons falling into the water were lost for want of proper treatment."[8] This was the first organized effort to deal with sudden and unexpected death. In this regard, 1767 is a watershed year. For the first time in history there existed an organized will to respond to sudden death. It would take exactly 200 years before successful resuscitation was an accepted reality.

One year after the Amsterdam Rescue Society was established, magistrates in Milan and Venice began similar societies. In 1769 the City of Hamburg passed an ordinance requiring notices to be read in churches describing assistance to be given to the drowned, strangled, frozen, and those overcome by noxious gases. Paris started a rescue society in 1771, and London and St. Petersburg in 1774.[9] Within four years of its founding, the society in Amsterdam claimed that 150 persons, ages two to seventy-two, were saved by their recommendations.[10] Supposedly the victims had been immersed from fifteen minutes to an hour and a half.[11] The members of the Society recommended (1) warming the victim; (2) removing swallowed or aspirated water by positioning the victim's head lower than the feet, applying manual pressure to the abdomen, and tickling the victim's throat; (3) stimulating the victim by such means as rectal and oral fumigation with tobacco smoke; (4) using a bellows or mouth-to-mouth method (mouth-to-mouth or mouth-to-nostril respiration are described, including the advice that "a cloth or handkerchief may be used to render the operation less indelicate"); (5) rubbing the body with woolen cloths ("wetted with brandy and strewed over with dry salt"); and (6) bloodletting. There was no time limit on these treatments. Efforts continued until either the victim revived or it was plainly evident that rescue was impossible. In general, six or more hours were considered a reasonable resuscitative effort.[12] For persons attempting a resuscitation the reward of six ducats was offered.[13]

Tobacco was widely known as a stimulant and this feature was the basis for its use in resuscitations. David Hosack wrote about tobacco's stimulating properties in his 1792 book, *An Enquiry into the Causes of Suspended Animation from Drowning with the Means of Restoring Life:* "There is scarely a substance in nature which so immediately stimulates the moving fiber, as is evidenced from its immediate efficacy when taken into the stomach, or thrown into the bowels by clyster, in case of costiveness (constipation). I am acquainted with a lady, who when occasionally costive, has recourse to a pipe of tobacco; and before she uses it one minute, it has the desired effect—a proof of its stimulating effects upon the nervous system."[14] An earlier publication, *A Physical Dissertation on Drowning* (1746), described a drowned woman resuscitated with tobacco smoke. According to the account, immediatiely after the drowning, a soldier happened by and, with the consent of the distraught husband, placed his pipe in the victim's anus and blew "the smoke of the tobacco into her intestines, as strongly as he possibly could." After the fifth blast the woman's abdomen was heard to rumble, "she discharged some water from her mouth, and in a moment after returned to life." The author claimed that tobacco worked by "irritation of the intestines, excited by the heat and acrimony of the smoke of the tobacco, produces in the muscles subservient to expiration, such a reflux of the animal spirits, as induces a contraction of them sufficient to surmont that resistance which the air contained in the breast, found it to discharge."[15]

Cases of tobacco's stimulating properties can be found in the early annals of many rescue societies. The Amsterdam Rescue Society reported the following successful resuscitation: "At Rotterdam, on the 8th of April, 1769, the daughter of Meindert den Broeder, a girl of ten years of age fell into a stagnant pool, near the rampart of the town, and stuck in it for some time. When she was taken out of it, she seemed to be absolutely dead, and looked as black as if she had been hanged. She was immediately stripped, put between warm blankets, and rubbed. After the introduction of some tobacco-vapor into the intestines, a bleeding was attempted, and only about four ounces of blood obtained. Three persons then continued to rub, and inject smoke, for the space of an hour, when a faint yawning, gave the first small sign of life. In an hour and a half some slight pulsation was discovered and she then began to move her legs and arms."[16]

Many of the Amsterdam Rescue Society's recommendations did not stand the test of time. In 1811, Benjamin Brodie in England denounced fumigation after demonstrating that four ounces of strong tobacco inserted into the

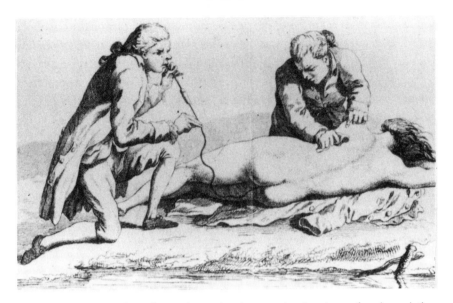

FIGURE 10. *Rectal smoke used to stimulate respiration in a drowning victim. (Courtesy of Wood Library-Museum of Anesthesiology, Park Ridge, Illinois)*

intestine would kill a dog within eight to ten minutes and one ounce would kill a cat. The practice of blowing smoke in the rectum seems bizarre today, but it is possible that the dilatation of the anus by the tube provided some reflex stimulus of respiration.[17] Hundreds of anecdotal reports testifying to the benefit of tobacco could not overturn the power of Brodie's crude experiments. The practice ceased almost overnight.

Royal Humane Society

News of the success of the Amsterdam Rescue Society soon reached England and, in 1774, Thomas Cogan (1736–1818) and William Hawes (1736–1806), both London physicians, founded the Society for the Recovery of Persons Apparently Drowned. In 1776 the Society renamed itself the Humane Society, and in 1787 adopted its present name, the Royal Humane Society, a result of the royal patronage of King George III.[18] In 1773 Dr. Cogan had obtained a copy of the memoirs of the Amsterdam Society and translated them into English to share with the medical community. Cogan's wife was Dutch and he had trained in the Netherlands. Dr. Hawes was sufficiently impressed with what he read that he offered rewards for personal accounts of drownings and rescue attempts. The 1788 annual report listed 410 pounds paid for reports of "restorations, preservations of life, and unsuccessful cases" representing almost 45 percent of the society's annual budget. Another 157 pounds were allocated for "apparatusses and drags" to be placed in "several parts of the kingdom," presumably on waterways and in ports.[19] The charter membership had thirty gentlemen, half who were friends of Cogan and the rest of Hawes.

The Royal Humane Society bestowed medals on individuals who attempted to save drowning victims. The medal reads on one side: Lateat scintillula forsan ("Possibly a little spark may yet lie hid") And on the reverse: Hoc pretium cive servato tulit ("He has obtained this reward for having saved the life of a citizen").

The Royal Humane Society had considerable influence. Its annual reports, which recounted in anecdotal fashion all the cases of attempted resuscitation, were widely circulated to the medical profession both in England and throughout the world. Pocket-sized cards containing "Directions for the Recovery of the Apparently Dead, Etc." were printed and widely disseminated. The Society established contacts with physicians in over thirty cities from Prague to Philadelphia, and helped spawn twenty-seven Rescue Societies throughout Great Britain. Typical of the British Societies, the Bath Humane Society was founded for the purpose of paying attention to "one of the greatest calamities that can befall mankind, *the danger of Sudden Death,* particularly by DROWNING" (italicized in the original). The Bath Society, like most others in Britain, inaugurated itself with appropriately high-sounding poetic words of inspiration:

> Resuscitation Hail! whose potent breath,
> Can wrest the Victim from impending Death . . .
> And, list'ning to the Widow's piercing cries,
> Command to life her bier-stretch'd Son to rise.[20]

There was a moral, as well as a lifesaving, side to these societies. Perhaps as a reaction to the negative aspects and moral dislocation associated with the Industrial Revolution, the founders of the various humane societies argued that "the glow of satisfaction at having done good" stimulated moral growth. Rescuers often refused the proferred award, a sign of "disinterested benevolence." The moral arguments were probably a reaction to the cultural and physical dislocation of the times. Indeed, the height of the Industrial

Revolution (1760–1840) coincided with the burgeoning formation of rescue societies. The disruption of society, with migrations to the industrial towns, weakened the moral fiber of the times. The rescue societies offered a moral antidote. It was argued that seeing good conduct would "shame the indifferent and lukewarm out of their supineness." In the final analysis, "It is probable that the moral benefits resulting to the community from these Institutions, may rival the advantages conferred upon the numbers who have been saved from destruction."[21]

The initial annual reports of the Royal Humane Society advocated numerous techniques, usually based on a single episode. The Society made no attempt to study or verify the effectiveness of any method. An individual would try a technique, find success, and report it to the Society. Realizing the limitations of such anecdotes, the Society began to seriously assume its mission of defining the most effective means of resuscitation. It solicited investigations by the most renowned scientists to determine the benefit of various treatments. The Society kept statistics on each reported rescue attempt and summarized them in its 1795 annual report. Until that year 2572 cases had been reported and investigated. A total of 959 lives had been saved by the Society's medical assistants; 876 were saved by the use of the Society's apparatus; and 747 cases were unsuccessful.[22] The Society also did much to ban what it believed were archaic or dangerous methods. For example, it strongly opposed the use of bleeding (though it was recommended in earlier years) and prohibited the inversion method for drowning, where the victim is hung from the feet to allow water to drain out.

The Royal Humane Society established eleven receiving stations near waterways throughout London. These stations were stocked with bellows, tubes, and other resuscitation devices. The most elaborate was located near the Serpentine, an artificial lake in Hyde Park, on a plot of land that had been granted to the Society by the King in 1790. In 1834 an even more elaborate station was constructed with recovery rooms and accommodations for a resident superintendent. The station was destroyed by a German bomb during the Battle of Britain in 1940.[23]

American Rescue Societies

The Royal Humane Society attained international prestige, and eventually American physicians who had trained in London formed humane societies in Philadelphia (1780), New York (1784), and Boston (1786).[24] The Humane

Society of Philadelphia posted signs along the waterfront telling where life-saving equipment might be found. However, often these societies seemed to function more as social clubs than rescue organizations. This led Benjamin Waterhouse to declare that "to blow one's own breath into the lungs of another is an absurd and pernicious practice!!" Gradually, the American humane societies were absorbed into philanthropic leagues. In New England, for instance, grants-in-aid created for seamen eventually resulted in the formation of the United States Life-Saving Service in 1871, a precursor of the Coast Guard.

Bellows and John Hunter

Among the instruments of resuscitation, bellows were the most widely advocated for artificial respiration, perhaps because they were readily available in the hearths of most homes. But there may have been a more intuitive reason—blowing air into the lungs of a nonbreathing person was a relatively simple operation. Its use also obviated the need to risk contagion from the victim's mouth. Furthermore, several scientists had demonstrated that exhaled air contained poisonous gas. This component of air was called "fixed air" and is today known as carbon dioxide. The discovery of increased carbon dioxide in exhaled air lent support to the belief that mouth-to-mouth resuscitation might not provide enough oxygen (oxygen had been discovered in the 1770s)[25] to the victim. Sophisticated means for answering these concerns were not available, making it all the easier for advocates of bellows to argue about the inadequacies of exhaled air. Consequently, in 1782, the Royal Humane Society recommended inflation by bellows over mouth-to-mouth ventilation.

Complicated directions accompanied the recommendations of some rescue societies. The Humane Society of the State of New York wrote in 1795, "As soon as possible a bellows which must be clear of all dirt and dust should be applied to one nostril, while another person should close the other nostril and the mouth, and at the same time press back the lower part of the wind pipe. The person who holds the bellows must then blow gently, and repeat the blowing five or six times; when this is done and the breast is a little swelled, a third person must press the belly up so as to force the air out."[26]

The English surgeon, John Hunter (1728–1793), was a particularly strong advocate of bellows and recommended them for administering stimulating vapors. He also suggested using a two-chambered bellows, one chamber to inspire, and the other for expired air. He wrote: "First, a pair of bellows, so contrived with two separate cavities, that by expanding them, when applied to the nostrils or mouth of a patient, one cavity may be filled with the common air, and the other with the air sucked out of the lungs be discharged into the room." Hunter was aware of a major problem with bellows, namely air entering the stomach instead of the lungs and offered a simple solution, "If during this operation the larynx be gently pressed against the oesophagus and spine, it will prevent the stomach and intestines being too much distended by the air."[27] Almost 200 years later, the same maneuver was rediscovered and is now a routine procedure in anesthesia.[28]

Hunter's key contribution to resuscitation science was to demonstrate that deprivation of breathing was the "first cause of death." The cessation of heart activity was the "second or consequent cause of death" and the result of insufficient respiratory activity. Hunter's conclusions were elegantly drawn from dog experiments in which artificial respiration was induced and then stopped. The animal had been prepared with its sternum removed so the heart's activity could be observed. When the respiration stopped, activity continued for minutes, gradually weakening until the contractions ceased completely. Hunter considered the process identical to what occurred in drowning. Therefore, he argued, if the respirations can be restarted, the heart activity will regain its normal force.

Hunter can also be considered the father of cardiovascular epidemiology. He wrote, "I shall conclude this account by proposing that all who are employed in this practice (the practice of resuscitating drowned individuals) be particularly required to keep an accurate journal of the means used, and the degree of success attending them; whence we may be furnished with facts sufficient to enable us to draw conclusions, on which a certain practice may hereafter be established."[29]

Copenhagen Rescue Society

The Society for the Rescue of Drowning Persons, the Copenhagen equivalent of the Amsterdam and London Societies, was established in 1796 as a result of an influential book published in the same year by John Daniel Herholdt (1764–1836) and Carl Gottlob Rafn (1769–1808). It was titled *Life-Saving Measures for Drowning Persons*[30] and it made some convincing arguments while summarizing the prevailing wisdom about resuscitation. Herholdt and Rafn gave what may have been one of the first cost-effective arguments in health care. They claimed that approximately forty-five people drowned each year in Copenhagen and a rescue society "might save the lives of thirty fellow townsmen." If each of these lived another twenty years, within twenty years there would be 600 more people (not counting their offspring) within the community. They "would yield to the State better return than the life-saving measures would cost." They also argued that older doctors are not aware of the resuscitation techniques and younger doctors cannot learn if the older ones don't show them.

Herholdt and Rafn summarized thirty steps that should be followed in dealing with drowned victims. Their list of remedies is typical for resuscitation art at the end of the eighteenth century. The first eight steps can be performed by laypersons. Ideally, a physician and four or five helpers are sufficient to carry on the resuscitation. Here is their list:

1. Remove the victim from the water with due caution.
2. Carry to the nearest convenient place.
3. Remove the clothes.
4. Wipe the body well.
5. Place the victim on a bed of straw.
6. Carefully cover him.
7. If he is stiff with cold, rub him with snow or ice-water.
8. Cleanse the mouth and nose.
9. Compress the chest. [Compression is recommended to remove the foul air and water from the lungs and allow fresh air to enter.]
10. Insufflate the lungs with air. [Tubes and bellows are recommended.]
11. If no air enters the lung, use a catheter.
12. If this proves impossible, perform a tracheotomy.
13. Apply electric shocks to the heart. [Electrical therapy in resuscitation is extensively covered in later chapters.]
14. Coax the blood toward the chest.
15. Continue for 15 minutes.
16. Ascertain the body temperature.
17. Administer an invigorating stimulant into the stomach.
18. Place bladders filled with hot water on the stomach and feet.
19. Administer a stimulant clyster [tobacco smoke in the rectum].
20. Continue rubbing the surface of the body.

21. Shake the victim vigorously.
22. Place in a suitable hot bath.
23. Stimulate the senses of smell and hearing [strong odors and loud noises].
24. Remove from bath and dry.
25. Continue insufflation of air into the lungs.
26. Apply electric shocks to the heart again.
27. Apply electric shocks to the spinal cord and neck.
28. Give the Drip Bath a trial [drip ice cold water on the abdomen or neck].
29. Continue the above remedies for several hours.
30. Finally, apply red-hot irons to the feet or other sensitive places.

Resuscitative efforts may be abandoned at this stage. However, every encouragement must be used during the attempt. Herholdt and Rafn noted, "During the procedure the unskilled helpers should be encouraged to unremittent diligence, and one should not entertain any doubt of seeing one's endeavors being crowned by a successful outcome. No one should believe that he had done his duty until he had rendered all the help he owes the victim."

Step 10 in their list involves insufflation of the lungs. Hernholdt and Rafn acknowledge mouth-to-mouth ventilation, but quickly dismiss it. They wrote, "But as the insufflation of air by mouth is a very toilsome and loathsome act, and since accordingly an otherwise laudable delicacy of feeling usually prohibits both the physician and other people of propriety from using this method . . . it is only of little use."

Amazingly, all the modern elements of resuscitation are present on this list. Admittedly, there are also a few that would not be part of accepted medical practice today. What was lacking was not the creativity of devising rescue techniques but the ability to separate effective from ineffective therapies. Anatomic understanding of the heart, lungs, and capillary exchange of oxygen was well understood. Not appreciated, however, was the rapid destruction of brain function within minutes of oxygen deprivation. And, most important, there was no awareness of the heart's rhythm disturbances, especially ventricular fibrillation. Much attention was given to the diagnostic significance of pulses and variations from normal, but without the electrocardiogram there could be no appreciation of fibrillation, nor any rational approach to the problem.

The rescue societies of Europe and the United States were ever mindful of opportunities for publicity and political goodwill. Not unlike today's large philanthropic societies, such as the American Heart Association or the American Red Cross, these societies produced widely circulated annual reports, gave medals and certificates to honored citizens, enlisted dues-paying members, and generally took advantage of fortuitious situations for self-serving promotion. One such opportunity involved the Emperor of Russia, Alexander I (1777–1825). The episode, reported to the Royal Humane Society by a member who had heard the story in St. Petersburg, occurred on April 15, 1806. It appeared that while the Emperor was traveling in Lithuania he encountered a drowned peasant. According to witnesses, "Prompted by humanity alone, and without any other assistance than that of the ignorant boors around him, he . . . immediately proceeded, with his own hands, to assist in taking off the wet clothes from the apparent corpse, and to rub his temples, wrists, etc." The effort continued for over three hours and, despite the advice of a surgeon to cease, the Emperor persisted. His perseverance was rewarded, and, following a fresh bleeding, a groan was heard from the victim. The Emperor was emotionally overcome and tearfully exclaimed in French, "Good God! this is the brightest day of my life!" To stop the blood, Alexander removed his own royal handkerchief, tore it into strips, and "with his own hands, bound the poor fellow's arm with it." The peasant survived and, needless to say, was astonished to learn the identity of his rescuer. The Emperor ordered the peasant a considerable present of money and then continued on his journey. On learning of this remarkable royal resuscitation, the Royal Humane Society issued a special account of the event. It also awarded the Emperor a gold medal. The accompanying florid letter stated that because of the perservering efforts of His Imperial Majesty, "life was, under Divine Providence, restored to one of his subjects, who, otherwise, would have been prematurely consigned to the grave."[31]

Resuscitation in London, *1820*

If John and June Colven had lived during this time in history, John's experience with sudden death would at least have had a chance of ending in a more fortunate fashion. Let us imagine the two in London in 1820. Average life expectancy by then has reached forty, the highest ever. The increase, though, was not progressive. During the Dark Ages the average life expectancy fell to thirty because of ravages of famine and plague that periodically swept through Europe. The leading cause of sudden and unexpected death remained accidents, with drownings near the top of the list.

John and June live near each other in the High Street Kensington part of London. He is a clerk for Lloyds of London; she works in a millinery shop. It is winter and he is courting her. John asks June to go ice skating on the lake at Hyde Park. John shows off by skating around the thin-ice warning flag. As he does, he hits a rut and falls down. The ice begins to crack and John panics. Instead of lying flat, he struggles to get up on his feet, causing him to slip through. John cannot swim and his clothing drags him under. Horrorstruck, June lets out a scream.

Others have also witnessed the accident and come running. The Royal Humane Society staffs a warming hut and someone grabs a long-poled hook from inside. The volunteers from the Humane Society are not physicians, but they have all read the Society's recommendations for dealing with drownings. After several minutes of fishing, the rescuers hook John's coat and drag his limp body onto the shore. He is not breathing.

Several men carry John to the warming hut. First they undress him and cover him with blankets. Next the rescuers press down on John's stomach in an attempt to remove swallowed water. A small amount appears to gurgle up. One of the attendants grabs a tube attached to a bellows, inserts it in John's throat, and begins vigorously squeezing the bellow. After about two minutes they hear a small cough. John starts to gag on the tube. The attendant quickly removes it and John begins to breathe on his own. The attendant later writes a full description of John's rescue. The Royal Humane Society receives the report the following day and enters it as case 763 for 1820.

Premature Burial and the Rise of Mortuaries

Concurrent with the rise of Rescue Societies was a growing dread of being buried alive. The numerous accounts of miraculous resuscitations publicized by the Societies helped convince the general public that people could literally be snatched back from the grave. But if such miracles could occur, then so could the opposite. A person could be buried *while still alive*. The dread of being buried alive seemed particularly widespread in the latter part of the eighteenth century. Popular fiction, particularly the works of Edgar Allen Poe, did much to reinforce this dread. Legislation was passed in Germany,

Austria, Holland, England, and France requiring some delay—as much as three days—before burial. The only exceptions were after executions and for threats to public health such as epidemics.[32]

Medical historian Maria Trumpler describes widely circulated stories of premature burial during the late 1700s and throughout much of the 1800s. These stories led to ingenious devices allowing a buried person to signal that he or she had revived. The U.S. Patent Office awarded patent number 81,437 in 1868 for a coffin with a superstructure protruding from the ground. Inside the above-ground portion was a ladder for the person to climb up. Should the individual be too weak to use the ladder, a bell could be rung, alerting a cemetery visitor. The patent specification reads in part, "Should a person be interred ere life is extinct, he can, on recovery to consciousness, ascend from the grave and the coffin by the ladder; or, if not able to ascend by said ladder, ring the bell, thereby giving an alarm, and thus save himself from premature burial and death." The coffin had a sliding door atop so that if the corpse is confirmed dead, the superstructure portion could be pulled up and the sliding door closed—permanently one would hope. The ladder portion could be used again.[33]

Dr. Benjamin Rush, writing in the annual report of the Royal Humane Society for the year 1805, noted, "If we for a moment contemplate the dreadful situation of a human being, not really dead, hurried to the grave, and thus rashly precipitated into the arms of death; can we too highly appreciate . . . (such) a fear, which surpasses even the fear of death itself?" Dr. Rush once recounted the story of an eighty-year-old patient of his who begged that he not be interred for seven full days after his death. The reason for the request was that as a young man he had died "to all appearance of the yellow fever in one of the West India Islands." The man heard the people who attended him fix on the time and place of his burial, and the horror of this information caused "diffuse motion throughout his body, and finally excited in him all the usual functions of life."[34]

In 1869 Charles Dickens, writing in his weekly journal, *All the Year Round,* alludes to a technique for preventing premature burial. He advocated the placement of atropine drops (which would lead to pupil dilation in a live person) in the corpse. A camera obscura with photographic film was used to take repeated photos of the eye over thirty minutes. If the film revealed no pupil dilation, the person was presumed dead. Apparently, Dickens was serious in his suggestion. There is no record of anyone using this complicated method.

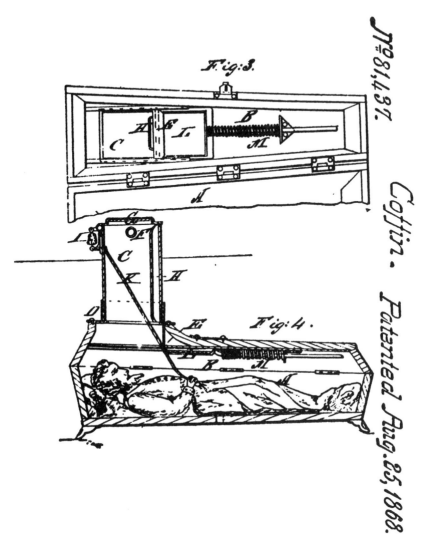

FIGURE II. *Device to allow a prematurely buried person to pull a rope and signal a bell above ground. (Courtesy of Dover Publications, Inc.)*

It's doubtful that a physician who accidentally declared a live person dead would be in much demand. The only way to be absolutely certain of death was for the onset of putrefaction to occur. This was aesthetically as well as olfactorily not a very attractive option. What's more, infectious disease could easily spread to bystanders as the body began to decompose. Some people suggested that towns build morgues where the dead could be kept for several days until definitive death was ascertained by the stink of putrefaction. In 1791, Christoph Hufeland proposed that the morgue logically be located next to the graveyard. He also advocated that a small adjacent apartment be built for a watchman who could look through his living room window directly into the room with the bodies. He could then both smell the sign of definitive death as well as observe someone coming back to life.[35]

In Weimar, Germany, the first elaborate mortuary was constructed in 1792 and other cities throughout Europe and Scandanavia proposed or built similar ones in the following years. One plan called for a mortuary with forty-six cells clustered around an observation window. Attached to the hand of each corpse was a string, which, if moved even slightly, would trigger a loud alarm. A guard was on duty twenty-four hours a day and physicians made rounds on the dead patients from time to time. One writer compared this plan to a intensive care unit for patients without vital signs.[36] It is very likely that many alarms were heard since the watchmen received extra pay when they attempted resuscitations.

Relating the fear of premature burial to rescue societies is a bit like the origin of the chicken and the egg. Did the fear of being buried alive stimulate rescue societies to attempt new methods for revival, or did the new methods of revival activate a deeply felt primeval fear? It is, of course, impossible to say. The increasingly common reports of resuscitation from drowning or suffocation must have paradoxically fueled the fear of premature burial. What is clear is that both phenomena coincided in time.

The ability to recognize death was the subject of many scientific treatises of the late eighteenth and early nineteenth centuries. In his essay of 1788 Charles Kite proposed that an electric shock should be given to apparently dead persons and, if the muscles did not twitch, the person was dead. Kite wrote, "Electrical shock is to be admitted as the test, or discriminating characteristic of any remains of animal life; and so long as that produces contractions, may the person be said to be in a recoverable state; but when that effect has ceased, there can be no doubt remain of the party being absolutely and positively dead."[37] James Curry, writing in 1815 in his book *Observations on Apparent Death from Drowning, Hanging, Suffocation by Noxious Vapours, Fainting-fits, Intoxication, Lightning, Exposure to Cold, etc, etc.*, offers some indicators of death. He ghoulishly describes that the Vital Principle (modern equivalent terms are spark of life or essence of life) is extinguished when the body is cold and rigid, livid and contracted, or of black and swollen countenance. None of these findings, however, either singly or in combination, is an infallible indicator. He writes, "A beginning putrefaction of the body is perhaps the only unequivocal proof of death..."[38]

Not until our own century did physicians distinguish between clinical death and biological death. What added to the confusion was the awareness that muscle contractions were possible with electrical stimulation for hours after death. This is why the effort to revive Mary Macintyre continued so long, as we saw earlier. The assumption, given muscular contractions plus observations that some drowning victims were revived after long periods of submersion, was that life extinguished slowly. If hours, why not days? In reality, the journey from clinical death to biological death is traveled in minutes, not hours.

Out goes the bad air, in goes the good air.

A BETTER MOUSETRAP

« »

In the middle of the nineteenth century a major departure occurred in artificial respiration. Until this time most techniques advocated warming, direct stimulation, or fumigants to stimulate the body. Marshall Hall (1790–1857), a London physician, took issue with these methods and ushered in an era of mechanical expansion and compression of the chest wall. For the next 100 years this approach would define artificial respiration, with dozens of methods advocated. It was an era devoted to creating a better mousetrap—even though the jaws of death were far too large to be harnessed by this technique alone.

Hall, during his career, was apparently both loved and hated. The founder and editor of the prestigious medical journal *The Lancet* claimed that the stature of Hall's work equaled that of Harvey. Most of Hall's research and 150 published papers involved the study of spinal cord reflexes. Like many learned men of his day, his writings were often far afield from medicine, and he wrote on such diverse topics as geometry, Greek grammar, and social ills. He campaigned to abolish slavery in America and stop flogging in the British army. Others were not impressed and considered him insufferably conceited.[1]

In 1857 Hall published his paper, "Prone and Postural Respiration in Drowning," and criticized the Royal Humane Society's techniques. He believed that valuable time was lost in transporting the victim; that restoration with warmth without artificial ventilation was dangerous and too time consuming; that exposure to fresh air was beneficial; and that in the supine position, the victim's tongue and larynx fell back and blocked the airway. He favored shifting a victim's position from stomach (to cause expiration of air) to side (to cause inspiration of air) fifteen times per minute. He also suggested applying expiratory pressure to the victim's back while the victim was prone. Air-exchange volumes of 70 to 240 milliliters were reported with this technique, which was accepted by the Royal Humane Society and other rescue societies including the National Life Boat Institution. Hall called his technique the "ready method" because no equipment or complicated training were required. Charles Hunter, a contemporary surgeon, wrote, "no greater practical benefit has been conferred on mankind than this ready method of Marshall Hall."[2] Hall's technique recognized two aspects of resuscitation that any effective method must address: airway obstruction and the need to institute aid instantly.

FIGURE 12. *Marshall Hall's technique of artificial respiration, 1856. Top figure shows inspiratory phase and bottom figure depicts expiratory phase. (Courtesy of* The Lancet*)*

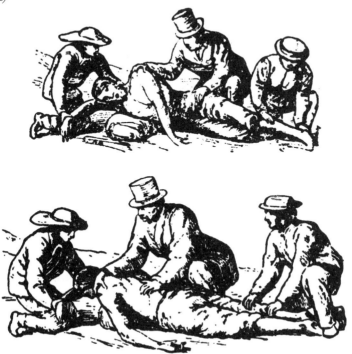

One year later, Henry R. Silvester, another London physician, advocated raising the victim's arms above the head, thus expanding the upper rib cage and facilitating inhalation. The rescuer would then put the victim's arms on his or her chest and apply pressure, causing exhalation. Silvester felt Hall's method was too cumbersome and objected to the "trundling" of patients, as he called it. Silvester believed his method produced more air exchange than Hall's technique and could be performed in a warm bath. He also claimed that Hall's method moved less than twenty-five milliliters of air. Silvester introduced his paper of 1858 by saying that "inducing respiratory movements, by which air is drawn into the lungs without apparatus . . . is of universal application, easy of performance, entirely in harmony with that of Nature."[3] To Silvester, the essential part of respiration was alternate compression and relaxation of the chest to induce expiration and inspiration. After pointing out the risks of inducing respiration by placing the patient prone or on the side, Silvester describes his own method, "a simple imitation of natural deep respiration . . . effected by means of the same muscles as are employed by nature. Therefore, in my method we lift the ribs and sternum by the pectoral and other muscles . . . by extending the arms up by the side of the patient's head, which elevates the patient's ribs, creates a vacuum and allows a rush of air into the lungs. Expiration is brought about by simple compression of the sides of the chest by the patient's arms. . . . The arms of the patients are to be used by the operator as handles to open and close the chest. . . . The patient is on his back."[4] When it was applied expertly, an air exchange of 300 to 500 milliliters was purportedly accomplished.[5] In 1858 Silvester's method was published in the *British Medical Journal* under the title "A New Method of Resuscitating Still-born Children, and of Restoring Persons Apparently Drowned or Dead." At the article's conclusion, he lists twelve advantages for his method, among them: "It may be adopted when the patient is in the warm bath," "The contents of the stomach are not liable to pass into the windpipe," "This process is entirely in harmony with that of nature," "This method is the most easy of adoption," and, perhaps the coup de grace, "A larger amount of air is inspired than by any other method."[6] Indeed, Silvester was prominent enough to be featured in the *London Illustrated News*. A spoof of one of his resuscitation ideas shows various dogs, cattle, and boys being blown up with air to prevent drowning.

Shortly after Silvester's method was published the battle began. His method was critized for causing possible dislocation of the arms as well as leading to inadequate ventilation. Advocates of the new method argued just

FIG. 3.

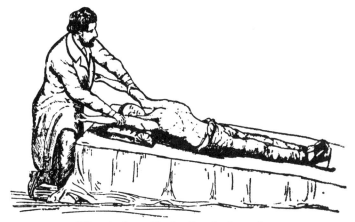

Silvester's method. Inspiratory phase.

FIG. 4.

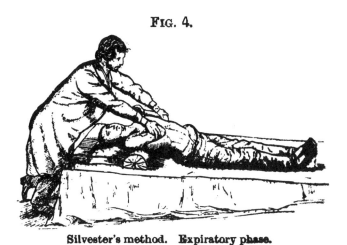

Silvester's method. Expiratory phase.

FIGURE 13. *Henry Silvester's technique of artificial respiration, 1858. Top figure shows inspiratory phase and bottom figure depicts expiratory phase. (Courtesy of* The Lancet*)*

as vehemently that Hall's technique was grossly insufficient in the amount of air it supplied to the victim's lungs. The Royal Medical and Chirurgical Society finally settled the matter in 1862. A committee convened by the Society recommended Silvester's method after performing experiments on cadavers. It was accepted as the preferred method by the Royal Humane Society, and it remained popular well into the first half of this century.[7]

The most famous person to receive Silvester's method of artificial respiration was Abraham Lincoln. Within seconds after the assassin's bullet struck, Charles Augustus Leale, an army surgeon, tended to the mortally wounded president. At first glance, Leale saw the extremis condition of Lincoln and, on attempting to locate the source of blood, quickly found the bullet wound in the back of Lincoln's head. His effort to remove the obstructing clot and thereby relieve pressure on the brain (or so he reasoned) was easily accomplished but without result. Leale next tried to revive the president using artificial respiration. According to the account he later recorded, "I leaned forward, opened his mouth and introduced two extended fingers of my right hand as far back as possible, and by pressing the base of his paralyzed tongue downward and outward, opened his larynx and made a free passage for air to enter his lung." Leale used an assistant to apply the Silvester maneuver. Lincoln's arms were repeatedly raised to expand the thorax, then slowly brought to his side to force air out of the lung. Leale pressed on the diaphragm to facilitate air movement. Though he thought temporary signs of recovery resulted from his efforts, he concluded that "something more must be done to retain life." Acting out of desperation, the surgeon "leaned forcibly forward directly over his body, thorax to thorax, face to face, and several times drew in a long breath, then forcibly expanded his lungs and improved his respiration."[8] It is not clear if Leale performed mouth-to-mouth resuscitation as it is done today, but, whatever he did, Lincoln's heartbeat improved in strength and spontaneous breathing occurred. The resuscitation was short-lived, however. Lincoln died the next day.

A New York physician, Benjamin Howard, surgeon and professor at the Long Island College Hospital, criticized both Hall and Silvester in describing his own method in 1869. His publication, "Plain Rules for the Restoration of Persons Apparently Dead from Drowning," is a modest five-page pamphlet specifying six rules of artificial respiration. His instructions included the following: "Rule 3. (to open the airway) Patient is on his back. Let some bystander hold the tip of the tongue out of one corner of the mouth with a dry handkerchief. Rule 4. (to produce respiration) Kneel astride the patient's hips, and with your hands resting on his stomach, spread out your fingers so that you can grasp the waist about the short ribs. Now, throw all your weight steadily forward upon your hands, while you at the same time squeeze the ribs deeply, as if you wished to force everything in the chest upwards out of the mouth. Continue this while you slowly count one-two-three; then, SUDDENLY, let go, with a final push, which springs you

FIG. 5.

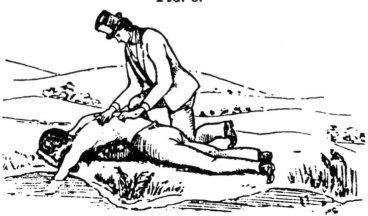

Howard's method. Preliminary compression.

FIG. 6.

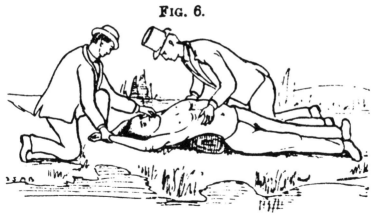

Howard's method. Posture of patient and of operators.
(From Howard's original paper.)

FIGURE 14. *Benjamin Howard's technique of artificial respiration, 1871.*
(*Courtesy of* The Lancet)

back to your first kneeling position." The process is repeated initially at the
rate of five times per minute, but gradually increases up to fifteen. In Step 5,
Howard recommends continuing this treatment, if needed, for two hours.[9]

In a later article published in *The Lancet* in 1877, Howard gives the reason
for naming his method. "This method is called the 'direct method' because

by it the few things needed to be done are, simply, done. The tongue needs holding forward—it is held; the ribs, pressing—they are pressed. It is so simple that a Harbour policeman, after a single lesson, has done it as well as I . . . can do it. Adjunctive measures as friction, electricity, insufflation, or even tracheotomy, can be used simultaneously."[10]

Indeed, many physicians and inventors tried to develop their own new and improved method, among them Alexander Graham Bell. After Bell had invented the telephone at age thirty, he continued to pursue innovative ideas, often failing to bring them to fruition. After he had taken courses in anatomy and physiology at University College in London in 1868, he became interested in the physiology of respiration and asphyxia, and began working on the construction of an apparatus that would resuscitate by assisting the victim's breathing. He called this a "vacuum jacket," which would mechanically produce expansion and contraction of the thoracic cavity. It was rigid and airtight, and connected to a piston pump. He argued that manual techniques did not allow sufficient expansion of the thorax. When Bell moved to Ontario in 1870, he left his vacuum pump jacket with a Professor Minchin at the Alexandria Hotel for further experiments. Twenty-two years later (!) when Bell wrote to find out what had happened to the jacket, it was still located at the hotel "with no evidence that it had been disturbed for experimentation." After some further misadventures, the jacket finally came to rest in the Alexander Graham Bell Museum at Baddeck, Nova Scotia.

By 1890, the Royal Medical and Chirurgical Society in England felt it was time to form another committee to reevaluate current methods of artificial respiration, and appointed Edward A. Schafer its chairman. Schafer immediately pointed to the inadequacy of testing the various techniques on dogs and cadavers, and introduced the novel idea of suspended respiration. By having his subjects hyperventilate Schafer could test the various methods after a period of hyperventilation when the subject had little desire or need to breathe. His experiments found the Silvester method the least effective, the Hall method a little better, and the Howard method the best of the three, but still far below normal ventilation. Schafer considered them all inadequate and of course developed his own. His procedure consisted of intermittent pressure on the back of the prone victim, a technique he called the "prone pressure" technique. Schafer believed this afforded gas exchange, maintained an open airway, and allowed water and mucus to drain from the airway. He felt it posed no risk to other organs, was easy to learn, and could be performed without fatigue.

Not surprisingly, many of the old guard resisted Schafer's method. Silvester led the opposition, objecting to the suggestive posture of a male rescuer "athwart the (female) patient." Despite this opposition, the Schafer method gradually became the standard in the United States and throughout Europe, and, by 1910, the American Red Cross began teaching it. Julius H. Comroe, writing in 1979 says: "When I was a boy, there were only three things for sure in medicine: (1) if you had tonsils, they had to come out; (2) if you had TB, you went to bed for two years; and (3) if you drowned, the first person to reach you applied Schafer's prone-pressure method of respiration." Millions of Boy Scouts and Girl Scouts learned the Schafer technique along with the rhythmic chant, "Out goes the bad air" (as the back is pressed) "and in comes the good air" (as the pressure is released). One historian claims a more appropriate chant would have been, "Nothing is going out and nothing is coming in."

For the first several decades of the twentieth century advocates for either the older Silvester method or Schafer's newer prone-pressure technique argued. These two methods defined the debate, though occasional critical voices could be heard. In 1906, the Irish surgeon Robert Woods rejected both methods and revived the long neglected mouth-to-mouth technique. He wrote, "It seems to me to be clear from every consideration that the

FIGURE 15. *Edward Schafer's technique of artificial respiration, known as the prone pressure method, 1903. (Courtesy of The Royal Life Saving Society UK, Warwickshire, England)*

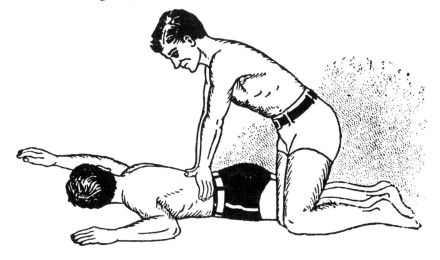

mouth-to-mouth or nose method gives the patient the best chance, for to recapitulate: (1) The quantity of tidal air is greater than by any indirect method . . . (2) The impurities, if present at all, are neglible, (3) The method can be applied without a moment's loss of time."[11] But his voice was stifled in the maelstrom over Silvester's and Schafer's techniques.

There was also widespread geographic variation in which technique was preferred, with Silvester's method popular in Germany, Holland, and Russia, and Schafer's in England, France, and Belgium.[12] Colonel Holger Louis Nielsen (1866–1955), in Denmark, was well aware of the controversy. He believed the best resolution was to develop a synthetic method that combined the optimum features of both. His original plan was to have two rescuers—one to perform prone pressure on the lower back to cause exhalation while the other lifted the arms above the victim to facilitate inhalation. But this method was rejected by the Danish Red Cross in 1930 because it required two rescuers. Back to the drawing board.

Nielsen's breakthrough came when he visited a masseur for relief from rheumatic pains in his shoulders and noticed that when the masseur pressed down on his shoulder blades, he experienced a forceful expiration. This experience led him to suggest one rescuer positioned at the head of the victim, who alternates pressure on the upper back for expiration and lifts the arms for inhalation. Nielsen described his prone back-pressure arm-lift methods in 1932, and presented physiologic data to support the superiority of his method. Tidal volumes of 450 to 1750 milliliters were measured in relaxed, hyperventilated subjects, a much better performance than other methods of artificial ventilation.

Acceptance of Nielsen's method by Red Cross and rescue societies was rapid in Denmark and other Scandinavian countries. Over the next two decades instruction in the new artificial respiration spread throughout Europe and then to the United States. In 1953 the International Red Cross conference in Toronto adopted Nielsen's method as its standard in first-aid teaching.

Yet before the 1950s ended, a truly effective method of artificial respiration would resurface. Nielsen's place in the history of resuscitation would be maintained as a historical footnote, yet there was no indication of his disappointment. On learning of an improved method of artificial ventilation, he said, "I am only too pleased if there is another method more efficient than mine."[13]

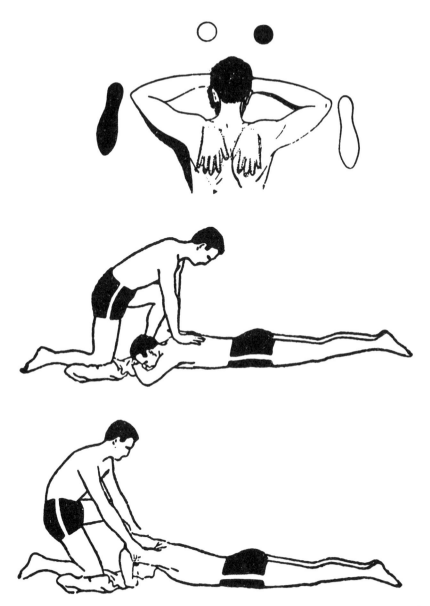

FIGURE 16. *Holger Nielsen's technique of artificial respiration, known as the back-pressure arm-lift method, 1932. The top figure shows hand, feet, and knee placement of rescuer, middle figure depicts expiration; bottom figure shows inspiration. (Courtesy of Danish Red Cross, Copenhagen)*

Archer S. Gordon and the Search for the Best Method

Archer S. Gordon first became involved with resuscitation in 1949, when he began research under the mentorship of Andrew Ivy. A well-known physiologist, Ivy was then vice-president of the University of Illinois Medical Center in Chicago. Under his direction, Gordon evaluated different methods of artificial respiration to determine the most effective one. This was work that Ivy and two colleagues had begun a few years earlier when Ivy had used human corpses immediately after death to measure how well different manual methods of ventilation worked.

Gordon enlarged the research's scope and included corpses from all the adult wards of Cook County Hospital, running the program on a twenty-four-hour-a-day basis. With no research funds available, Gordon worked without a salary and slept on a cot in Ivy's office.

Cook County Hospital was across the street from Ivy's office. "When I received a call that a patient had expired," Gordon later recalled, "I rushed across the street, got my cart of equipment, rushed to the ward, moved the corpse to a secluded examining room, and proceeded with my studies." Gordon would insert a tube into the corpse's trachea and hook it up to a machine to measure air volume. As Gordon performed the various manual methods, he would determine which pushed the greatest volume of air into the lung. This was long before the days of sophisticated electronic measuring devices. He recorded the results of his experiments on paper-covered drums in a spring-loaded machine called a kymograph. He personally prepared the paper by coating it with a fine layer of soot from a burning candle. After each case, he would shellac the tracing in order to preserve the record.

Gordon soon discovered that others had tried similar research with corpses, but had not fared well. Yet he pressed on. "After about five months I had collected useful data from over a hundred corpses. That's when the American National Red Cross got interested in the project. They provided me with a small grant of $5,000," that enabled Gordon to give himself a small monthly stipend of $150. Meanwhile, his research had taken a physical toll. Gordon had to quit his studies and undergo surgery to repair a hernia caused by lifting so many corpses.

By now Gordon had gotten a general surgery residency at Hines Veterans Administration Hospital. That was later followed by a thoracic surgery residency at Hines and a cardiovascular surgery residency at Rush-Presbyterian-St. Luke's Hospital in Chicago. Over the next several years he obtained his master's and doctorate in physiology, married, and started a family. Through it all, he continued his research on manual ventilation methods. Gordon's early results were published in December 1950 in the *Journal of the American Medical Association.*[14]

Meanwhile, the U.S. Defense Department became interested in Gordon's work. The Army was particularly worried about the effects of nerve gas on its troops, and wondered if some form of manual resuscitation might help stricken soldiers. They also wondered if Gordon's corpse-based studies really applied to nonbreathing living humans. Their question led Gordon to begin working with living bodies—anesthetized medical students. Gordon asked for volunteers and followed a procedure that paralyzed their respiratory systems with curare injections. He would quickly carry out the same set of procedures and measurements he had done on the corpses, and then revive the volunteers. Despite the potential danger of these experiments, Gordon proceeded carefully and meticulously. There were no complications or problems, and a paper based on this research appeared in the same issue of *JAMA* that reported his work on corpses.

By the end of 1951, Gordon had produced considerable data on the relative effectiveness of currently used methods of artificial respiration—the Silvester method (Arm-Lift Back-Pressure), the Schafer (Prone Pressure), Eve (Rocking),[15] Nielsen (Arm-Lift Back-Pressure), Emerson (hip-lift), and Schafer-Emerson-Ivy (a combination of the Schafer and Emerson methods). His work indicated that a modified Nielsen method of manual respiration surpassed all others in efficacy, ease of performance, and simplicity of learning. Gordon urged that an hoc Conference on Artificial Resuscitation be convened by the National Research Council and National Academy of Sciences, and in fall 1951, the meeting took place. Its recommendation was that the modified Nielsen method become the preferred method of resuscitation. Gordon presented the results of his research at this meeting and later published his work in the December 6, 1951, issue of *JAMA*. In this article he alludes to mouth-to-mouth and mouth-to-nose artificial respiration, but because of the "difficulties involved in studying and teaching the method, it has not been included in these tests."[16]

In 1952 Gordon encountered James Elam. Gordon was speaking at a meeting in Chicago of the AMA Council on Medical Physics and gave a presentation on his research, focusing on the relative efficacy of the Nielsen method. By that time Elam had had six years of private experience in reviving people using mouth-to-nose resuscitation and could no longer contain his sarcasm. "Didn't they rotate you through anesthesia, Dr. Gordon?" he inquired. After Gordon's talk, Elam rose and remarked that manual resuscitation methods "were doomed." Mouth-to-nose worked; he'd been doing it for years with polio patients.

At the time, Gordon was apparently not convinced by Elam's extemporaneous proselytizing. He continued to champion the Nielsen method of manual resuscitation, and pursued his research. Not long after, however, Gordon and Elam met again at the Edgewood Army Chemical Center. "Why don't you give expired air resuscitation [as Elam then called mouth-to-mouth] a chance; go home and try it," Elam urged. Gordon did just that, beginning a series of studies of mouth-to-nose and mouth-to-mouth resuscitation.

Gordon's research on Nielsen's and other manual techniques represented the concluding chapter in hundreds of years of experimentation and development on artificial respiration. All the methods worked to some degree, but what was shown to be moderately effective in the laboratory would be worthless in the real world.

Peter Karpovich's book, *Adventures in Artificial Respiration*, written in 1953, lists 105 published methods of artificial ventilation for adults and twelve for infants.[17] He divides the adult methods into thirty-seven expiratory, eighteen inspiratory, and fifty combined methods. With such a deluge of techniques and the cacophony caused by their numerous advocates, it is no wonder that confusion, argument, and controversy reigned. The world awaited a better method, one that would take into account adequate air exchange, ease of application, and also facilitate artificial circulation.

God blew into his nostrils the breath of life, and man became a living being.
—Genesis 2

THE KISS OF LIFE

《 》

As the germ theory of disease gained acceptance in medicine, mouth-to-mouth respiration fell into disrepute and then near-oblivion. It seems self-evident today that blowing air into someone's lungs is effective—it is the logical thing to do for someone not breathing. Yet mouth-to-mouth ventilation has only been reconsidered in the past fifty years and officially sanctioned since 1958. Even as recently as 1935, some zany (by today's standards) recommendations were made in the medical literature. For example, for non-breathing newborns one authority proposed plunging the baby into cold water. In another technique, "the large finger of the obstetrician is thrust into the tiny anus of the infant. Like a badly adjusted motor it is 'cranked' so vigorously that, if there is any vitality, a gasp results."[1]

Several people in the 1950s and early 1960s played a vital role in rediscovering and reviving this ancient and effective method of resuscitation. They included a former Boy Scout, a survivor of the Nazi occupation of Austria during World War II, and a Baltimore, Maryland, fire chief.

Jim Elam and the Method of Elisha

For Jim Elam, the journey that led him to mouth-to-mouth (or, to be more accurate in his case, mouth-to-nose breathing) may well have begun on a

football field. In the fifth grade Elam was the mascot for the local high
school football team. "Mascot" meant "water boy," but young Elam did get
to wear "a little bitty football uniform" (as he called it) like the other players.
He got his first glimpse of a form of resuscitation during this time. "When a
guy got the wind knocked out of him," Elam recalled, "the coach would
come out and pick him up by his belt, raise his chest about a foot in the air,
and drop him. It really worked! I'd see this prostrate guy get up on all fours,
and breathe and he was OK. That impressed me." The memory of those inci-
dents stuck with him.

So did the rescue training he would later receive: "In the Boy Scouts I
learned the Schafer method. And at Scout camp I learned a lot of Red Cross
lifesaving stuff." Another important influence was something he saw as a
medical student at Johns Hopkins University. "Sometimes residents would
get called to the side of a patient who had collapsed and had no pulse or was-
n't breathing. I'd see them pushing on the patient's chest a few times. They
didn't take the pillow out from under the person's head, not realizing that
flexion of the head meant airway obstruction. They would just push a few
times, then turn around and sign the death certificate," he said. "I couldn't
help but wonder whether what I had seen attempted were maneuvers for
artificial respiration. It sure seemed a hopeless picture, though." Just as hopeless was a procedure used at another hospital. "I heard Bob Dripps describe
that at the University of Pennsylvania Hospital, before he began a program
in anesthesiology, that when a patient stopped breathing they called the fire
department to come to the hospital with their equipment. I thought that was
kind of ludicrous."

Elam discounts the influences of football mascot or Boy Scout training on
his lifelong interest in resuscitation. He attributes the reason to his own
resuscitation—at his birth. Elam was born prematurely and weighed less
than two pounds. Few "preemies" that small survived in 1918. According to
Elam, the general practitioner in Austin, Texas, who delivered him told his
mother to "spank him every time he stops breathing." She did just that and
years later would often tell the story to her son. During a poliomyelitis epidemic in Minnesota in 1946, Elam first tried mouth-to-nose breathing on
patients with acute poliomyelitis paralysis. These episodes invariably
occurred at times of equipment failure or when patients arrived in the hospital with acute respiratory paralysis. According to Elam, he performed mouth-
to-nose ventilation because it seemed the obvious thing to do.

Polio was a terrifying disease in the 1940s and 1950s, usually striking children and young adults. Though present for centuries, it reached public consciousness during a large epidemic in New York City in 1916 when 9000 cases were reported. The disease spread throughout the country with small and large epidemics usually occurring in the summer months. The epidemic peaked in the early 1950s with 50,000 cases per year. Ironically, the disease is very mild in infants and leaves no residual paralysis. When it strikes older children or adults, the result is permanent paralysis in 10 percent of cases and death in 1 percent. Death occurs from paralysis of the swallowing and breathing muscles; the person suffocates because he or she can't inhale air or is unable to swallow and chokes on saliva. Iron lungs allowed the lung to expand. The patient lay inside the tubular machine with only the head sticking outside. Negative pressure, sufficient to cause the lung to passively expand, is cycled inside the machine at a rate of fifteen times per minute. The principle is similar to how a vacumn cleaner operates, except air instead of dirt is sucked in. If assisted breathing kept the person alive, after a while he or she might partially recover and not require the iron lung. Unfortunately, some individuals did not readily recover and needed the iron lung for years.[2] Elam treated the worst variety of polio, the type known as combined spinal bulbar paralysis. This form affected both the spinal cord (resulting in paralysis of the arms, legs, and breathing muscles) and the bulbar part of the brain (causing paralysis of the swallowing muscles). The patient couldn't move, couldn't breathe, and couldn't swallow. The mortality from this severe form of polio was almost 50 percent.

Elam describes the first time he tried mouth-to-nose breathing. The year was 1946. Having completed an internship at Bethesda Naval Hospital, Elam traveled to Minneapolis for graduate work in respiratory physiology. His graduate professor suggested he apply oximetry (determining the level of oxygen reaching the blood) to acute polio patients. The University of Minnesota Hospital was in the middle of a raging epidemic. "I had a copy of *Medical Physics*, edited by Otto Glasser," Elam recalled. "I was reading the ten-page chapter in it by Dr. Hart Ellis Fisher on the history of resuscitation. I had just gotten to Minneapolis, and had settled in and was reading this Fisher chapter. It impressed me." The chapter detailed eighty-four manual methods of artificial respiration. Mouth-to-nose and mouth respiration were mentioned as early techniques especially for midwives delivering infants. The method was dropped as a reliable method of resuscitation largely because "the medical profession considered it a vulgar act."[3] Fortunately Elam was not dissuaded.

"A few days later," Elam continued, "I reported to the polio ward and was being shown around by the head nurse when along the corridor came a gurney racing—a nurse pulling it and two orderlies pushing it. The kid on it was blue. I went into total reflex behavior. I stepped out in the middle of the corridor, stopped the gurney, grabbed the sheet, wiped the copious mucous off his mouth and face and tilted his head back, took a big breath, sealed my lips around his nose, and inflated his lungs. In four breaths he was pink. I kept on because they had to do a tracheotomy. He was just totally unable to swallow; he had bulbar polio. While we were waiting to do the trach, the nurses and interns gathered around the gurney where I was inflating his lungs and someone said, 'Dr. Elam, you're going to get polio.' 'Well, it's possible, but I kind of doubt it since I was exposed to a lot of polio at Hopkins and I reckon I have immunity. Besides, I'm doing mouth-to-nose on a dry face and if anybody gets bugs transferred it'll be him not me.' To make a very long three weeks short, I saved probably twenty or so teenage kids who came into the ER and I got paged instead of them paging anybody else."

There was no polio vaccine in 1946; the Salk vaccine would not become available until 1957. While Elam probably did have immunity (most cases of polio occurred in infancy or childhood and conferred lifelong immunity), there was of course no way of knowing. In fact, some epidemics resulted in the spread of polio to doctors and nurses. In 1934 during an epidemic in Los Angeles, 5 percent of doctors and 11 percent of nurses contracted the disease.[4]

At that time there was no squeeze bag for emergency ventilation. The only thing available to Elam was his own mouth and chest. As an anesthesiology resident in Iowa City in 1949, he frequently did the procedure on patients being induced for anesthesia after insertion of the endotracheal tube while waiting for the anesthesia machine.[5] To demonstrate that expired air was sufficient for oxygenation, Elam asked residents to draw blood gas measurements from the patient's wrist artery. The level often came back 100 percent. Elam had his confirmation that expired air could oxygenate a non-breathing person. Such "experiments" were done in an era when informed consent was considerably different from today's complex regulations and written documentation. Then consent was verbally obtained. Elam saw no risk to the patient.

Elam's next move was to Boston. In 1949, while at Massachusetts General Hospital where he was training as an assistant resident, Elam wondered why no one officially recommended mouth-to-mouth emergency ventilation. He did a literature search and found 108 techniques in use between 1850 and

1950. These were manual methods and mouth-to-mouth was used, primarily by midwives on newborns. One article totally ignored by the medical community was a paper in the October 30, 1943, issue of *JAMA* by Ralph M. Waters. Entitled "Simple Methods for Performing Artificial Respiration," the paper argued that mouth-to-mouth or mouth-to-nose ventilation was easy to perform and expired air was sufficient to ventilate a nonbreathing person. Waters writes, "Direct inflation of the lungs is always at hand. Either the nose or the mouth may be blown into while one hand of the rescuer holds the other portal closed. The other hand, resting on the subject's chest, perceives the point at which the chest moves; in other words, when the lungs are sufficiently inflated." The figure accompanying the article is remarkable in its resemblance to contemporary mouth-to-mouth ventilation. It even includes a handkerchief to guard against infectious diseases. In 1943 the major infectious killers were polio and tuberculosis.[6] The article may have been ignored because of its lack of experimental data—it reads more like an editorial with no objective proof to support the author's conclusion.

Another article unknown either to Waters or Elam had been published in the *Transactions of the Royal Academy of Medicine—Ireland*, in 1906. The author, Robert H. Woods, a throat surgeon at the Richmond Hospital in Dublin, recognized that manual methods of artificial ventilation were ineffective. Instead, he recommended mouth-to-mouth respiration at a rate of once every five seconds. Four cases are described; two survived respiratory arrest. Perhaps the journal's obscurity prevented anyone else from picking up on the idea.[7]

Elam had become convinced of the value of mouth-to-nose ventilation; he spoke out whenever he could, noting the ineffectiveness of the Nielsen method. Elam recalled his comments to a 1952 meeting on medical ethics of the American Medical Association in Chicago: "It was fresh on my mind that midwives had never abandoned the method in Europe, that it had fallen into disrepute with the advent of the germ theory, and that there were religious, cultural and all kinds of objections of which the medical profession had virtually been unaware. When I first did it, I behaved reflexively; it may be that I recalled what I had read about mouth-to-mouth. At the time I thought to myself, 'Why the mouth'? It would be a lot easier to ventilate through the nose because that's what we ordinarily breath through and besides it probably wouldn't blow up the stomach. I never did blow up the stomach. Besides, if you're dealing with a kid that's just pouring out saliva, very copious stuff, you're much better off to make a seal around the nose—really dry off the mouth and then close the lips with two fingers."

To prove the value of mouth-to-nose breathing, Elam first had to show scientifically that exhaled air was adequate to oxygenate a nonbreathing person. It was widely believed that exhaled air, with 16 percent oxygen, was too low compared to air, which contained 21 percent. His personal observations while on the polio ward in Minnesota and during his anesthesiology residency, though compelling, were not reported to the medical world. Elam needed irrefutable data collected in a rigorous fashion. The year was 1952 and Elam was an assistant professor in the Division of Anesthesiology at Barnes Hospital in St. Louis. He obtained permission from his chief of surgery, Dr. Evarts Graham, to do studies on post-op surgical patients before they recovered from ether anesthesia. The endotracheal tube was left in place and succinylcholine (used to keep the patient paralyzed) was continued as a drip. By blowing into the tracheal tube with his expired air, Elam found that total arterial oxygen saturation could be maintained at 100 percent. Nine patients were studied and the results were unequivocal: expired air was able to maintain adequate oxygenation. In his scientific writings Elam called his technique expired-air resuscitation, but he always thought of it as the "method of Elisha."

From Barnes Hospital Elam was recruited to direct a new anesthesiology department at Roswell Park Memorial Institute (a cancer research hospital) in Buffalo. Elam arrived at his new job in May 1954, the same week his article was published in the *New England Journal of Medicine*[8] proving the usefulness of expired-air resuscitation.

Elam barely unpacked his boxes before he began proclaiming the benefits of mouth-to-mouth and mouth-to-nose breathing. Elam realized that expired-air resuscitation was most useful for drownings, smoke inhalations, and other breathing emergencies. He therefore began a series of Saturday morning lectures and demonstrations for rescue personnel. Up to 200 attended these seminars; they undoubtedly must have left an indelible impression. Elam used a volunteer medical student, Jim Doyle, to demonstrate the superiority of mouth-to-mouth respiration over the back pressure-arm lift methods. Doyle was anesthetized and paralyzed with succinylcholine and an oximeter attached to his earlobe to measure the oxygen content of his blood. This was no ordinary oximeter—it had a dial big enough to be seen from the back of the room. When Elam performed the Schafer and Nielson methods, the amount of oxygenated blood fell toward a dangerous 70 percent. The plunge in oxygen saturation would have continued with these methods. But with a magician's dramatic flair Elam began to breath into Doyle's mouth and the audience could see the immediate increase in oxygen saturation reflected on the oximeter. After a few breaths, the level approached a normal 100 percent. Elam and Doyle put on their Saturday show a dozen time, and if the rescue personnel couldn't travel to Buffalo, he would go to them—he once demonstrated rescue breathing before 1200 members of the New York Police Department.

A fortuitous sequence of events brought Elam to the Army Chemical Center in Edgewood, Maryland, only twenty miles from Baltimore and close to the nation's capital. A military obligation, partially interrupted by his anesthesiology training, had to be completed. The Army Chemical Center was the perfect assignment. It allowed Elam to continue his research and demonstrate to the Army the benefits of mouth-to-mouth breathing. It was close enough to Washington, D.C., that he could lobby the Surgeon General's office and the Red Cross. And the job supported his travel to Buffalo every other week to collect data on anesthetized patients using expired air. The Army Chemical Center learned firsthand of Elam's findings and became interested in it as a method for ventilating victims of nerve gas (anticholinesterase) poisoning. They invited Elam to present his results. Though impressed, particularly because it required no respiration equipment, the Army could not endorse the technique without the blessing of the National Research Council. The Red Cross, meanwhile, was unconvinced that expired-air resuscitation was the superior technique. Manual methods continued to prevail.[9]

Elam never let up in his efforts to convince the medical world. At every opportunity and every scientific meeting, he spoke up and argued passionately. Throughout 1954 and 1955 he literally knocked on doors jawboning whomever would listen in the Surgeon General's office or at the Red Cross headquarters. The method of Elisha had become an obsession. According to Elam, he even "told them that Elam was a biblical name and that I might be a prophet disguised as a major."[10]

Perhaps it would have ended there—a person can take only so much rejection. He certainly had the support of leading physiologists and it's likely that his scientific data would eventually prevail. What did happen was a fateful encounter with Peter Safar.

Peter Safar and the Angel of Death

In 1978, at the founding of the International Resuscitation Research Center at the University of Pittsburgh, Peter Safar said: "Resuscitation implies a commitment on the side of life. To devote one's energies to the restoration of lives cut short before fulfillment is to declare that life is intrinsically valuable, that it is worth living."

That was Safar's feeling from the beginning, when he founded the University's Department of Anesthesiology and Critical Care Medicine in 1961. And an argument can be made that, for Safar, it's in the genes. He is the child of two doctors—his mother, Vinca Safar, was a pediatrician, and his father, Karl Safar, the ophthalmologist who developed the method of repairing detached retinas with electrocoalgulation. Born in 1924, he and his parents lived in Vienna. His mother would later write that Safar was "impulsive and hot-tempered, like me." The young Safar was active in sports and mountain-climbing, despite problems with allergies and asthma. In 1938 his carefree living came to an end when the Nazis rose to power. His mother was half-Jewish and both parents were anti-Nazis in a city and country where many people were strongly pro-Nazi and anti-Semitic. In 1942 Peter spent six months doing forced labor, and was then drafted into the German army. After two months when he was about to be forced as a simple soldier into the battle of Stalingrad, he "disappeared" in Vienna with the help of resistance physicians. He spent the rest of the war staying one step ahead of the Nazis and pursuing medical studies as best he could. "Ever since 1945 I have considered myself extremely fortunate," Safar later said. "Thirty million Europeans lost their lives in World War II. Fifty percent of my schoolmates, including my two closest friends, died in that war, along with many Slavs and Jews. It could easily have been me."

Safar and his parents survived World War II. He received his M.D. at the University of Vienna in 1948, and spent an additional year training in pathology and surgery. In 1949 he came to the United States on a surgery fellowship to the Yale University School of Medicine—with five dollars in his pocket. After two years of residency at the University of Pennsylvania Hospital in Philadelphia, Safar headed south. He and his wife Eva needed to leave America temporarily in order to change their visas. Instead of returning to a Europe of bad memories and tragedy, they "decided to make an adventure of it," as Safar later remarked. "We wanted to do some good," he continued. "So we accepted an offer to go to Peru for a year." He founded the first academic Department of Anesthesiology in Peru at the National Cancer Center in Lima. During that year, Safar carried out "a fair amount of resuscitations, which included, of course, open-chest CPR." In 1954 he returned to the United States to set up the anesthesiology department at Baltimore City Hospital and take teaching positions at Johns Hopkins University and the University of Maryland.

In the early 1950s Safar had become fascinated by what happens to a patient who has been anesthetized. Essentially, an anesthesiologist places the patient in a controlled coma, a state at the edge of death. With vital protective reflexes abolished, the anesthesiologist has to support airway, breathing, and circulation. When the surgery is over, the patient is brought back from death's borderland. Safar began to wonder if it might be possible to carry out the same process—bring a person back from the edge of death—when the initial conditions have not been quite as controlled, when the patient has "died" as a result of illness or injury.

The initial answer came from Jim Elam. It was pure chance that threw Safar and Elam together. On October 13–14, 1956, the two drove together from Kansas City to Baltimore after an anesthesia meeting. They debated about resuscitation the entire trip while Peter's wife did all the driving. Elam clearly wanted to convince Safar—he certainly could use an ally, and sensed Safar's readiness to shift career gears, perhaps because he recognized Safar's drive to succeed. Elam writes of this trip: "I decided there had to be more prophets, and during that two-day conversation, Peter became interested in resuscitation problems."[11]

Safar also noted the catalytic role of the information he had learned during the car ride from Kansas City to Baltimore. "Jim Elam's published proof that exhaled air is an adequate resuscitative gas inspired me," Safar remarked. "His work was then not widely known. I was surprised to learn that first-aid agencies still jealously adhered to the teaching of back-pressure arm-lift."

For Safar, something clicked: breathe life into them. Beginning in the winter of 1956, with support from the Office of the Surgeon General, Safar initiated a series of experiments to study both the manual chest-pressure arm-lift methods of artificial ventilation and mouth-to-mouth breathing to see which would best keep someone alive who had stopped breathing. Elam was invited to join the experiments and contributed his expertise, not to mention some vital pieces of scientific equipment. Most important, Elam shared his results with paralyzing subjects. Safar recalls that they carried out their experiments mostly on weekends, when time and operating room space were available. The real problem, though, was with the subjects. It was fairly easy and morally acceptable to experiment on unconscious, nonbreathing animals. However, it would have been unethical to use dying, nonbreathing people. And conscious people and animals simply would not provide Safar and his team with the answers they needed. Safar knew from laboratory experience with dogs and pigs that their airways are straight, and thus the problem of obstruction by the tongue does not arise. Because the human airway is kinked, the tongue obstructs the passage as soon as consciousness is lost. Therefore, the subjects had to be unconscious and nonbreathing humans.

The result was a daring effort by a handful of doctors, nurses, and medical students. They allowed themselves to be sedated and then totally, but temporarily, paralyzed with a powerful drug, to simulate a nonbreathing patient. Once they were paralyzed, a dozen or so laypersons tried various techniques of artificial ventilation on them. At the time of Safar's experiments, review committees did not exist. Thus, it was up to the chief investigator to ensure the safety of his or her subjects and guarantee the experiment's ethical undertaking. If Safar had conducted his work today, the only way he could have convinced a human subjects review committee to authorize the experiment would be if the safety of his subjects could reasonably be assured, if the findings were sufficiently crucial to justify the risk, and if there was no animal model available. Safar was well aware of the potential risks and went to great lengths to explain the experiment to the subjects. He instituted multiple safeguards for the volunteers and personally supervised each experiment. Volunteers were heavily sedated and not conscious of their paralysis. They were generally paralyzed for one to three hours. Devices continuously monitored their breathing volumes and the oxygen and carbon dioxide content of their blood. They all breathed a combination of 50 percent oxygen and 50 percent nitrous oxide. One hundred percent oxygen was used just before the manual methods. No one was allowed to remain in a nonbreathing state for more than 90 seconds and the high oxygen content in the lungs made this safe.[12]

His experiments began in January 1957 at Baltimore City Hospital, funded with a $10,000 Army grant. Safar later recounted the process. "Thirty-one physicians and medical students and one nurse volunteered for forty-nine experiments following an announcement spread by word of mouth. They probably volunteered for mixed motivations, including helping science and getting a modest stipend. Consent was very informed: all volunteers had to observe me ventilate and life-support anesthetized and curarized patients or other volunteers without tracheal tube. I tried the analgesics and muscle relaxants on myself, but I did not go through an entire experiment as a victim." The payment for volunteering was $150 dollars, a substantial sum considering a resident's monthly salary was then less than $100.

Safar wrote, "Although the U.S. Army supported this research, even Lloyd's of London refused to insure it.[13] Of course, I was concerned about using volunteers, but knew it was the only way to get to the truth. I was confident that I could make it safe. Indeed, there were no cerebral or other sequelae, except for one case of aspiration in a volunteering physician who did not reveal a pre-existing gastroenteritis; he recovered. By then the required series of experiments was essentially completed."

The experiments convincingly demonstrated that the manual methods of artificial respiration (Silvester's, Schafer's, and Nielsen's) were virtually worthless and mouth-to-mouth ventilation the most effective means of respiration. And, perhaps most important, anyone (his rescuers ranged from ten years to old age) could perform effective mouth-to-mouth respiration, even on adult victims, after only minutes of instruction. No bags, masks, or tubes were required.

The Fire Captain from Baltimore

Martin McMahon was a captain in the Baltimore City Fire Department, in charge of the department's ambulance service. One morning in December 1956, while he was teaching at the Fire Academy, McMahon received a phone call from Safar who wanted to know if McMahon would help develop a new resuscitation method.

McMahon wanted to improve the department's ambulance service and welcomed anything that could enhance emergency medical service for the people of Baltimore—and anything that would help firefighters do a better job. As he later recalled, "I thought we should be a little more (medically) educated than the people we picked up." Until this point the two main methods of resuscitation had been the Schafer and Nielsen techniques. McMahon had been trained as a first aid instructor and knew the American Red Cross advocated the Schafer method. He admits he was not as skeptical then as he is now of its efficacy. "The Red Cross was gospel," he noted. "If you were an instructor and you varied in the way you were teaching the prescribed method, and the Red Cross found out, you could really get chewed out.

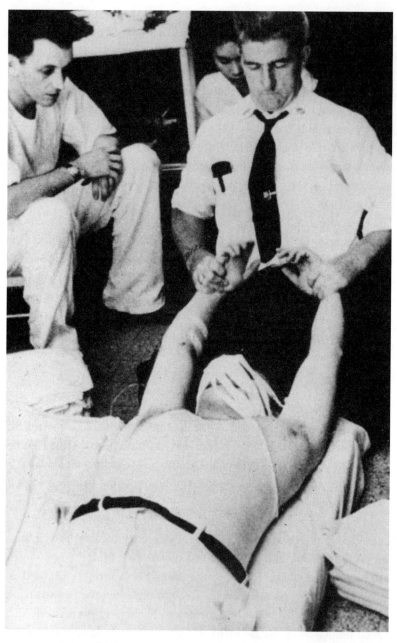

FIGURE 17. *Fire Chief Martin McMahon performing artificial respiration on volunteer subject. Peter Safar, MD (sitting), is looking on. The subject is temporarily sedated and paralyzed in order to measure the effectivness of the various methods of respiration. (Courtesy of Peter Safar)*

Basically, you accepted what came down the line, and did what you could, not knowing any better." Safar showed McMahon something better.

In 1956 McMahon joined forces with Safar in testing various methods of artificial respiration and discovered the uselessness of the Schafer method and other manual ventilation techniques. He also witnessed the difficulty these methods had in keeping the victim's airway open. When McMahon saw the ease of mouth-to-mouth respiration and how quickly it could be learned, he was converted. "Once you started to see the chest rise . . . then you knew damn well that you were making an exchange of air," McMahon said.

With McMahon's help, Safar began enlisting firefighters and ambulance personnel from throughout Maryland to perform as operators in his volunteer experiments and learn the new method. "I started bringing in some of my people," McMahon recalled. "I'd tell them, 'For the next couple of sessions you'll be at the City Hospital,' and give them the date and time. We began to teach our people. And as soon as the first ones got back to their quarters, the word began to spread. The first thing I knew, I was getting calls from other firefighters and ambulance people asking when they could go."

McMahon knew this would not be enough. "I told Safar," he said later, "that before the American Red Cross would accept [mouth-to-mouth], he would have to prove that women and children could do it. So we started bringing in civic groups. We'd keep them in the hallway and bring them in one at a time and give them instructions." McMahon vividly recalled one occasion. "We had Dr. Steichen who was a barrel-chested individual of about 200 pounds. We had him down as a victim and we brought an 85-pound Boy Scout in who proceeded to successfully ventilate him. Safar was most amazed."

A Willing Volunteer

Dr. Felicien Steichen remembers Safar's experiments well. Today Steichen is a practicing surgeon in New York City renowned for his development of surgical stapling techniques. At the time of Safar's experiments, Steichen was a third-year surgical resident at Baltimore City Hospital. Steichen describes Safar as a strong force, one difficult to resist: "Peter was a little like the Pied Piper, and he attracted a lot of young people around him, and some of those volunteered."

Steichen stepped forward as a volunteer, though his motives were partly prompted by monetary considerations. Steichen recalls: "I also wanted to go and visit my parents, whom I had not seen in four years, and my salary was only $50 a month. In those days residents would sell a pint of blood now and then when they wanted to do something special or take their wife or girl-friend out for supper." Steichen volunteered twice, which gave him enough money to visit his parents in Luxembourg. "My other motive," he later recalled, "was to do something that was exciting, that was proposed by a man who led by example." Fear never entered Steichen's mind, "I had seen Peter at work for over a year before, at night, seen him intubate, so I had absolute confidence in Peter. To me, there was no way this could go wrong." Eva Safar, in commenting on Steichen's trust and Safar's confidence, remarked, "Both were young and cocky."

As predicted by Safar, Steichen remembers nothing of the actual experiments, "I remember going to asleep, and in order to do this experiment right, we would lie on the floor on a small mattress, a camping mattress. The Baltimore fire chief was there and a lot of his people. I remember going to sleep, and I remember waking up. I tried to remember right afterwards and people would ask me, but I could not remember a thing. Ultimately they escorted me to my room—I was a bachelor then, and I was living in the hospital—and they stayed with me apparently until I was fully awake. And I must say, the following day I went to work as if nothing had happened." The only side effect Steichen recalls is slightly swollen lips.

Convincing the World

By the spring of 1957, Safar had conclusively documented three essential points for mouth-to-mouth respiration. First, simply tilting the person's head backward would remove obstruction in the airway. Second, most manual ventilation techniques then in use actually provided no air at all, while mouth-to-mouth offered excellent artificial ventilation. Finally, Safar and his team of volunteers and researchers showed that anyone could easily and effectively perform direct mouth-to-mouth resuscitation, without the need for gadgets, even on adults.[14]

By 1958, Elam, Safar, and Gordon were well on their way to convincing the world to switch from manual to mouth-to-mouth methods. According to Safar's recollections, acceptance was extremely rapid. "In 1957," he recalled,

"David Dill [Deputy Director of Medical Research at the Chemical Warfare Laboratories of the Army Chemical Center] held a decision-making meeting in his home outside the Army Chemical Center concerning endorsement of mouth-to-mouth breathing by the Army." After that meeting the Armed Forces convened a conference on "Artificial Respiration and Nerve Gas Poisoning" at Denver on May 9–19, 1957, and adopted the method. With Army help, Safar made documentary films of his experiments.

Elam was also in the filmmaking business. Since moving to the Roswell Park Memorial Institute in Buffalo in 1954, Elam increased the pace of his resuscitation research. Whereas Safar's films were targeted toward physicians, Elam's intended audience was the general public. In 1959 he produced *Rescue Breathing,* a twenty-seven-minute film demonstrating expired air resuscitation. Several thousand prints were distributed or sold for $38 thanks to support of the Army's Walter Reed Movie Group.[15] Governor Nelson Rockefeller and the New York Commissioner of Health learned of Elam's work and asked that an instructional pamphlet on rescue breathing be distributed throughout New York schools. Over one million copies were printed and given to students.

Elam, Safar, and Gordon used every opportunity to educate physicians and the public. Safar vividly recalls his first public scientific demonstration of mouth-to-mouth respiration. It occurred at a national anesthesiology meeting in Los Angeles the same week *Sputnik* was orbited, October 4, 1957. He likes to relate how they were both launched at the same time. Two months later, Elam and Safar presented their research findings at the New York Post Graduate Assembly of Anesthesiologists and somehow a local TV station learned of their work. Elam and Safar readily agreed to demonstrate mouth-to-mouth, with Safar's wife Eva as the victim. Safar performed mouth-to-mouth on Eva while Elam simultaneously narrated the technique on live TV. It must have been quite a show.

The following year, in May 1958, the AMA unequivocally endorsed mouth-to-mouth artificial respiration in adults[16] and urged that "information about expired air breathing should be disseminated as widely as possible."[17]

Given the endorsement of the American Medical Association and the ever growing body of scientific data, not to mention the personal lobbying done by Elam, Safar, and Gordon, the National Research Council/National Academy of Sciences endorsed mouth-to-mouth respiration in adults. With this announcement, in November 1958, mouth-to-mouth respiration became the official, nationally sanctioned method of resuscitation. The American Red Cross eventually followed with its endorsement. The Canadian Red Cross, however, stood tough. As late as 1959, it stated that the disadvantages of mouth-to-mouth resuscitation outweighed the advantages and refused to endorse the technique in adults. The commissioner of the organization remarked that it would be difficult for "a layman to place his lips against the lips of a corpse." By May 1960, its endorsement finally came through.

In September 1958, Safar presented the Baltimore data at the Scandinavian Society of Anesthesiologists' meeting in Gausdal, Norway—the first presentation of mouth-to-mouth resuscitation to a professional European audience. Norwegian anesthesiologist Bjorn Lind was in the audience during Safar's talk and almost immediately approached doll maker Asmund Laerdal (1913–1981) of Stavanger, Norway, about creating a training manikin. Laerdal was a logical person to ask, given his experience with plastic manufacturing; he also had a connection with the Red Cross and was working with them to create simulated plastic wounds for first-aid training. Laerdal's ready acceptance of such a need undoubtedly was colored by his personal brush with tragedy four years earlier. In 1954 his two-year-old son, Tore, was found in the sea in front of their summer house floating face down. When retrieved from the water he was comatose and blue in appearance but fortunately was revived.

Along with Hans Dahll, the Secretary-General of the Norwegian-American Chamber of Commerce, Laerdal visited Safar in November 1958 to learn about the requirements for a realistic artificial ventilation manikin. The mouth and airway had to move in a lifelike way and the chest needed to rise and fall as air passed in and out. Laerdal's challenge was to create a manikin resembling an unconscious person that did not appear too frightening. In 1959 he returned with a prototype. Laerdal was particularly obsessed with the appearance of the manikin's face. He wanted the expression to be realistic and appealing, yet impersonal. After much searching he happened to see a death mask hanging on the wall of his in-laws' home of a young woman who drowned herself in the river Seine. He was moved by her enigmatic yet peaceful gaze and decided it was what he needed for the training manikin. Laerdal named his manikin "Resusci-Anne." (The name Anne was chosen in honor of his first line of dolls, the Anne dolls.) Resusci-Anne was ready for production in May 1960 and was unveiled in New York to the Red Cross as well as to Safar and Gordon. Within two years, Bjorn Lind, who had worked with Laerdal in developing the training manikin, documented that schoolchildren could learn mouth-to-mouth ventilation,[18] and was instrumental in introducing compulsory training in mouth-to-mouth breathing in Norwegian schools. Resusci-Anne became the forerunner of a series of manikins that have been used worldwide to teach CPR to millions.

Throughout his experiments on mouth-to-mouth ventilation, Safar worked very closely with Fire Chief McMahon. This partnership led Safar to the conviction that emergency treatment must reach people "on the streets" and in their homes. Few people wait until they get to a hospital to have a heart attack, stroke, or be accidentally electrocuted. Then, as now, most such events and accidents happen at home or in the workplace. In Baltimore, the fire department supplied most of the ambulance services. So Safar decided to concentrate on firefighters as the "vector of life" for his vision. Before he could begin, however, he got a professional offer he could not refuse. In 1961 the University of Pittsburgh asked him to set up a Department of Anesthesiology at the School of Medicine and its five hospitals. Safar accepted, and shifted his base of operations. Starting in 1967 he worked with medical personnel and ambulance leaders in Pittsburgh to establish the city's first paramedic service, known as Freedom House. This service is itself a unique footnote in the annals of resuscitation. Safar realized that Pittsburgh needed a quality ambulance program. Simultaneously, representatives of Pittsburgh's black community wished to set up a transport system for the Hill District. The two needs meshed. With foundation funding, Safar helped train forty-four inner-city unemployed blacks in advanced prehospital emergency care. The program went on-line in 1968, several years before the federal government developed guidelines for community prehospital emergency programs.

By the 1960s it seemed the fear and tragedy of Safar's young adult life were far behind. In 1966, however, tragedy struck again, in a most ironic fashion. His oldest child Elizabeth, then twelve, suffered a severe asthma attack while her parents were out of town. When they arrived at Children's Hospital, Elizabeth had gone into cardiac arrest. Safar helped to successfully restart her heart and lung function. However, she never woke from the coma she had fallen into, and died a week later with brain death. For many years Safar, with the unstinting support of his wife Eva, had labored to relieve the agony of those whose relatives had crossed the line between life and death. He and Eva now had to endure that same terrible anguish, but with no happy ending.[19]

While much progress had been made, Safar knew that the target organ for resuscitation must be the brain, and began working on techniques to reduce permanent brain damage after cardiac arrest. For Safar, the brain is the organ that makes us human; the heart is merely a pump to nourish the brain. The death of his daughter from associated brain damage was a powerful current in Safar's life. Permanent brain damage from delayed resuscitation or other causes was costing families and communities millions of dollars each year. In 1978 Safar gave up the chairmanship of the Department of Anesthesiology and Critical Care Medicine and consolidated and expanded his resuscitation research by founding the International Resuscitation Research Center at the University of Pittsburgh. He and his research teams would explore the reversibility of various acute dying processes with particular emphasis on ways to delay, ameliorate, or even reverse brain damage.

The Missing Component

The history of mouth-to-mouth artificial respiration has been a circuitous one. Although described in the Bible, it would require millennia before it was rediscovered in the Enlightenment, only to be lost. Through the dogged efforts of several physicians, it was recovered yet again in the 1950s. Today we speak of the ABC's of resuscitation. But while "airway" and "breathing" were well understood, artificial circulation was not. Credit for the development of modern mouth-to-mouth respiration justly goes to Jim Elam and Peter Safar. Yet mouth-to-mouth ventilation alone is not sufficient for victims of sudden cardiac arrest. "Rescue breathing," as Elam called it, will save some drowning and suffocation victims and all who are temporarily comatose (those in whom the heart is still beating), but it will do little for true cardiac arrest when both the heart and lungs are stilled. The "C" for "circulation" was still waiting to be discovered.

Cardiac Arrest, 1958

John Colven survived his cardiac arrest in 1991, and still lives near Seattle with his wife June. What if these two were residing in Baltimore in 1958? If John had a sudden cardiac arrest, would he survive? Imagine a Saturday afternoon in August, hot and muggy as only Baltimore can be at that time of year. John and June are having a small party for their neighbors. Adults stand around the barbeque grill and chat, while children rush in and out of the house and run around the yard. With no warning, John suddenly collapses. He gasps for air a few times, then falls ominously silent.

June rushes into the house and looks up the seven-digit phone number for the fire department. When she finally places the call, the dispatcher provides her with no instructions for resuscitation. She hangs up and races outside. Neither she nor any of the adults can provide John with any assistance. They don't know what to do, and surround him helplessly. One of the neighbor's boys is a Boy Scout who knows the Nielsen method of resuscitation. The adults stand aside as the youngster works on John.

By 1958, fire department rescue personnel had learned mouth-to-mouth respiration and were proficient in its application. When they arrive, they apply mouth-to-mouth resuscitation to John. But they do not use any chest compression; it hasn't yet been rediscovered. John's heart and brain therefore do not receive any oxygenated blood. The rescue squad loads John into the ambulance and take him to Baltimore City Hospital.

But it's far too late. The intern feels for a pulse and perhaps attaches an electrocardiogram; it shows a flat line. The epidemic of heart disease has tallied another victim.

The problem in 1958 was that artificial respiration alone can do nothing for sudden cardiac death except allow pooled blood in the lungs to take up oxygen. That oxygen, however, will go nowhere unless it is propelled forward. Thus, only half of the puzzle had been solved. But just across town from Safar, the other half was soon to be put in place—again accidentally.

Part III

THE PULSE OF LIFE

« »

I send it through the rivers of your blood
Even to the court, the heart, to th' seat o' th' brain
—William Shakespeare, *Coriolanus*

THE SEARCH FOR ARTIFICIAL CIRCULATION

《 》

Anecdotal reports on the use of chest compression appeared throughout the late eighteenth and nineteenth centuries.[1] But what is thought to be the first report of external heart massage was published October 4, 1858, by Janos Balassa, a professor of surgery at the University of Pest in Hungary. (Buda and Pest were separate cities on opposite sides of the Danube until around 1900.) Balassa had been called to the bed of an eighteen-year-old woman suffering from ulcerated laryngitis. During preparations for a tracheostomy, the woman collapsed, stopped breathing, and her heartbeat ceased. Balassa hastily performed the tracheotomy, while at the same time exerting "bellows-like rhythmic pressure to the front of her chest imitating breathing." After about six minutes, the woman gave some sigh-like inspirations; after fifteen minutes she recovered consciousness. Though often cited as the first case of CPR, it is that likely Balassa simply attempted to simulate respirations.[2]

The problem with many of these early accounts is ascertaining whether the heart had in fact stopped beating. If the cases merely involved problems with respiration alone, then mechanical pressure on the chest made sense. It would assist breathing and be sufficient to resuscitate the patient. If the heart had truly stopped beating, though, it was unlikely that only chest compression would save the patient.

Nineteenth-century physicians quickly grasped the relationship between anesthesia (specifically chloroform) and cardiac arrest. The first case reports of chloroform-associated sudden death began to appear rather soon. In fact, it was only two months after chloroform was introduced in late 1847 that the first death from chloroform occurred. The unfortunate patient was a fifteen-year-old girl named Hannah Greener who was having a painful ingrown toenail removed. During the inquest the surgeon, Dr. Thomas Meggison of Wickham, England, reported being completely surprised by the patient's collapse. He had given her brandy in an effort to revive her and then, in a last-ditch effort, attempted to bleed her in the arm and jugular vein. "But (I) only obtained about a spoonful," he reported. "She was dead, I believe, at the time I attempted to bleed her."[3]

At first, few studies were done to define how to deal with the problem. One of the first scientists to study chloroform-related deaths was Professor R. Boehm at the University of Dorpat in present-day Estonia in 1878. Boehm observed the resuscitation of cats that he placed in cardiac arrest using overdoses of chloroform and noted that side-to-side compression of the cat's thoracic cage or downward compression of the thorax could produce blood pressures of 50 to 120 millimeters of mercury. This procedure was effective for up to thirty minutes or until the chloroform wore off and the cat's normal heartbeat returned. Beohm confirmed that forward flow of blood occurred with his technique. When he opened the carotid artery, he observed a vigorous spurting of blood with each chest compression. He also noted that arterial blood remained bright red even after an hour of chest compression, something that could only happen if the blood was circulating through the lung. Boehm called his technique of chest compression "a kind of emergency circulation."[4] It is doubtful, however, if many physicians knew of Boehm's work.

Not surprisingly, many surgeons and anesthesiologists wrote reports describing their successful techniques in dealing with cardiac arrest. Howard Atwood Kelly (1858–1943), a professor at Johns Hopkins Hospital and Medical School, described his own method, used successfully on fifteen patients. "An assistant steps on the table, takes one of the patient's knees under each arm and thus raises the body from the table until it rests upon the shoulders. . . . The patient's clothing is pulled down under her armpits, completely baring the abdomen and chest. The operator, standing at the head, institutes respiratory movements as follows: inspiration by placing the open hands on each side of the chest posteriorly over the lower ribs, and drawing

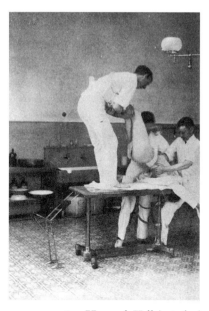 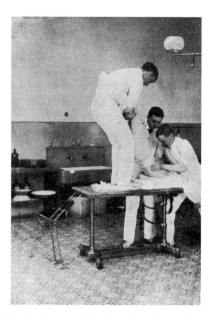

FIGURE 18. *Howard Kelly's technique of inducing artificial respiration using chest compression, 1895. Left photo shows inspiration, right photo expiration. (Courtesy of Johns Hopkins Hospital, Baltimore)*

the chest well forward and outwards, holding it thus for about two seconds; expiration, reversing the movement by replacing the hands on the front of the chest over the lower ribs and pushing backwards and inwards, at the same time compressing the chest. The success of the manoeuvre will be demonstrated by the audible rush of air in and out of the chest."[5]

Dr. Kelly passionately felt that every surgeon should be able to handle chloroform-related respiratory and circulatory catastrophes. He wrote, "Any surgeon having a death from chloroform should be indicted for murder."[6] Strong words indeed. The implied admonishion to "learn resuscitation" was unfortunately not heeded at the time.

In 1891 Dr. Friedrich Maass performed the first unequivocally documented chest compression in humans. The recipients were two patients with cardiac arrest resulting from chloroform anesthesia. Maass was a surgical assistant working in Göttingen under the supervision of Professor Franz Koenig. In his 1883 textbook of surgery, Koenig had proposed using compression in the heart region to artificially ventilate a patient. Though the position was the correct one for CPR, it is clear that Koenig was describing a means of assisted ventilation.[7] As Koenig's assistant, Maass was undoubtedly aware of this recommendation.

Maass's first case, in 1891, involved a nine-year-old boy being operated on for a repair of a cleft palate. The child could not be easily anesthetized with chloroform and the procedure had to be repeated several times before the child lost consciousness. Maass recognized the dangers of chloroform and knew it could on rare occasion induce shock and death. There was no way to predict which patients would react negatively to the anesthetic agent—it seemed to happen spontaneously with little warning. Today we give a name to such an awful event. It is called an *idiosyncratic* reaction—a multisyllabic phrase to describe a bad outcome without known or identifiable causes. To the surgeon it was terrifying. Surgeons like to control a situation—clamp the artery, stop the bleeding, cut out the diseased organ. With chloroform-associated death, the surgeon stood by helplessly. Just such a nightmare happened to Maass as he was about to operate. The boy's normal breathing stopped suddenly and only shallow ineffective attempts at breathing were present. The pulse disappeared and the child began to turn blue. His pupils opened wide, a sign of insufficient oxygen to the brain and a harbinger of impending death.

Maass recognized what was happening and attempted to support respirations by applying his professor's method of compression in the center of the chest. Maass pressed at the rate of thirty to forty times per minute and achieved some success. He watched the child's color improve from the corpse-like bluish shade to a healthy pink. He also saw the child's pupils constrict again, evidence of oxygen reaching the brain. Things looked promising except for one crucial fact: Maass could not find a pulse. The surgeon stayed at it for thirty minutes and even performed a tracheostomy (a surgical opening made in the windpipe just beneath the Adam's apple) to aid in artificial breathing. Yet without a pulse, the boy was doomed. In order to free up the operating room for the next patient, the boy was moved to an adjoining room where he could quietly expire. "Due to the completely dilated, reactionless pupils, the corpse like appearance, the absence of respiration and pulse, I now had to regard the patient as dead," Maass later wrote.[8] But Maass was not willing to let the child go quite so easily. He continued to administer chest compressions, and increased the rate. He wrote, "I returned immediately to the direct compression of the region of the heart and, indeed, in my excitement applied it very rapidly and forcefully. The pupils again became rather quickly constricted . . . a few gasping respiratory movements too returned."[9] Maass persisted and at approximately fifty minutes from the moment of the boy's collapse, he perceived heart movement. One hour after he had begun, Maass felt a pulse in the carotid artery in the boy's neck. Maass recorded that, after ninety minutes, the radial pulse returned in the wrist. According to the account, the boy slept until the next morning and slowly recovered so that he could be discharged. After five weeks, he was "completely well."[10]

The second case involved an eighteen-year-old young man being operated on for a hip inflammation resulting from tuberculosis. As with the nine year old, the young man lost blood pressure and pulse during induction of anesthesia with chloroform. Maass initially tried the slower rate of chest compression to simulate respirations, but, when the situation did not improve, increased the rate to 120 compressions per minute. He noted a carotid pulse and within twenty-five minutes the patient achieved a spontaneous pulse and blood pressure. After the man recovered, Maass again operated on him—this time successfully and without complications. Maass concluded, "So long as compression is applied at the speed of the patient's breathing, slow deterioration. When compression is speeded up, gradual improvement follows."[11]

Describing his technique, Maass wrote, "One steps to the left side of the patient facing his head, and presses deep in the heart region with strong movements . . . the frequency of compression is 120 or more a minute. The effectiveness of the efforts is recognized from the artificially produced carotid pulse and the constriction of the pupils."

Maass did not neglect the need to maintain an open airway. "In order to . . . ensure that the air passage remains open, someone stands at the head of the patient. As long as the condition has not essentially improved, it is expedient to make as few and as short pauses as possible."[12] Maass advised that it was safe to stop the chest compressions "as long as the pupils remain constricted and spontaneous breathing continues."[13] Those are in fact reasonable criteria for successful resuscitation.

In 1904, the first American case of closed-chest cardiac massage involved George Crile, a well-known surgeon in Cleveland, who resuscitated a twenty-eight-year-old woman undergoing an operation for a large goiter. During surgery the woman's heart activity ceased completely and Crile sprung into action: "Rhythmic pressure upon the thorax over the heart was at once made. . . . After an interval of between five or six minutes the heart slowly began to recover its beat and circulation was re-established."[14] Crile believed that thoracic pressure caused blood to flow through the heart's valves. In his book *Anemia and Resuscitation* (1906), Crile wrote, "The person who exerts the rhythmic compressions [on the thorax] causes an external pseudo-cardiac movement. The author was able, personally, to produce on a recently deceased person, a total circulation which caused a pulse in the radial artery and bleeding of the peripheral vessels."[15]

The occasional case report of closed-chest massage was rare throughout the nineteenth century and the first sixty years of the twentieth. Far more common was open-chest massage. Moritz Schiff, a professor of physiology in Florence, Italy, provided a description of the earliest demonstration of the effectiveness of open-chest cardiac massage in 1874. Schiff wrote of his experiments with dogs, "By rhythmical compression of the heart with the hands . . . it is possible to re-establish the heart beat even up to a period of eleven and one-half minutes after the stoppage of that organ."[16] Because most cardiac arrests under medical supervision occurred during chloroform anesthesia, the surgeon had the opportunity to open the chest and directly observe the heart and its response to massage.

In 1906 T. A. Green, a British physician, reviewed the animal experiments with heart massage done by doctors in Europe from 1874 to 1906, including Schiff. Green's article, published in *The Lancet*, provided a synopsis of forty cases involving humans that had been reported in the medical literature. Thirty of the reported heart stoppages were related to anesthesia and chloroform was the agent in twenty-four cases. Nine of the forty patients described in Green's report recovered. Green also gave a detailed description of two of his own patients. His first case involved a nine-year-old boy being operated on to close and repair a draining wound of the naval. Shortly after chloroform anesthesia, the boy had difficulty breathing. Although artificial respiration began and strychnine and ether were administered, there was no recovery by twenty-five minutes. Green cut into the upper abdomen, reached under the diaphragm, and performed manual heart massage. Eventually, the respirations and heart began functioning, but the patient was still unconscious. The patient received enemas of salt water and brandy several times, but never recovered. Green's second case involved a child of three with diphtheria who suddenly stopped breathing. Green began artificial respiration, and then opened the abdomen and compressed the heart through the diaphragm. When he suspected air was not reaching the lungs, another doctor did a tracheostomy and cleared the trachea with a feather, then continued respiration through a cannula. Green could not feel heartbeats and opened the pericardium. None of these methods, however, was successful.[17]

The distinction of performing the first successful open-heart cardiac massage goes to the Norwegian physician Kristian Igelsrud (1867–1940). In 1901 a patient being operated on for cancer of the uterus went into cardiopulmonary arrest as the operation was nearing completion. Doctors tried artificial respiration and electrification of the phrenic nerve for several minutes. The phrenic nerve, which innervates the diaphragm, was easily reached through the abdominal incision and this was an effort to induce respiration by causing the diaphragm to contract. Igelsrud then cut into the chest between the third and fourth ribs and opened the sac surrounding the heart. He compressed the heart using his hands for one minute until the heartbeat returned. The patient recovered.[18] It is doubtful that the patient had ventricular fibrillation since electricity is mandatory for reversing this fatal rhythm and, even though the heart sits atop the diaphragm, the current Igelsrud used to stimulate the phrenic nerve would not be enough for defibrillation. More likely, she had an extremely faint pulse and might have revived merely with artificial ventilation. Whatever her heart rhythm may have been, she became the first patient to survive open-chest cardiac compression. A visiting physician from Philadelphia happened to be assisting Igelsrud during the arrest. He published an account three years later in 1904 in the *Philadelphia Therapeutic Gazette*, a journal with only a small regional circulation.

One wonders why closed-chest massage, well described in several case reports, did not catch on. One can only surmise that the reports—like the one about Igelsrud's success—never made it into the general medical literature. Those few clinically relevant case reports, such as Maass's accounts, appeared only in German and French publications. Not even Green knew about them when he wrote his 1906 review of heart massage.

Perhaps the more likely possibility is that physicians easily accepted chest pressure as a means of aiding ventilation, but may have found it hard to visualize a dual cardiac and respiratory role. Physicians also faced a seeming contradiction: how could chest compression at the rate of twenty per minute assist in circulation and a compression rate of 120 assist in ventilation? The answer, of course, is that chest compression alone cannot fill a dual role. But this physiology wasn't understood for another fifty years.

During the late 1950s, Peter Safar and others had recognized the need to find an effective means of artificial circulation short of open-chest cardiac massage. By 1958, most knowledgeable individuals realized the effectiveness of mouth-to-mouth ventilation. It was simple to do, and maintained adequate oxygenation in someone with isolated respiratory arrest. But sudden cardiac arrest involves both the heart and the lungs—air and circulation must be supplied. Mouth-to-mouth alone will not maintain life. Safar had helped solve the problem of an obstructed airway and mouth-to-mouth breathing, but recognized that circulation still needed to be addressed. Just across town at Johns Hopkins University, a researcher well known to Safar, William B. Kouwenhoven, was about to serendipitously make the discovery.

The Engineer from Brooklyn

Kouwenhoven was born January 13, 1886. There never was any doubt about where he came from—his thick Brooklyn accent said it all. He did his undergraduate and graduate work at Brooklyn Polytechnic and received his master's degree in electrical engineering in 1908. As a graduate student, he was assigned the task of assisting—mostly setting up equipment for—Charles Steinmetz, the legendary head scientist of General Electric, who was a regular lecturer at the Poly. Steinmetz liked what he saw. He encouraged Kouwenhoven to pursue an engineering doctorate in Germany. Armed with a letter of introduction from Steinmetz, and accompanied by his young bride Abigail, Kouwenhoven did just that. In 1914, as the storm clouds of World War I gathered, he returned to the United States.[19]

After a short stint at Washington University, Kouwenhoven went to Johns Hopkins. The university was forming its School of Engineering, and Kouwenhoven soon was engaged in numerous engineering research projects. Nearly all focused on high-voltage electricity and the development of electrical measurement devices. Kouwenhoven never out-Steinmetzed Steinmetz— but he certainly followed in the great man's footsteps. Kouwenhoven also taught power engineering in the department and eventually became a full professor and Dean of the School of Engineering. His research on cardiac problems began in 1929 when he was invited to join a team studying defibrillation in animals. He continued until funding dried up because of the war. After spending World War II engaged in engineering education programs, Kouwenhoven resumed his contacts with the university hospital in 1950. Although he was now sixty-four and nearing retirement, his skills were still in demand. Alfred Blalock, then Chief of Surgery at Johns Hopkins, persuaded Kouwenhoven to work in his department.

Kouwenhoven was given space on the top floor of the old Hunterian research building where he began experiments involving electric currents as high as 4000 volts. The staff on the floor below was told to rush upstairs with airway tubes and respirators if they heard anyone collapse above them. Though half said as a joke, there was no denying the great danger involved. Fortunately no one was ever electrocuted.[20]

Kouwenhoven plunged into several fascinating research projects. One involved the risk of accidental electrocution to TV repairmen, and was largely funded by the then-burgeoning television industry. Another, a contract with the U.S. Navy, involved the electrical and mechanical properties of certain laminated plastics. And then there was the project to develop what can only be called a portable heart defibrillator. Kouwenhoven had returned to the work he had started and then abandoned back in the 1930s. His objective was twofold: first, to develop an external heart defibrillator for hospitals; and second, to find ways to treat power utility linemen accidentally electrocuted in the field. The Edison Electric Institute funded much of his work on defibrillation and, with Blalock's consent, he continued to run his lab at the University Hospital.[21]

Even when Paul Zoll successfully demonstrated the clinical application of closed-chest defibrillation, Kouwenhoven continued focusing on the development of a portable unit. Closed-chest defibrillators at that time were large, ungainly units that had to be wheeled around hospital corridors and up and down elevators to reach the dying patient. But it was not a portable heart defibrillator that catapulted Kouwenhoven to worldwide fame—it was his work on dogs. Enter Guy Knickerbocker and James Jude, the two other actors to make CPR a reality.

The Engineer with the Bow Tie

The 1977 book *Advances in Cardiopulmonary Resuscitation*, edited by Peter Safar and James Elam, contains a photograph of three men who changed the world. The caption, as befits a no-nonsense medical volume, says simply, "Dr. James R. Jude (left), Dr. William Kouwenhoven (center), and Dr. Guy Knickerbocker (right)." Knickerbocker is the one smiling and wearing a bow tie. Both may be clues to his character—especially the bow tie. He is a shy, soft-spoken man. A colleague once said of him, "When he walks into a room, he brings peace with him."

Born in 1932, Knickerbocker began working in Kouwenhoven's lab at Johns Hopkins in 1954, after finishing his bachelor's degree. Kouwenhoven

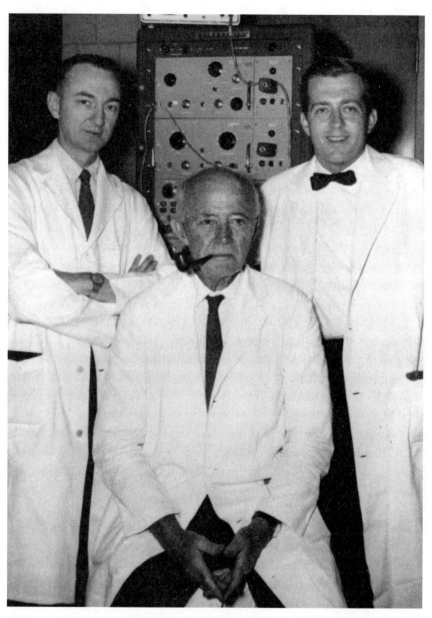

FIGURE 19. *James R. Jude, MD (left), William Kouwenhoven, PhD (center), and G. Guy Knickerbocker, PhD (right), in Kouwenhoven's laboratory at Johns Hopkins Hospital, 1961. (Courtesy of Peter Safar)*

was sixty-nine and semi-retired; Knickerbocker remembers attending his last engineering lecture. He was twenty-two, and had no firm idea about what he wanted to do after graduation. Living at home in Baltimore with his parents, he finally decided to go for a graduate degree in electrical engineering. William Kouwenhoven needed someone to work on an engineering project and Knickerbocker fit the bill. Kouwenhoven had taken over management of a contract with the U.S. Navy, evaluating the electrical and mechanical properties of certain laminated plastics. The research dollars being pumped into this and other projects enabled scientists like Kouwenhoven to carry on related research projects.

"I actually did my master's work on that particular project," Knickerbocker later recalled. "That work gave me the opportunity to see what was going on at the hospital and at the school of medicine." Knickerbocker was particularly interested in studies that involved the development of the closed chest defibrillator and evaluation of electrical variables leading to ventricular fibrillation.

During his senior year, Knickerbocker recalled, he had dropped by the university hospital several times and had seen Kouwenhoven's work on closed-chest defibrillation. "I guess I began getting an interest in and taste for it then," he says. "It became kind of natural for me, while I worked on the Navy contract stuff, to go to the hospital one or two afternoons a week and help Kouwenhoven with his experiments down there. That's really how it all got started."

Although Kouwenhoven was not a medical doctor, Knickerbocker says that Alfred Blalock—the Chief of Surgery for Johns Hopkins who had enticed Kouwenhoven into the hospital—"was always open to Kouwenhoven's suggestions." "It was remarkable," Knickerbocker notes today, "the openness with which we were treated in that department." Knickerbocker—also not an M.D.—was a self-described "real neophyte" at the Hopkins hospital, as much of an outsider as anyone could be in that environment filled with doctors and medical researchers. "The surgical fellows in the department who worked in the research lab liked to have regular meetings to talk about various subjects," Knickerbocker recalls. "Once I did a series of talks for them on basic electricity and electronics, and Blalock came and sat in on one of them. He seemed interested.

"In fact, I recall him asking a rather insightful question. I was explaining the relationships among energy and power, and work, and how work is force times distance. And Blalock said, 'You mean if I hold a twenty-five pound sack of potatoes out at arm's length, but it isn't moving, that I'm not doing any work? Why do I feel I'm getting tired, then?' It was a good question. The point is, he took the time to come and see what was going on." In Knickerbocker's opinion, the relationship between the non-M.D. researchers and the medical personnel was "marvelous. We always had open interchanges. I don't think we were ever looked down upon."

The Surgeon Who Wondered

The third member of "The Big Three" at the beginning of artificial circulation was James Jude, a resident in surgery at Johns Hopkins. Hypothermia brought Jude into the world of CPR, deliberately induced hypothermia. In the early 1950s, when he was in medical school at the University of Minnesota, Jude had worked with a professor named John Lewis who wanted to use hypothermia as part of the surgical treatment of congenital heart disease. Lewis's idea was that by cooling the heart down, he could stop blood circulation for a few minutes, and carry out some surgical procedures.

Several years later, Jude was in the middle of his medical residency at Johns Hopkins and he continued to do medical research in his spare time. He met Kouwenhoven, who was working on the effects of electricity on the heart, along with Guy Knickerbocker. Jude was naturally drawn to Kouwenhoven's work. As he explained, "The thing is, sometimes, during the use of hypothermia you get ventricular fibrillation. As you cooled the heart down, it would fibrillate. I talked to Kouwenhoven and his staff about what kinds of treatment to apply, how to use a defibrillator in such cases." Kouwenhoven was then only working experimentally with animals, mostly dogs. He had not yet begun applying his work to humans.

In 1956, after a year working on and off with Kouwenhoven and Knickerbocker, Jude went into the Public Health Service at the National Institutes of Health in Bethesda, Maryland, but remained in contact with the two researchers.

According to Knickerbocker's recollections, Jude's involvement began when Jude was working with Don Proctor in the department of anesthesiology. Jude was deeply into his research on hypothermia for cardiac bypasses. "Pump bypassing was really being worked on at that time, too," notes Knickerbocker. Surgeons doing certain cardiac procedures on children would often use hypothermia because Knickerbocker explained, "It cooled them down; temporarily occlude the vena cava, dry up the heart, plop a patch in there real fast, close it up and get out of there before the heart got so deoxygenated they couldn't get a return."

Proctor was carrying out related experiments in dogs, and Jude was the resident assigned to the project. The two realized that dogs—like people—frequently would go into ventricular fibrillation when they were cooled. "And Jude started getting interested in what 'these guys'—us—were doing around the corner with electrical defibrillation," Knickerbocker noted. "That's how we came to know each other." He was there when we found out that we could support circulation in a dog by pushing on its chest. He was convinced that what we were doing with the dogs was important."

Jude was in a unique position to connect the research being done in Kouwenhoven's lab with real people in the real world. As a cardiac resident, Jude had the responsibility to do follow-up closures—sew up the chest—in those cases where the chest had been opened by others on the clinical floor. It was a messy business, fraught with complications, performed as a desperate act of last resort. Surely there had to be a better way.

By contrast, according to Knickerbocker, Blalock was interested in their work on dogs, but "didn't express any confidence in any practical application—certainly not in adults, though possibly in kids. But Jim believed the techniques had widespread application. He kept an eye on what we were doing."

An Accidental Discovery

The actual discovery came about by accident—actually, two accidents. The first involved Kouwenhoven and was later described by an associate, Claude Haggard. Kouwenhoven had been preparing to defibrillate a dog and was holding the paddles. According to Haggard, "Kouwenhoven appparently nodded or grunted, and one of the young assistants thought he meant to turn the power on. Kouwenhoven, who was about seventy at the time, took the charge full bore across his chest. He swore in seventeen languages." Kouwenhoven then redesigned the paddles to make them safer. He arranged it so they would require fifteen pounds of pressure to trip a microswitch that would discharge the capacitor. In other words, it became impossible for the paddles to be discharged while merely holding them or even exerting light pressure. This safety feature set the stage for the second accident.

It was a routine day in the laboratory—Kouwenhoven and Knicker-bocker wanted to determine how long they could leave a dog's heart fib-rillating and still successfully defibrillate it. They had taken an anesthe-tized dog and inserted a catheter into the femoral artery to measure its arterial blood pressure. While observing the dog's steadily decreasing pres-sure, Knickerbocker applied the defibrillator paddles to the animal. Because they now had the built-in safety feature, strong pressure was required to get the charge to transfer. As Knickerbocker pressed down, he noticed a blip in the blood pressure. The application of the paddles to the dog's chest had apparently caused the heart to circulate a pulsation of blood and momentar-ily increase the arterial pressure. It was not one of those ah-ha! moments—there was no shout of "Eureka." But Knickerbocker was intrigued enough to call Kouwenhoven over and they both observed the phenomenon. By repeat-edly applying the paddles, they were able to extend the period of time the dog's heart was in fibrillation from a minute or so to several minutes, and still successfully defibrillate it. (Today's defibrillators are designed differently. Instead of a pressure requirement, the two paddles each contain a discharge button that must be pressed simultaneously. Had Knickerbocker used a modern defibrillator he probably would not have seen the dog's pressure rise.)

These experiments and observations played out over a period of weeks, and Jude became more involved during this initial period. All three soon realized they could use their hands to apply pressure to the heart externally instead of relying on defibrillator paddles, obtain the same blood-pressure results, finally defibrillate—and get a surviving animal.

Knickerbocker recalls one incident where a dog was not expected to fib-rillate. They had been caught without a defibrillator in their twelfth-floor lab. He remembers saying to one of the medical students in the lab that day, "Go ahead and do [chest compression on the animal]; I'll go and get the defibril-lator." Adds Knickerbocker, "I think I can say honestly that I said that with a pretty good feeling. I didn't think their work would be futile." At that time the defibrillator was kept on the fifth floor at the heart station. Knicker-bocker ran down seven flights to get it and rode the elevator back since the defibrillator was a large, heavy machine on wheels. "The Hopkins elevators were not famous for their speed," he recalls wryly, "but I did eventually get back to the twelfth floor. I don't know how long it took—five minutes, seven, eight." Since he had done studies on the effects of delay on defibrilla-tion without circulatory support, Knickerbocker knew that the odds of a successful defibrillation fell rapidly after four minutes. He also knew that if the dog did survive, it would be a real struggle to keep it going. As Knickerbocker had anticipated, his medical student's external chest compression worked. The dog was shocked into a normal rhythm when he finally arrived with the defibrillator. "I remember that it was fairly remarkable, the rapidity with which the animal's circulation came back. That seemed to me to be pretty striking evidence that its blood was moving and respiration in its true sense was taking place."

According to Knickerbocker, the dogs in their experiments were strapped to a V-shaped table. The animal lay with its back in the bottom of the V, with its sternum straight up and its four legs tied to the two sides of the V. This allowed researchers to push down on the animal's sternum when doing external chest compression—"just like in humans." Some dogs had pointed chests, and the researcher's hands would often slip when he or she pressed down. Other dogs had fairly flat chests and were easy to massage. Knickerbocker and his colleagues monitored the animal's heartbeat with an ECG[22] and kept track of blood pressure with special electrodes attached low to the animal's chest.

"The point, though, was that they came back," says Knickerbocker. "They'd bounce right back—defibrillate on the first shock and come back with vigorous circulation. Many of them we'd put back in their cages and then look at them again after a couple of days. . . . They appeared to be the same animal afterwards as they were before."

They always intubated their experimental dogs. "We were really aware that there were significant puffs of air moving in and out when we compressed the chest." At the time, Knickerbocker assumed, falsely it would turn out, that these puffs of air achieved adequate ventilation. Chest compressions can produce a suboptimal level of ventilation but only in intubated persons—not a realistic scenerio for individuals collapsing suddenly in cardiac arrest.

At first, it was not at all self-evident where the chest should be compressed. Should it be side to side? Front to back? On the upper chest? Lower chest? Through a series of experiments in late 1958 the team discovered that the best procedure was to apply rhythmic pressure on the lower part of the sternum and press straight down using the heel of the hand. Other locations led to higher rates of complications, including lacerations of the liver, stomach, or lungs. They repeatedly measured actual arterial pressures and through trial and error discovered that the optimal depth of compression should be one and one-half to two inches and the best rate of compression was approximately sixty to eighty per minute.

Laboratory researchers before Knickerbocker certainly must have observed that chest compression maintains artificial circulation. However, Knickerbocker, Kouwenhoven, and Jude recognized its *importance*. They were the first to realize that chest compression was the means for delaying the dying process and thus allowing definitive therapy, such as defibrillation, to restart the heart in cardiac arrest. With his colleagues, Kouwenhoven was able to refine and document in dogs the rediscovery of chest compression — the missing ingredient in CPR. Measurements with a device called a rotameter showed that arterial pulse waves did indeed reflect some (although low) carotid-artery blood flow. The question was whether the chest compression merely produced pressure waves, like pushing on a balloon, without causing a forward flow of blood. "The hand was substituted for the defibrillator electrode and rhythmic pressure given on the lower sternum over the heart." The investigators could show repeatedly that when chest compressions were begun shortly after onset of ventricular fibrillation and continued uninterrupted for twenty minutes, they could successfully defibrillate dogs without brain damage.[23] Later, when asked how he knew the dogs personalities were unaffected, Jude succinctly noted, "They bit us the same afterwards."[24]

Ready for Humans

By early 1958, Kouwenhoven, Knickerbocker, and Jude realized they were onto something important. Their experiments convincingly demonstrated that external chest compression resulted in artificial circulation. Now the interval of cardiac arrest could be prolonged before defibrillation had to occur. Chest compression slowed down the dying process and thus made defibrillation more likely to succeed. Without circulating blood, the heart's fibrillating muscle cells weaken and stop completely. Within minutes a defibrillatory shock will not work — unless artificial circulation keeps oxygenated blood bathing the heart cells. So long as the fibrillating cells are oxygenated, defibrillation can be delayed up to ten or twenty minutes and still be successful.

Flushed with success, Kouwenhoven believed it was time to have his technique used on humans and Jude was given the assignment. The first patient to have this life saving procedure was a thirty-five-year-old woman in July

1959. She was, recalled Jude, "rather an obese female who was to have a cholecystectomy (gall bladder removal) and was being held in the pre-op room just before surgery. The patient went into cardiac arrest as a result of halothane. This was the new anesthetic that had started being used. People didn't yet understand it completely, as you would expect. It had a fairly low tolerance; it was an excellent anesthetic but it could move very quickly from not enough to thorough anesthesia and to depression of myocardium and cardiac arrest.

"Anyway, this woman had no blood pressure, no pulse, and ordinarily we would have opened up her chest and done direct cardiac massage. Instead, since we weren't in the operating room, we applied external cardiac massage and they immediately switched back to straight oxygen in ventilation. Her blood pressure and pulse came back at once. We didn't have to open up her chest. They went ahead and did the operation on her, and she recovered completely."

Jude and his colleagues did not have the equipment in the pre-op room available today to monitor patients. He was sure the women had gone into cardiac arrest and that external cardiac massage had brought her back—but he couldn't prove it. Shortly after this incident, Jude began doing heart surgery. During surgery and in recovery these patients were well monitored, with an electrocardiogram and devices for measuring arterial blood pressure. Among the patients who unexpectedly went into cardiac arrest, Jude found his proof. "Now we were able to see immediately that we were getting a pulse [with external heart massage], an arterial pulse, and they recovered," Jude recalled. "We were able to get the heart started and didn't have to open the chest for internal heart massage."

Jude and his colleagues now extended their practice even further. "We had a patient who went into ventricular defibrillation right in the emergency room," Jude said, "and we gave him cardiac massage while we were getting an external defibrillator. [That technology was in its infancy then, too.] The patient was defibrillated and survived. There was another patient who came to the hospital's outpatient clinic with chest pain. While he was in the clinic being examined, he went into cardiac arrest. The cardiologist who was examining him called us up and asked us what to do. When we got there, he was giving him cardiac massage and mouth-to-mouth ventilations. We got an electrocardiogram hooked up to the patient and later determined that he had indeed gone into fibrillation. We defibrillated him and he survived."

News of the chest compression and the "miracles" it performed spread throughout the hospital. The interns and residents in training were skeptical and wanted to see it for themselves; one intern soon got his chance. On January 6, 1960, Henry Thomas was on duty in the emergency department tending to Eugene Barnes, a forty-five-year-old man experiencing crushing chest pain, which radiated down both arms. Barnes was probably terrified about the pain, what it meant, hoping it would soon diminish so he wouldn't have to be admitted. While he was removing his clothes prior to being examined, his heart suddenly went into ventricular fibrillation and he collapsed. Dr. Thomas had his chance. "What the hell," he said to himself, "let's try Jude's closed chest approach." So he began chest compression while someone went to retrieve a defibrillator. Twenty-two minutes later the machine arrived. Barnes was successfully defibrillated after the second shock and made a full recovery. His only minor deficit was a two-hour period of amnesia following his temporary death.[25]

Jude, Knickerbocker, and Kouwenhoven eventually compiled an impressive list of similar cases. They began presenting their reports at local and national medical meetings, and writing them up in published papers. Their first major presentation was made to the American Surgical Association meeting in Boca Raton in 1960. That same year the entire medical community became aware of the new discovery when *JAMA* published an article describing their work. This first publication, dated July 9, 1960, reported the use of external cardiac massage on twenty cases of in-hospital cardiac arrest. Fourteen of the twenty patients, 70 percent, survived and were discharged. The patients included an age range of two months to eighty years. The duration of chest compression varied from less than one minute to sixty-five minutes. All twenty patients were in ventricular fibrillation. The *JAMA* article was very straightforward: chest compression buys time until the external defibrillator arrives on the scene. As the authors wrote, "Anyone, anywhere, can now initiate cardiac resuscitative procedures. All that is needed is two hands."[26]

The public first learned of the new procedure several days before the article appeared. *The Sun*, a Baltimore daily newspaper, scooped the medical journal by printing a story with the headline "Easy Method: Press Chest, Start Heart" on July 5, 1960. The article, not quite front-page news, appeared on page 32 and opened with the prediction that this "simple method to restore heart action" would be adopted all over the world. The article described the technique of chest compression in detail, but it was not picked up by the Associated Press or any other news service, so news of the procedure did not leave the Baltimore area.

In 1961, the three colleagues reported a larger series of 138 episodes of cardiac arrest in 118 patients. About 55 percent of these episodes occurred outside the operating and recovery areas, and the majority of patients were in ventricular fibrillation. In 78 percent of 138 cardiac arrests, cardiac action was restored. However, respiration or ventilation received relatively little attention.[27] The reason, Jude said, was simple. "Most of these patients would breathe," he said. "Or else they were being ventilated because we were doing surgery on them. Or they were intubated if they were in post-op, like a cardiac surgery patient. But we soon found that you needed to give them ventilation, so we started paying more attention to that and spoke more about it."

Meanwhile, James Elam and Peter Safar at Baltimore City Hospital were carrying out their research on the effectiveness of mouth-to-mouth resuscitation. Jude admits that he was not aware at that time of the work going on across town. "We were basically working on the cardiac end. The idea we had was that patients got enough oxygenation from intubation." Using mouth-to-mouth ventilation happened only slowly at Johns Hopkins Hospital, and at others as well. Quick intubation of a nonbreathing patient was the preferred method of getting enough oxygen into them. In hospitals, it still is. However, Jude and his compatriots eventually found that it was difficult to intubate a patient quickly enough to prevent oxygen starvation.

It wasn't until 1960 and 1961 that the work by Kouwenhoven, Jude, and Knickerbocker was combined with that of Safar and Elam. Chief McMahon played a crucial role in merging mouth-to-mouth respiration with chest compression—he was the conduit between Safar's and Kouwenhoven's labs. For all of 1957 and well into 1958, McMahon had worked with Safar on the mouth-to-mouth experiments and demonstrations. In mid-1958 Jude invited McMahon to observe their technique of closed-chest cardiac compression. McMahon watched the procedure in the dog laboratory and recalled his reaction. "They had a tube down the throat of the animal, but nobody was blowing. There was no air exchange being made. I told them, you've got to supply air at the time you're compressing the chest." As he did with Safar, McMahon began bringing in his crews to see and learn the technique of chest compression.

It was not long before chest compression was utilized in prehospital settings. The date was May 1, 1960. The lucky recipient was a man named Bertie Bish, age sixty-eight. By then McMahon had trained all his firemen in mouth-to-mouth respiration and chest compression and had warned his men, "If you ever do any of these techniques, get them to Johns Hopkins

Hospital, where they know what's going on and can continue them." They followed his advice.

"Bish was the first rescue-squad resuscitation," Jude later recalled. "In those days a guy who had a heart attack was sent home after about four or five weeks—they kept heart attacks forever back then. So he'd had a heart attack earlier, and finally he went home." Bish and his son, a coal miner trained in the arm-lift chest-pressure version of artificial respiration, were together having dinner at home. Bish suddenly developed chest pain and shortness of breath. His wife called the Baltimore fire department and Bish collapsed shortly before its arrival. There was no pulse and his breathing ceased. He was clinically dead. The two fireman, Hubert Cheek and Marvin Burkendine, who arrived at the scene, had just received their training in closed-chest compression four days earlier. They immediately applied their newly learned skills and, after one minute, put Bish in the ambulance and raced for Johns Hopkins. Cheek continued with ongoing chest compression while his partner drove hell-bent to the hospital.

"They'd always call me to the emergency room when they'd get some-thing like this," Jude said, so he was there when the squad arrived. Nearly twenty-five minutes had elapsed since Bish had his attack. The technicians continued mouth-to-mouth and chest compression until the defibrillator was wheeled into the emergency room and Jude applied it. Bish's heart was successfully defibrillated. The *Readers Digest* wrote up the event and called it "the first case of cardiac arrest to be snatched from death by laymen [refer-ring to the rescue crew] using the closed-chest method."[28]

It was an astounding event, Jude recalled, and everyone realized it. All the firemen involved received commendations. "This was the beginning," said Jude. "I think that was really the start of all the 911 and everything else." For many years thereafter, Bish called James Jude on the anniversary of the event and thanked him for what he termed his "second birthday." He also called McMahon. "Every year until he died, Bertie Bish would call me up and say, 'Chief McMahon, I just wanted you to know that I'm still alive!'"

The people in Baltimore were believers. Now it was time to inform the world. For Guy Knickerbocker, his work in developing modern CPR would take on a personal meaning. In 1963 his father had a heart attack and was in the hospital. "They were trying to regularize his rhythm," Knickerbocker remembers. "I don't remember if it was with epinephrine or what. Dr. W. R. Milnor had taken over his care. He was a cardiologist at Johns Hopkins who was interested in pulmonary blood flow and had done a lot of basic research.

Because of the close ties we'd had with him over the years, it was natural to turn to him when my dad had his heart attack."

"Milnor and another doctor named Henry Thomas were there when my dad went into cardiac arrest. They did closed-chest heart massage on him, and then defibrillated him." Knickerbocker's father returned to consciousness the next morning to see the huge defibrillator sitting next to his bed. He had closely followed his son's career—it was difficult not to, since Knickerbocker had been living at home all this time. "He knew enough about what I'd been doing to know what the gadgets were," recalls Knickerbocker. "He had seen pictures of them." His father never returned to work after his heart attack, Knickerbocker says, and, after two more heart attacks, died in 1968. "But he did live for four more years and had a lot of good times through that."

Knickerbocker is objective about what he helped accomplish. "I had this very clear view that we were slowing down the dying process. We weren't necessarily holding them—we weren't providing for them something that was as good as or better than they could do on their own. I remember saying this again and again in presentations I made: 'You are slowing down the dying process.' And that bought us time to get a defibrillator there."

Looking back, Knickerbocker says that he is "still in awe" of how CPR has developed in the years since his early work in the late 1950s. "You can't step aside from the fact when you hear about some person out there who's had CPR, and somehow or other you were part of the beginning."

Where, however, the cessation of vital action is very complete,
we ought to inflate the lungs and pass electrical shocks through the chest.
Practitioners ought never, if death has been sudden and the person
not very advanced in life, to despair of sucess. . . .
—Allan Burns, 1809

THE BIRTH OF CPR

« »

The period between 1958 and 1961 began with demonstrations of the effectiveness of mouth-to-mouth for artificial respiration and chest compression for artificial circulation. All that was needed was the formal connection of the two techniques to create CPR as it is practiced today. That connection took place at the scientific level when Peter Safar and William Kouwenhoven presented their findings to the Maryland Medical Society on September 16, 1960. That meeting, held in Ocean City, can rightly be considered the birth of CPR.

The late Donald Benson, then Professor of Anesthesiology at Johns Hopkins University, moderated a panel that included Safar, Kouwenhoven, and James Jude. In his opening remarks Benson said, "Our purpose today is to bring to you, then, this new idea." It was so new it didn't even have a name. Benson stated that the two techniques of closed-chest massage and artificial respiration "cannot be considered any longer as separate units, but as parts of a whole and complete approach to resuscitation."[1]

James Jude then showed a film demonstrating chest compression on a child and an adult and recounted several cases in which it had saved lives. William Kouwenhoven was the second speaker. He described ventricular fibrillation and the technique of electric defibrillation. He used the metaphor of an eight-oared racing shell to portray what happens when the heart changes from normal rhythm to fibrillation. In normal rhythm, he explained, the coxswain calls "Pull" and the oarsmen heave in unison. In fibrillation, the oarsmen are working in an uncoordinated fashion and the forward motion of the shell ceases. Kouwenhoven showed two films. The first depicted a dog's heart in fibrillation and the application of electric shocks; the second demonstrated how to perform closed-chest defibrillation on a human. Kouwenhoven said that he saw the real benefit of chest compression as a means "to keep the patient alive until a defibrillator can be made available."

Benson next introduced Safar. He prefaced his introduction with the comment that full resuscitation required both artificial circulation and artificial respiration. Benson remarked to the audience, "Early on we thought that simple pressing on the chest would obviate . . . the need for artificial respiration. Gradually it has become apparent that this is not necessarily true and must not be counted on."

Safar began his talk by stressing the need to maintain an open air passage. If the head and neck are not positioned properly, he said, it becomes impossible to blow air into the lungs. To drive home his point, Safar projected three slides depicting X-rays of the neck and air passage. Not to be outdone in the film business, Safar brought a film demonstrating mouth-to-mouth artificial respiration on a paralyzed volunteer. He emphasized the importance of combining ventilation and circulation, and presented convincing data (later published in *JAMA*) that chest compression alone did not effectively ventilate a person.

Benson then called on Paul Hackett, anesthesiologist at the University of Maryland, to summarize the previous speakers. Hackett laid out in simple terms the sequence of resuscitation steps.

- First, open the airway.
- Second, provide ventilation. Hackett remarked, "We have many gadgets. If we have no gadgets available, we have a pair of lungs, a mouth, and some fingers."
- Third, perform chest compression.

If this meeting had been some kind of made-for-TV movie, the audience's reaction would have been rather predictable and the groundswell would be duly dramatized. But the Ocean City gathering was not a catalyst for action. The assembled audience appeared unimpressed by Jude, Kouwenhoven, and Safar, and seemed not to realize that a new lifesaving technique had just been presented. Nor was anyone aware to what extent this new technique would define the standard of resuscitation. No one, not even the speakers, realized that Baltimore had become the birthplace of modern CPR and this meeting was the public announcement of its birth.

All that remained now was to spread the word. Jude, Kouwenhoven, Knickerbocker, and Safar did just that through nationwide and world speaking tours. Archer Gordon chose a different means to educate with his film, *The Pulse of Life*. It soon became the standard for CPR training films, and was ultimately dubbed into eight languages and followed by a series of similar training films.

As a means of simplifying the instructions in the film, Gordon devised the mnemonic ABC for the sequence and steps of cardiopulmonary resuscitation. A stands for airway, B for breathing, and C for circulation. Though ABC seems so intuitive today as a memory aid, it was not immediately obvious at the time—the prevailing terms in 1961 were artificial ventilation and artificial circulation.[2]

In these early talks and films,[3] cardiopulmonary resuscitation as a label didn't exist. The Los Angeles County Heart Association called the procedure Respiro-Cardiac Resuscitation.[4] Gordon referred to it as Heart-Lung Resuscitation, and from 1960 to 1963 that term was widely used. The American Heart Association suggested a more medical sounding name, "cardiopulmonary" (or CP) instead of "heart-lung." The AHA Ad Hoc Committee on Closed Chest Cardiac Resuscitation first proposed the term cardiopulmonary resuscitation in February 1962, and thus the abbreviation CPR came into being.

It was relatively easy for Elam, Safar, and Gordon to advocate CPR. They represented themselves and were not speaking on behalf of any national organization. The American Heart Association, on the other hand, like most large, complex, inherently conservative organizations, moved much slower and more cautiously. In November 1961, the Professional Education Committee of the AHA considered closed-chest cardiac massage and agreed that it should be brought to the attention of physicians throughout the country.[5] Despite the lack of an endorsement, the committee recommended that training institutes be put on for physicians. In the course of six months, ten such programs were conducted and over 1000 physicians trained.[6]

The key issue before the American Heart Association in the early 1960s was who should be taught CPR? The potential risks of its being improperly performed were already well documented. These risks included lacerated liver, spleen, ruptured stomach, or punctured lung, not to mention broken ribs. Fractured ribs, though often an inevitable complication, were considered non-life-threatening. There were sizable pressures on the association to endorse training for nurses, rescue personnel, and even the general public. News of chest compression had reached the public mostly through newspaper and magazine stories.

In February 1961, the AHA, mostly because of concern about potential for harm, stated that the public and rescue personnel should not be taught closed-chest cardiac compression. Furthermore, dentists and nurses should also not learn the procedure until "clinical experience makes it more medically acceptable."[7] The well-documented experience in the Baltimore Fire Department, the work of Con Edison's Medical Department, and dozens of anecdotal "saves" were compelling enough to overcome any lingering caution. By April 1962, the AHA Council on Cardiovascular Surgery recommended CPR training for rescue groups. The following year, in September 1963, CPR was sanctioned with the formation of the Committee on Cardiopulmonary Resuscitation. Cardiologist Leonard Scherlis was its first chairman. On the committee were Elam, Gordon, Jude, and Safar. Early deliberations centered about whether CPR was a medical procedure (and thus taught only to doctors) or first aid (and thus taught to nurses and rescue personnel). The committee came down on the side of first aid, but continued to stop short of endorsing CPR for the general public.

No sooner had the Committee on CPR been formed than the spectre of lawsuits loomed. The committee, at its first meeting, heard about a Veterans Administration hospital nurse who, through the application of closed-chest compression, saved a patient's life. That's the good news. The bad news is that he remained in a vegetative state. The family sued the nurse and the Veterans Administration. The case was either dropped or settled out of court since no further information was contained in the committee minutes. To this date, there has not been a successful suit against someone performing CPR.

If the American Heart Association was cautious, the American Red Cross was downright ossified. The Red Cross, perhaps worried about potential harm, perhaps thinking it had too much of a training investment in artificial respiration, or perhaps concerned about added expense, did not want to get into the active business of teaching chest compression and looked to a national endorsement before they would totally revamp their training program. Gordon, Safar, Jude, and Elam worked behind the scenes to arrange such an endorsement. They reasoned that the Red Cross would take medical direction only from an entity as prestigious as the National Research Council. The AHA hoped to catalyze such a meeting by mid-1965, but large bureaucracies cannot move that fast. On May 23, 1966, the National Academy of Sciences' National Research Council convened an ad hoc Conference on Cardiopulmonary Resuscitation. Its goal was to establish standardized training and performance standards for CPR. Over thirty national organizations were represented. Elam, Safar, Gordon, and Jude were conveniently in attendance on behalf of the AHA. Recommendations from this conference appeared in the October 24 issue of *JAMA* in 1966[8] and the National Research Council published the full proceedings in 1967. The results were almost anticlimactic. CPR worked—there was little doubt about that. The conference provided an impartial, scientific imprimatur and the Red Cross finally began to teach chest compression.

The May 1967 Second International Symposium on Emergency Resuscitation in Oslo, Norway, again initiated and hosted by Asmund Laerdal, increased international awareness[9] and the proceedings, published the following year, documented the new techniques.[10] The American Heart Association convened another national conference on CPR in May 1973. Subsequent national conferences took place in 1980, 1986, and 1992.

Who, then, should receive credit for discovering CPR? Medical history credits Kouwenhover, Jude, and Knickerbocker as the discoverers. For example, almost every research article referring to modern CPR cites the 1960 *JAMA* issue where the three describe chest compression. Kouwenhover received the distinguished Albert Lasker Clinical Medical Research Award in 1973 for his discovery of CPR. The Lasker Foundation citation reads in part: "Dr. Kouwenhover devised the simple technique of external chest massage which makes it possible to sustain by hand the circulation through the body long enough to get the patient to a defibrillator." Today such an award would refer to getting the defibrillator to the patient. The award citation continues: "This technique, so simple that anyone who cares to, can learn it, and so effective that ambulance drivers, firemen, and policemen the world over are trained to use it, initiates cardiac resuscitation wherever the cardiac crisis occurs, and has saved the lives of thousands of heart attack victims."

Strong words—and words that clearly identify Kouwenhover as the inventor of CPR. What about Elam and Safar? Why aren't they referred to in the same breath as the numerous references to Kouwenhover? Several reasons can be offered, though none are entirely convincing. Kouwenhover's

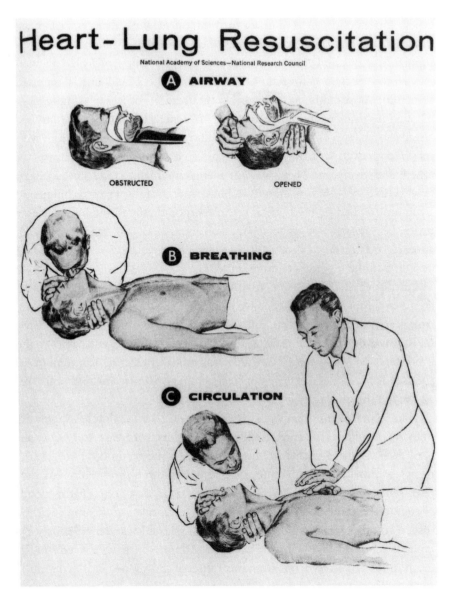

Heart-Lung Resuscitation

National Academy of Sciences—National Research Council

Ⓐ AIRWAY

OBSTRUCTED

OPENED

Ⓑ BREATHING

Ⓒ CIRCULATION

FIGURE 20. *Heart-lung resuscitation (today known as cardiopulmonary resuscitation) showing the ABC steps of Airway, Breathing, and Circulation, from the 1966 issue of the* Journal of the American Medical Association. *(Courtesy of the* Journal of the American Medical Association, *October 24, 1966;198:372–379, Copyright 1966, American Medical Association, Chicago)*

article appeared in *JAMA*, a major medical journal with a very wide circulation. Though Elam and Safar had published in the equally, if not more, prestigious *New England Journal of Medicine*, the circulation of *JAMA* in 1960 was almost 200,000, four times larger. Also, the *JAMA* article reported something apparently new—namely, the benefit of chest compression. Though it virtually ignored ventilation, the benefit of mouth-to-mouth had already been reported and was well known. Artificial ventilation with mouth-to-mouth ventilation was demonstrated in the medical literature over a period of five years. There was not a single dramatic article announcing a new technique. Mouth-to-mouth respiration was hardly a new technique; as Elam himself had pointed out, it was used sporadically throughout the centuries but mostly on infants. Chest compression, on the other hand, appeared to be new—though it was actually a rediscovery of a method obscured in the medical literature.

Putting chest compression together with mouth-to-mouth was considered a detail for improving effectiveness, not a new breakthrough. When the American Heart Association and American Red Cross formally endorsed CPR, it was done in their usual way, which was not to attribute names to the procedure. It would have been unseemly for Elam, Safar, Kouwenhoven, Jude, or Knickerbocker to attempt to attach their name to the technique. Yet all five are the inventors of CPR.

Had John Colven suffered sudden cardiac death in Baltimore in 1958, the outcome would have been inevitable death. A mere two years later, he would have had a fighting chance at survival. In 1960 the Baltimore Fire Department was providing chest compression as well as mouth-to-mouth resuscitation. Thus, the brain and heart could receive a trickle of oxygenated blood, enough to keep the body alive and the heart in fibrillation. If John could be rushed to an emergency room quickly enough, and if a defibrillator were immediately available, he might be saved. Admittedly, few survived sudden death in 1960. The epidemic from heart disease and sudden death continued to rage. But the impossible was becoming thinkable.

Part IV

THE SPARK
OF LIFE

《 》

Electricity, properly administered, is of use in a greater variety of diseases than any other single article in the whole Materia Medica.
—Frances Lowndes, 1787

EARLY CURRENTS

《 》

The discovery of CPR, as remarkable and improbable as it was, is only half the story of resuscitation. To treat sudden cardiac death, there must be a way to stop a fibrillating heart and a means to provide the therapy fast enough so that it is effective. The development of defibrillation—fundamentally an electric current applied across the heart—has its beginnings in the discovery and understanding of electricity itself.

In one of the Dialogues Plato mentions the ability of lodestones to attract iron, which then attracts more iron. "Sometimes there is formed quite a long chain of bits of iron and rings, suspended one from another; and they all depend for this power on that one stone."[1] Lodestone, actually magnetite, received its name from the Anglo-Saxon *laeden*, meaning to lead or conduct. The words *magnetite* and *magnet* in turn are derived from the city, Magnesia, in Asia Minor, where lodestones were first found in abundance. Chinese, Venetian, and Florentine mariners all had magnetite compasses. Around 1000 B.C. early Greeks used a magnetite effigy of a man whose outstretched arms always pointed south to find their way back to the Peloponnesus.[2]

For 2000 years, no progress was made in the understanding of magnetism or electricity. Superstition and the occult ruled. There were stories of gigantic magnetic mountains so powerful that nails would be torn out of sailing ships. Some believed that a star in the Great Bear constellation held the compass needle pointing to the north.[3] Magnets were said to protect against witches. And ground-up lodestones were administered as medicines for certain diseases.[4]

With the Renaissance and the beginnings of true scientific inquiry, superstitions slowly began to crumble. William Gilbert (1544–1603), physician to Queen Elizabeth I, performed the first experiments that clarified the properties of magnets and electrostatic charges. He also invented the electroscope and gave us the word electricity.[5] Gilbert's book *De Magnete* was published in 1600 in Latin and summed up his discoveries and speculations about magnetism and the nature of lodestones. The book's full title, *On the Magnet, also Magnetic Bodies, and on the Great Magnet the Earth; a New Physiology, Demonstrated by Many Arguments and Experiments*, reveals Gilbert's belief that his discoveries represented an entirely new science. Several books had already been written about lodestones and magnets, chief among them the 1581 book by Robert Norman titled *The Newe Attractive*.[6] Norman's book, which first proposed that the earth was a giant magnet, was mostly anecdotal. Gilbert, on the other hand, was one of the first experimentalists of his era. He based his writing on observation and experiment and pleaded throughout for readers to confirm his findings by repeating the experiments themselves. In keeping with contemporary science, the book was also filled with speculation as well as astrological and alchemical references.

Electricity fascinated scientists. For many years it was used mostly for entertainment value—making luminous effects, creating sparks, setting fire to objects without using flames, ringing bells, and animating other mechanical contraptions. Debate raged about what objects might be electrified—and if humans could be. In 1730 the English amateur scientist Stephen Gray (1666–1736) devised an ingenious demonstration to lay the issue to rest. He used silk rope, known not to conduct electricity, to suspend a boy from the ceiling. He chose a boy simply because he couldn't afford enough of the expensive silk to suspend a fully grown man. The boy weighed only forty-seven pounds. Gray repeatedly electrified a metal rod, using a static electricity device, and touched it to the boy's leg. He then placed various substances under and close to the boy's hands or face. As the substances rose in the air attracted to the electrified boy, there was no doubt that humans could be electrified.[7] This supported the concept of living creatures being animated by a "spark of life."

Scientists began making serious attempts to create living organisms using mechanical and electrical principles. In 1738 Jacques Vaucanson exhibited

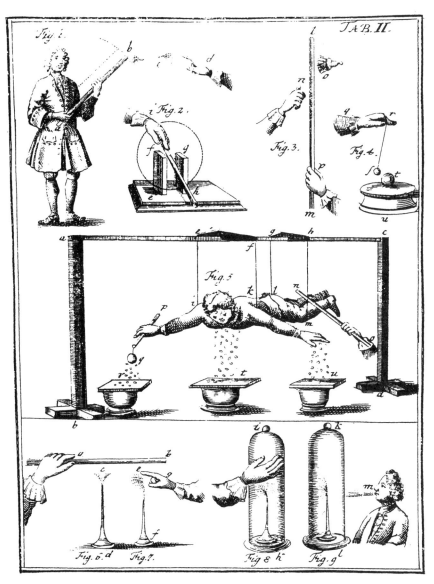

FIGURE 21. *Hanging boy experiments conducted by Gray. The boy is suspended by silk threads and electrified (middle). He can then attract lightweight objects to his hands or body. (Courtesy of The Bakken Library and Museum, Minneapolis).*

three automata, one of which was a mechanical duck that "drinks, eats, quacks, splashes about on the water, and digests his food like a living duck." The duck was built over a large wooden cabinet that contained the device's supporting gears and workings. Observers described their astonishment at the lifelike quality of the work.[8] Today it is easy to dismiss such a "toy" as an early precursor of animated figures such as those found in Disneyland. In Vaucanson's time, however, the device added more support to the belief that the ability to duplicate the spark of life would one day be discovered.

By the middle of the eighteenth century, electricity was thought to be so pervasive that it was considered the fifth element after fire, water, earth, and air. In 1743 the students of Johann Gottlob Kruger, Professor of Medicine at the University of Halle, asked him about the possible practical value of electricity. Their question posed in Latin was, "Cui bono?" (What good is it?)[9] They knew about the tricks and games one could play with it. But did electricity offer any benefit to patients? Professor Kruger replied in the affirmative and thus became one of the first to suggest that electricity might have medicinal properties and restore health. His conviction about the benefit of electrotherapy seems faint at best. Revealing his logic, he wrote, "For all things must have a usefulness; that is certain. Since electricity must have a usefulness, and we have seen that it cannot be looked for either in theology or in jurisprudence, there is obviously nothing left but medicine." Despite such lackluster enthusiasm, he omnisciently wrote, "Through electrification, changes in the deepest regions of the human body can be brought forth." Electricity, he claimed, would be "a new kind of cure," and he called for experiments to demonstrate its effect on life. Kruger predicted a benefit of electricity in the treatment of paralyzed limbs. Electricity would function, he predicted, "just as one uses flagellation with nettles to restore sensation and reestablish the power of motion." Kruger's lecture and subsequent publication on the application of electricity to medicine earns him the title of "founding father of electrotherapy."[10]

His contemporaries soon began to recommend electricity for many different ailments. A student of Kruger's, Christian Gottlieb Kratzenstein (1723–1795), reported the successful use of electrotherapy in paralysis in 1744. He wrote of "a woman who lost the paralysis in her small finger within one quarter of an hour by electrification."[11]

In 1752 the King of Denmark invited Kratzenstein to take a position at the University in Copenhagen where he could investigate the medical uses of electricity. He arrived with his electrical apparatus and, after some difficulty, found lodgings for himself and his large equipment. Kratzenstein then began advertising, inviting patients to visit between four and six in the afternoon. His therapeutic device was a large rotary static electricity generator. According to accounts, his treatment was associated with a smell of sulfur, which he attributed to unclean particles being driven from the body.[12]

Six years earlier the Leyden jar, named after the Dutch city where it was discovered, allowed the first convenient storage of large amounts of electricity. Pieter van Musschenbroek (1692–1761), a physics professor at Leyden, described the power of the jar in a letter dated April 20, 1746: "I wish to communicate to you a new but terrible experiment that I would advise you never to attempt yourself." He then reported how he accidentally discovered the principle of the Leyden jar and how the resulting shock led him to believe "it was all up with me."

Like many momentous discoveries, van Musschenbroek's was serendipitous. He had been experimenting with charged conductors and trying to find ways for a conductor to keep its charge. In the humid climate of Holland conductors rapidly lost their charge to the moist air. Using a rotating glass globe, he charged a gun barrel with static electricity. One end of the barrel had a brass wire leading through a cork into a bottle that was filled with water. When his assistant held the bottle and touched the wire with his other hand, he completed the circuit and received a massive shock.[13]

As scientists began experimenting with Leyden jars, they found that the stored charge could be kept for several days. Amazing demonstrations became possible. The same year the Leyden jar was discovered, the London Royal Society proceedings heard an account of a French demonstration in Versailles conducted by Nollet. One hundred-eighty guards were lined up before the King. Holding hands with the two individuals connected to wires from a Leyden jar, all 180 were made to jump simultaneously. On another occasion an entire community of 800 Carthusian Monks in Paris were linked by wires that allowed a shock to be transmitted over one and a half kilometers.[14] Given its amazing properties, it is not surprising that experiments were conducted to test electricity's benefit in every conceivable situation.

Jean-Antoine Nollet (1700–1770) performed experiments to determine the ability of electricity to stimulate life and growth in plants and birds and helped popularize electricity. He taught a course in physics in Paris that attracted wealthy, leisured students. Nollet's Cours de Physique (physics course) was a carefully prepared performance of 350 experiments, many involving electricity. Nollet also ventured to explain all physical properties,

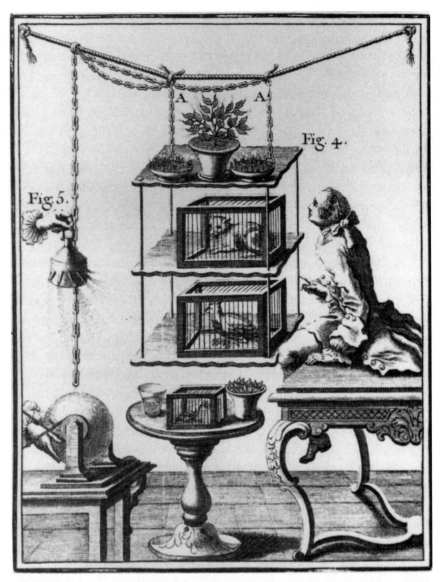

FIGURE 22. *Nollet's electrical experiments on animals and vegetables. A static electricity generator (lower left corner) electrified the silk-supported chain. Electricity stimulated growth "four-fold" in plants, but the cat and pigeon lost weight under its influence. (Courtesy of Burndy Library, Dibner Institute for the History of Science and Technology, Cambridge, Massachusetts)*

including motion, magnetism, vibration, hydrostatics, optics, and celestial motion. The course was extremely popular, and fit nicely into the Enlightenment mind. If the world could be described in a harmonious, rational way, then human life itself could become orderly and filled with happiness—and scientific knowledge was the means of achieving human harmony.[15]

Anecdotal reports did much to spread the interest in medical uses of electricity, though not all practitioners were converts. In 1748 Nollet concluded that electricity was not useful in treating paralyzed patients. The same year a French physician wrote, "I have electrified people attacked with gout and rheumatism with crippled extremities, and after exposure to electricity all were made more uncomfortable than before. Thus electric commotion can only increase the pains of the afflicted."[16]

Many distinguished scientists argued stridently for the medical benefits of electricity, yet other reputable investigators still questioned its healing properties. One skeptic was Benjamin Franklin. Writing in 1758 about the use of electricity in treating paralysis, Franklin declared, "In palsies, I never knew any advantage from electricity that was permanent." Franklin suggested that whatever temporary benefit occurred was probably from the placebo effect and noted that patients became discouraged from severe shocks.[17]

Franklin is, of course, better known for his 1752 experiment demonstrating the electrical nature of lightning. As he describes it, "The kite is to be raised, when a thunder-gust appears to be coming on (which is very frequent in this country). . . . The pointed wire will draw the electric fire . . . and the kite with all the twine will be electrified." To prove that the kite was electrified, Franklin held his knuckle next to a metal key hanging from the string. He wrote, "You will find it (the electric fire) stream out plentifully from the key on the approach of your knuckle."[18] Franklin was lucky his kite did not take a direct jolt of lightning since he would have surely died. He was apparently knocked senseless during one experiment, causing him to remark, "If there is no other use discovered for electricity, this, however, is something considerable that it may help make a vain man humble."

John Wesley (1703–1791), best known as the founder of Methodism, was also a great believer in the value of electricity. In 1760, he published *The Desideratum; or Electricity Made Plain and Useful, by a Lover of Mankind and of Common Sense* (London). In it, he offered case reports on the numerous conditions reported to have been cured by electricity. The alphabetical list started with ague (probably a severe cough) and ended with wens (benign surface tumors). Other medical conditions included blindness, consumption, cramps, deafness, dropsy, epilepsy, feet violently disordered, gout, headache, hysterics, King's evil (scrofula—otherwise known as monarchy malaise), leprosy, mortifications, palpitations, palsy, pleurisy, rheumatism, ringworm, sciatica, shingles, sore feet, swellings of all kinds, and toothache. One representative report was supplied by a doctor in Newcastle upon Tyne. "Last week a poor man in Sandgate, that had been blind twenty-four years, was led to the machine. I set him upon the electrical board, and drew sparks for about twenty minutes from the pupil of his eye. After he had rested himself a little . . . he told us he could see. He could also distinguish objects in the room and was able to walk home without a guide." In another case a women, aged eighty-six, who was afflicted with sciatica for twenty years "was electrified ten or twelve times and has been easy ever since." Wesley provides this physiologic reason: "It seems the Electric Fire in cases of this . . . dilates the minute vessels, and capillary passages, as well as separates the clogging particles of the stagnating fluids. By accelerating likewise the motion of the blood, it removes many obstructions."[19]

Wesley's comments on electricity and heart conditions are particularly interesting. Although the treatment of ventricular fibrillation would not occur for another 170 years, Wesley was able to show how electricity could benefit the heart condition of angina. Angina, pain caused by the narrowing of a coronary artery and only recently recognized, was described by Wesley in his 1774 journal as responding to electric shocks across the chest. "I was convinced it was . . . angina pectoris. I advised him to take no more medicines but to be electrified through the breast. He was so. The violent symptoms immediately ceased and he fell into a sweet sleep."[20] Perhaps anticipating skeptics, Wesley closed his book with the plea "that they would not peremptorily pronounce against Electricity while they know little or nothing about it. . . . Let him for two or three weeks (at least) try it himself for the above-named disorders. And then his own sense will show him whether it is a mere plaything or the noblest medicine yet known to the world."

The First Defibrillation?

Probably the first use of a portable electric device to save an individual was described in 1774 in a report issued by the Royal Humane Society of London: "Sophia Greenhill, on Thursday last, fell out of a one-pair-of stairs window, and was taken up by a man to all appearance dead. The surgeons at the

Middlesex Hospital, and an apothecary, declared that nothing could be done for the child. Mr. Squires, tried the effects of electricity. Twenty minutes elapsed before he could apply the shock, which he gave to various parts of the body in vain—but, upon transmitting a few shocks through the thorax, he perceived a small pulsation; in a few minutes the child began to breathe with great difficulty."[21] The child remained in a coma for several days but eventually her health was restored.

A similar case was reported in 1787. "A lad in perfect health, fell from a two-pair-of-stairs window into an area, and was taken up to all appearance dead. Upon the strictest examination, no mark of violence could be discovered either upon the head or upon any other part. After a variety of means had been tried by a surgeon without effect, the lad was pronounced dead, and sent home. A gentleman, past whose house he was carried, happening to inquire into the circumstances of the case, wished to try the effect of Electricity. After four small shocks had been given, the lad shewed some signs of life, and by continuing them he gradually recovered, so that in less than two hours he was able to walk about the house."[22]

The English physician, Charles Kite, in his 1788 *An Essay on the Recovery of the Apparently Dead,* comments on these cases, as well as ones he personally attended. "Do they not plainly point out that electricity is the most powerful stimulus we can apply? Is not the superior advantage of this stimulus evinced in the most incontrovertible and unequivocal manner?"[23] Well, yes and no. The accounts are certainly vivid and the use of electricity appears causally linked to the child's recovery. However, it is very unusual, (in fact, extremely rare) for a child's heart to fibrillate—develop a quivering, ineffective heart rhythm. Sudden death from ventricular fibrillation is an adult disease, primarily because the heart must be a certain minimal size for fibrillatory rhythm to be sustained—a child's heart is simply too small. The children who fell from the windows probably had a seizure (causing the fall) or a concussion (from the fall), or both, and may have appeared lifeless.

In his *Essay* Kite provides an illustration of the device likely used for resuscitating the two children. All the elements of a modern defibrillator are there: a source of energy, in this case a Leyden jar served as the capacitor; an electrometer functioned as the energy setting; brass knobs were the electrodes; metallic strings were equivalent to the cables; and glass or wooden tubes acted as insulators to prevent the operator from being shocked. As Kite so delicately put it, "In this manner, shocks may be sent through any part of the body . . . without a probability of the assistants receiving any inconvenience."

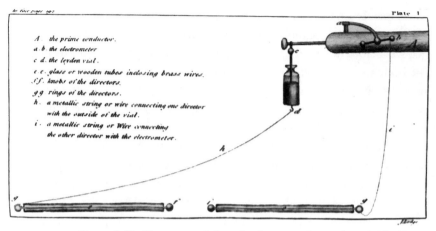

FIGURE 23. *Proto-defibrillator containing the elements of a modern defibrillator, from Charles Kite's 1788 essay. The leyden vial (d) is similar to a modern capacitor. The electrometer (a,b) regulates the current. The knobs of the directors (f) are equivalent to modern electrode paddles. The source of electricity is supplied by the prime conductor (A). (Courtesy of The Bakken Library and Museum, Minneapolis).*

Kite also distinguished between apparent (clinical) and absolute (biologic) death. The key was "the presence or absence of the principle of irritability." So long as the body reacted to an irritating stimulus, it could not be absolutely dead. Kite also talked about "vital heat" and how electricity could be used to test the presence or absence of life. "It appears to me," he wrote, "that the electrical shock is to be admitted as the test, or discriminating characteristic of any remains of animal life; and so long as that produces contractions, may the person be said to be in a recoverable state; but when that effect has ceased, there can be no doubt remain of the party being absolutely and positively dead."[24]

Although others were also aware of the benefit of electricity in reviving life, their understanding was superficial and based on observations of cause and effect. Electricity was applied across the chest and a lifeless creature came to life. How could one argue with such power? Writing in 1776, John Hunter (1728–1799?), a member of the board of the Royal Humane Society, in *Proposals for the Recovery of People Apparently Drowned,* said: "Electricity has been known to be of service and should be tried when other methods have failed. It is probably the only method we have of immediately stimulating the heart."

John Fothergill, another English physician, described a case in 1782 in which electrical therapy saved a man. "In a severe thunderstorm at a house in Gravel Lane, an elderly man was struck by lightning, thrown from his chair and taken up for dead. In this hopeless state, electrification was performed by a skillful practitioner of Guys Hospital, by which efficacious remedy the man was happily at length restored to life." Fothergill was a leading advocate of electricity for resuscitation. He wrote, "Instead of losing time in the application of several slight stimuli to the skin and intestines, why not have recourse to the most potent stimulus in nature, which can instantly pervade the inmost recesses of the animal frame."

Some physicians advocated that electricity was a more useful technique for resuscitation than the mechanical techniques then in vogue. Dr. William Henley, in an address to the Royal Humane Society, said, "I am of opinion that (together with warmth and friction) electrical shocks from a jar . . . passed in different directions through the body, but particularly through the heart and lungs, might produce the desired effect in a very short time. . . . In cases of apparent death from drowning, etc., wherein the organs are sound, and only their motion suspended . . . why not immediately apply electrical shocks to the brain and heart, the grand source of motion and sensation . . . ?"[25]

The ability to store electricity allowed it to be used for a variety of medical conditions, and special institutions offering electrical treatment opened in London in the late 1780s and 1790s. Calling himself a medical electrician, Francis Lowndes published a small book in 1787 titled *Observations on Medical Electricity*. Its subtitle was "A synopsis of all the diseases in which electricity has been recommended or applied with success, likewise pointing out a new and more efficacious method of applying this remedy by electric vibrations."[26] Lowndes freely admitted that electrotherapy had received a bad name by being touted as a remedy for every known human ailment. His book lists forty-three diseases that could be helped by electricity, among them tapeworm, tumors, locked jaw, epilepsy (sleeping sickness), urinary obstruction, cataracts, and amenorrhea (lack of menstruation).

Lowndes's practice was extensive and his electrical apparatus was said to be "the most complete and powerful in Europe." His technique of "electric vibrations" provided stimulation in a gentle fashion without pain. Lowndes treated over 300 patients per year and over half were said to be completely cured, with the remainder experiencing some benefit.

During the decades from 1750 to 1800, Luigi Galvani and Alessandro Volta, among others, made important discoveries about electricity. Galvani

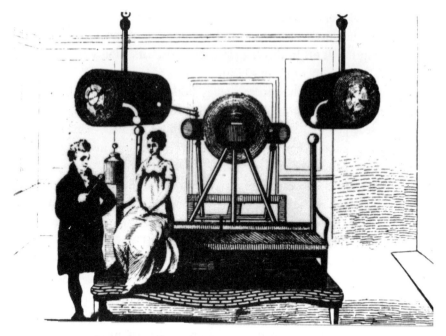

FIGURE 24. *Francis Lowndes's electrical machine used in therapy for a variety of ailments. (Courtesy of The Bakken Library and Museum, Minneapolis)*

(1737–1798) found that two different metals can generate a small amount of electricity. His interpretation of this phenomena, though erroneous, did much to stimulate the exploration of electricity and its effects on living organisms. Galvani, a professor of anatomy at the University of Bologna, conducted a series of experiments on frogs in which he used a brass wire placed in a frog's spine. When the frog's leg accidentally touched an iron plate, the leg twitched. Galvani had been using static electricity to induce a muscle twitch and recognized the twitches as identical. He believed that the frog's muscle contained its own source of power that he called "vital fluid." In this regard Galvani supported eighteenth-century theories that animals possessed subtle "fluids" that explained bodily functions such as muscular contractions.

Galvani's findings were published in 1791 in *De Viribus Electricitatis in Motu Musculari Commentarius* (*The Effects of Artificial Electricity on Muscular Motion*) in which he wrote, "It appears clear to me that electricity resides in all animals which we shall designate . . . 'animal electricity.'" The fifty-six-page book described a series of twenty-one experiments, twenty involving frogs and one with a sheep. He wished to show that his findings applied to warm-blooded as well as cold-blooded animals. Galvani believed that animal electricity was a new type of electricity, added to the forms of electricity then known as natural (lightning, electric eel, torpedo fish) and artificial (static electricity).[27] In a series of experiments he convincingly showed that nerves were specialized conductors for this animal electricity and speculated that animal electrical fluid is generated from the blood in the brain and passes through nerves to the muscles. The electrical fluid makes the core of the muscles positively charged and the outside surface negatively charged. A metal probe can carry the discharge from the inside of the muscle to its outside, thus causing a muscular contraction. The animal was supplying the electricity and the probe only served to release what was inherent in the animal. To some extent, Galvani's belief in animal electricity is correct. Nerve fibers *do* generate very small electric discharges when they are stimulated. He was completely wrong, however, in believing that muscles possess electricity. Electrical stimulation of nerves causes muscular contraction; the muscles themselves have nothing to do with electricity. Furthermore, there in no such thing as a unique substance called animal electricity—electricity is electricity.

The publication of Galvani's work caused a storm, as one commentator put it, and the population of European frogs probably hit an all-time low as experimenters replicated Galvani's observations and saw for themselves the remarkable properties of "animal electricity." Physicians believed Galvani had discovered a vital life-force. Some even suggested "galvanizing" corpses (the origin of the word "galvanize") to confirm death prior to burial.[28]

Volta and the First Battery

Galvani sent a personalized copy of his paper on the effects of artificial electricity to Alessandro Volta, a professor of physics at the University of Pavia in Northern Italy. Though he initially agreed with Galvani's conclusions, Volta soon speculated that electricity generated by the two metals was the cause of the muscular response—a conclusion just the opposite of Galvani's. There was no inherent animal electricity in the nerves and muscles, asserted Volta; the twitch was only the response to the electrical stimulation from two metals. Volta was aware of previous reports of two metals causing a bitter taste. He reproduced the effect by placing tinfoil on the tip of his tongue and a small silver spoon toward the back. When the handle of the spoon touched the tinfoil, he noted a strong sour taste. He also placed one form of metal on his forehead and a different metal on the roof of his mouth. When he connected the two metals with a copper wire, Volta's eyes perceived sensations of light. He concluded that the two metals were causing an electrical discharge that could stimulate muscular as well as sensory reactions.[29] He called this electricity "metallic electricity."

Volta used the principle of two dissimilar metals to generate electricity and created the world's first electrochemical battery. Known as Volta's pile, his battery consisted of alternating disks of copper and zinc separated by a piece of flannel soaked in saltwater. By connecting a wire to the end disks, he generated a considerable amount of current. The saltwater produced a chemical reaction between the different metals and caused electrons to flow from the copper to the zinc. The current of the battery could be crudely regulated by removing or adding disks to the pile. Volta fashioned an even stronger battery by using cups filled with dilute acid in which he placed copper and zinc strips.

By the second half of the eighteenth century, a number of people were experimenting with electrical shock for resuscitation. Among them were Alexander Humboldt (1769–1859) and Giovanni Aldini (1762–1834), Galvani's nephew.

Humboldt was in his library one day when a bird flew against his window and appeared to fall down dead. He ran into his laboratory and got a portable electric device (probably a Leyden jar) and attached the copper electrode to the bird's beak. Not knowing where to place the zinc electrode, Humboldt quickly shoved it in the bird's anus. He wrote in his journal in 1796, "To my amazement, at the moment of contact, the bird opened its eyes, raised itself on its feet by flapping its wings. It breathed anew for seven or eight minutes and then expired quietly." Humboldt was so impressed by what he saw that he decided to try the same oral-anal pathway on himself. He wrote that at the moment of contact, "I saw very vivid flashes before my eyes."[30] It's not known if he did this daily, but he lived to ninety.

Humboldt was particularly interested in the relationship of electricity to the heart's contraction, and, in 1797, conducted experiments on the hearts of carp, demonstrating that a mild shock could have a stimulating effect and speed up the heart's rate of contraction. But a large shock would lead to a completely stilled heart.

Volta described his discovery of the electrochemical battery in a letter to the president of the Royal Society of London in 1800 that was published in the *Transactions of the Royal Society*. He wrote: "I found myself obliged to combat the alleged animal electricity of Galvani, and to declare it an external electricity moved by the mutual contact of metals of different kinds." This announcement came exactly 200 years after Gilbert had published *De Magnete*. Volta was well aware that the amount of electricity generated by his pile was not so great that it could be stored in a Leyden jar. But the pile had the great advantage of offering a continuous supply of electricity. The importance of Volta's discovery was immediately appreciated. He was invited to appear before Napoleon, who presented him with an annual pension, and was elected one of the eight "foreign associates" of the French Academy of Sciences. A similar honor was bestowed on Benjamin Franklin. The principles behind this chemical battery are exactly the same as those used to manufacture modern batteries.[31]

It is perhaps ironic that Volta saw the new form of electricity honored with his rival's name. Galvanism was the label attached to this new source of electricity to distinguish it from the older form of static-generated electricity that was simply called electricity. To scientists around 1800, the two forms of electricity seemed entirely different and deserving of separate names.

Individuals soon recognized the potential therapeutic benefit of the voltaic pile. It was used to treat visual and hearing problems, and was even proposed for dissolving gallstones. The scientific basis was less important than that it offered a new means of delivering electricity to the body.

Electric fluid . . . wake the torpid powers to sudden life. Let fly the sudden shock.
—George Dyer, *Annual Report of the Royal Humane Society*, 1802

SEARCHING
FOR THE SPARK
OF LIFE

《 》

It was obvious that electricity could cause muscle contractions, and so it was not long before medical science thought that Galvani's work might shed light on the workings of the heart. The heart, after all, is a muscle. Was it possible for a stilled heart to be restarted? According to medical historian David Schechter, scientists working around 1800 believed "there might remain in the heart a flickering ember of vitality, which, if fanned by super-potent stimulation, could rekindle the flame of life in the entire organism."[1] This belief was hardly confined to scientists; musicians and novelists also referred to electricity and its lifegiving properties. In Mozart's wonderful opera *Cosi Fan Tutte*, written in 1790, Despina the maid uses a magnet to touch the heads of Ferrando and Guglielmo who have apparently been poisoned. Declaring electricity to be a great and mysterious invention, Despina revives the men from their stupor.

Mary Shelley produced perhaps the most famous example of electricity in literature. Writing in *Frankenstein* (1818), she described the scientist's attempt to create life in this way: "I collected the instruments of life around me, that I might infuse a spark of being into the lifeless thing that lay at my feet." Shelley was well aware of Franklin's experiments demonstrating that lightning was electricity since Franklin had been hailed throughout Europe as "the modern Prometheus." Indeed,the full title of Shelley's work is *Franken-stein, or the Modern Prometheus.*

Headless and Other Unwilling Subjects

At the beginning of the nineteenth century many studies were undertaken to determine if electricity could restart the heart, but results were contradictory and inconclusive. The French anatomist and physiologist Xavier Bichat (1771–1802) entered the controversy on the eve of the French Revolution, and found no dirth of subjects. What better laboratory specimens than guillotined bodies? With permission from the revolutionary authorities, Bichat conducted electrical experiments on freshly decapitated bodies using galvanism and chemical stimulants. His conclusion was a breakthrough for science: the heart could be reliably excited, but only by direct contact with a source of electricity.[2] When other French scientists performed similar experiments, however, they reached somewhat contradictory conclusions. The time interval from death to the actual experiment was often not taken into account and was, of course, the most significant factor explaining the heart's responsiveness.

The importance of time was intensively studied in a special commission formed in 1803 by the Academy of Turin in Italy. Its conclusion was that the heart lost its ability to contract in response to electrostimulation forty minutes after death.[3]

Perhaps the most bizarre experiments conducted on freshly decapitated bodies occurred in Mainz, Germany, on November 21, 1803. A band of twenty highwaymen were captured and condemned to decapitation. At the request of the town's physicians, authorities gave their permission for the unusual experiments. All twenty bodies and heads were to be brought to the eager physicians located only 150 feet from the execution site. A physician would lift every severed head as it fell into the basket and shout into each ear, "Can you hear me?" Since all the assembled agreed that no affirmative response was given, the bodies and "nonhearing" heads were rushed to waiting physicians who performed electrical stimulation experiments. Only four of the condemned were dissected and electrified, and the physicians were able to confirm that the heart was indeed a muscle and could respond to electric stimulation like any other muscle.[4]

Giovanni Aldini (1762–1834) also studied the effects of electricity on the body, especially the heart.[5] During a journey to England, Aldini received much attention from the local press when he used the "galvanic process" on a hanged criminal. According to the January 22, 1803, *London Morning Post,* an executed murderer who was taken to a nearby house immediately after hanging "was subjected to the Galvanic Process, by Professor Aldini . . . Aldini, who is the nephew of the discoverer of this most interesting science, showed the eminent and superior powers of Galvanism to be far beyond any other stimulant in nature. On the first application of the process to the face, the jaw of the deceased criminal began to quiver, and the adjoining muscles were horribly contorted, and one eye was actually opened. In the subsequent parts of the process the right hand was raised and clenched, and the legs and thighs were set in motion. It appeared to the uninformed part of the bystanders as if the wretched man was on the eve of being restored to life. This however was impossible, as several of his friends, who were near the scaffold, had violently pulled his legs in order to put a more speedy termination to his sufferings."[6]

Aldini outdid himself the next month, as the same paper reported. "Some curious Galvanic experiments were made by Professor Aldini. The head of an

FIGURE 25. *Aldini's electroresuscitation experiments on human cadavers. From* Essai theorique sur de la galvanism, Pt IV, *Paris, 1804. (Courtesy of The Bakken Library and Museum, Minneapolis)*

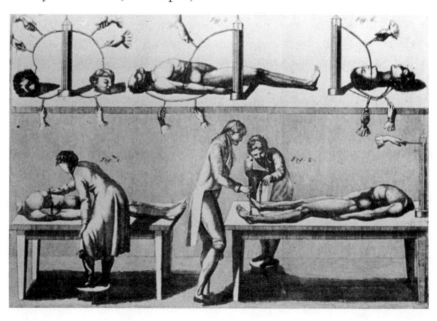

ox, recently decapitated, exhibited astonishing effects; for the tongue, being drawn out by a hook fixed into it, on applying the exciters, was retracted, so as to detach itself by tearing itself from the hook; at the same time a loud noise issued from the mouth, attended by violent contortions of the whole head and eyes." While Aldini held onto the ox's ear with one hand, he used the leg nerve from a dissected frog to serve as exciter. Aldini claimed the resulting evidence of contractions as support for the theory of animal electricity.

Like Humboldt, Aldini also personally tried the effects of electricity. Once he applied a very powerful current from a voltaic pile of several hundred pairs of metals through his own head just above his ears. This earns him the distinction of performing the first electroconvulsive shock therapy. According to his account, he became so excited he was sleepless for several days. He believed the technique would be useful for severe depression and treated two patients in just such a fashion with a resulting cure. Today electroconvulsive therapy is still used in treating intractable cases of severe depression.[7]

In 1804, while in France, Aldini wrote about the need to connect artificial respiration and electric therapy: "Galvanism is the primary means for cases of suspended animation." According to Aldini, electricity should be used immediately, not after a long period of artificial ventilation as recommended by most other scientists. Aldini wrote, "Artificial respiration ought to be attempted but it should be accompanied by the application of Galvanic power externally to the diaphragm and to the region of the heart." He was therefore one of the first to advocate a combination that presaged modern CPR and defibrillation. He freely admitted to ignorance about how electricity affects the heart, but "that it does affect it has, I trust, been sufficiently demonstrated by experiments. All that I maintain is that it produces an influence which, acting conjointly with the excitation given to the lungs, concurs in the work of reanimation." Without any understanding of ventricular fibrillation or heart disease (he was primarily concerned with drownings), Aldini had realized that ventilation combined with rapid electric therapy could reanimate the lifeless.

Spreading the Word

Experiments on executed criminals continued to occur. In Scotland, Matthew Clydesdale, thirty-five years old, was hanged for murder on November 4,

1818. His body hung for one hour. After being cut down, it was transported within ten minutes to James Jeffray, Professor of Anatomy at the University of Glasgow, and his colleague Andrew Ure, Professor of Natural Philosophy. Both had requested the body to further their work on resuscitation using battery-operated electrical stimulation. For the experiment, they constructed a giant battery consisting of 270 four-inch plates of zinc and copper bathed in acid. Ure was well aware of the moral dilemma he presented the people of Glasgow if indeed he was able to resuscitate a murderer, but the greater good would be served. "This event, however little desirable with a murderer, and perhaps contrary to the law, would yet have been pardonable in one instance, as it would have been highly honourable and useful to science."

Jeffray and Ure connected electrodes, one to the heel and the other to the spinal cord, and the result was such a violent extension of the bent knee "as nearly to overturn one of the assistants." Next, they connected rods to the left phrenic nerve and the diaphragm and "full, nay, laborious breathing instantly commenced. The chest heaved and fell . . . and the diaphragm widened and contracted as in natural respiration."

Clearly impressed with the potency of their stimuli, they then connected electrodes to the heel and nerve above one eye. The results must have been the talk of Glasgow for months, since as they varied the voltage, the "most extraordinary grimaces were exhibited. . . . Rage, horror, despair, anguish and ghastly smiles united their hideous expression in the murderer's face." According to Ure's own account before the Glasgow Literary Society five weeks later, "several of the spectators were forced to leave the apartment from terror or sickness, and one gentleman fainted"—not too surprising a response. Ure was convinced—electricity was the most promising means for restoring life to the dead.

Shortly after Jaffray and Ure's account of their experiment, phrenic nerve stimulation was reported as a way of resuscitating a drowning victim. The phrenic nerve travels along the esophagus and covers the diaphragm, causing it to contract. In one account, a drunken man fell into a body of water and remained submerged for six or seven minutes before being rescued and carried half a mile to a nearby house where his stomach was pumped and the usual means of resuscitation were tried without success. Dr. Ferguson, surgeon to the Westmeath Dispensary, cut into the chest below the seventh rib to expose the diaphragm. He attached a battery and repeatedly stimulated the diaphragm to mimic breathing. The patient soon began to breath on his own.

The use of electricity as a mean of resuscitation and the need to apply it

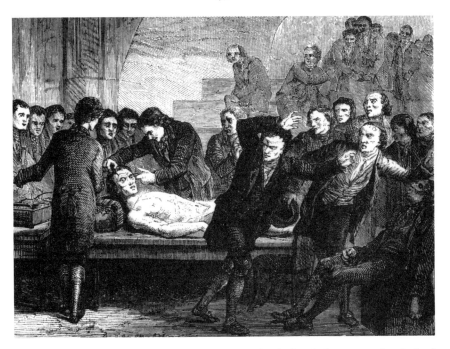

FIGURE 26. *Ure and Jeffray galvanizing the body of the executed criminal Clydesdale, Glasgow, 1818. (Courtesy of Hermiston Publishers, Ltd)*

rapidly were evident in the advice of Richard Reece, a London physician, who published *The Medical Guide* in 1820. He wrote, "In cases of suspended animation what is necessary to be done should be done quickly; therefore, on the first alarm of any person being drowned or suffocated, while the body is searching for, or conveying to the nearest house, the following articles should be got ready: viz. warm blankets, flannels, a large furnace of warm water, heated bricks, a pair of bellows, warming-pan, sal volatile, clyster pipes, and an electrifying machine."[8]

Reece's book provides an example of such an electric machine and a description by its inventor, Dr. de Sanctis. This device, called a reanimation chair, consisted of a voltaic battery, a bellows to ventilate the lung, and a metal tube to be inserted in the esophagus for delivery of stimulating vapors. The three resuscitation items were packaged in a carrying case and available for purchase in a London medical supply store. The bellows was to be inserted in the mouth and the nose clamped shut. An assistant pressed on the ribs to cause expiration after each ventilation with the bellows. The voltaic pile was to be suspended from a hook attached to the back of a chair.

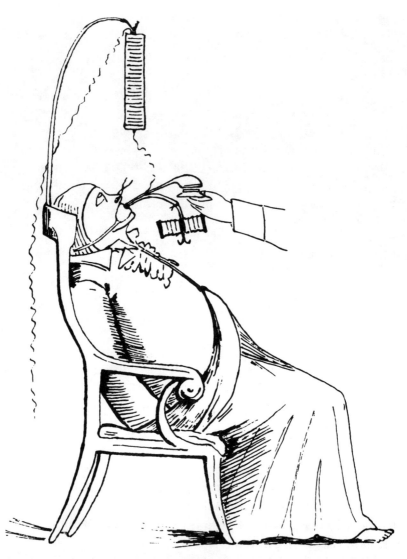

FIGURE 27.   *Reanimation chair. The patient's nostrils are closed with forceps and air is pushed by bellows into a silver cannula in the throat. Another metallic tube is inserted in the back of the throat and rinsed with stimulating fluid. Concurrently, one wire of a voltaic battery (hanging above the head) is fastened to the esophageal conduit, while the other wire is successively touched to different parts of the body. (Courtesy of The Bakken Library and Museum, Minneapolis)*

One wire from the battery was attached to the metal tube in the esophagus and the second wire successively touched to "the regions of the heart, the diaphragm and the stomach." There is no record of anyone being successfully resuscitated using the reanimation chair.

Electromagnetism

Twenty years after the discovery of the voltaic pile, Hans Christian Oersted (1777–1851), professor of physics at the University of Copenhagen, discovered the principle of electromagnetism. Oersted happened to place a conducting wire attached to a voltaic pile near a magnetic needle. He noticed the needle strongly deflected by the current in the wire and this observation led to his description of electromagnetism in *Experimenta circa effectum conflictus electrici in acum magneticam* (*Experiments of the Effects of a Current of Electricity on the Magnetic Needle*), published in 1820.[9]

Michael Faraday (1791–1867), the English scientist, extended and expanded Oersted's discovery, confirming Oersted's finding that electric current created a magnetic field. He also convincingly demonstrated that a magnetic field could create electricity. His article "On Some New Electro-Magnetical Motions, and on the Theory of Magnetism" was published in 1821 in the *Quarterly Journal of Science*. It contained an ingenious apparatus to illustrate the principle of electromagnetism. Though it involved only a small magnetic rod with a wire circling it, the apparatus was the first device to convert electrical into mechanical energy. Faraday's discoveries led to medical devices that were widely used throughout the later half of the nineteenth century.

Medical Electrical Devices

The earliest medical electrical devices were manufactured in the 1830s and used electrostatic-generated energy. Physicians, usually with an assistant in tow to help spin the glass globe, used these devices to treat a host of maladies. The patient would hold one electrode while the physician touched the diseased part of the body with the other electrode. These devices were widespread enough for Charles Dickens to allude to them in his novels. In the *Pickwick Papers* (1837), Sam Weller, Mr. Pickwick's trusty servant, remarks on

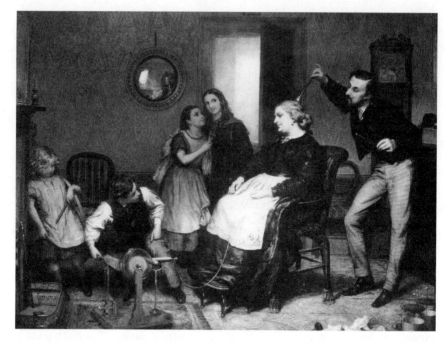

FIGURE 28. Treating Mother's Headache, *David Henry Friston, exhibited 1853–1869. The machine pictured is a cylinder electrostatic device for producing electricity. It was used by legitimate and quack doctors for treating mental disease of all kinds. Accessories on the floor include two Leyden jars, used for storing static electricity and a gold-leaf electroscope for measuring the electric charge. The woman is sitting on a chair with tumblers under the legs and with her feet resting on a stool with glass legs known as an insulating stool. (Courtesy of Spink & Son Ltd., London)*

encountering a lady who has fainted, "Here's a wenerable old lady a lyin' on the carpet waitin' for dissection, or galwinism, or some other rewivin' and scientific inwention."

Electromagnetic home electrical devices became popular in the United States beginning around 1840, and enthusiasm for medical uses of electricity blossomed after the Civil War. The home devices were advertised as beneficial for a constellation of diseases and ailments. Harvey Green, in his book *Fit for America: Health, Fitness, Sport and American Society*,[10] cites three reasons for this rising interest. First, the established medical community's credibility was at an all-time low with much internal disagreement and rancor among physicians, homeopaths, and herbalists. Second, new diseases such as neurasthenia, which was reported in almost epidemic proportions in the late nineteenth and early twentieth century, seemed particularly unresponsive to traditional medicine. (Today we would use the term psychosomatic illness, or anxiety, or depression.) Though effective therapies and medications exist today, at that time no one knew its cause, let alone an effective treatment. Thus, the opportunity for nontraditional therapies found a large market. Third, a growing number of scientists appreciated the connection between electricity and human physiology. The experiments of Galvani had convincingly demonstrated the relationship of muscle action and electricity, and the use of sophisticated machines that looked modern and contained dials and means of measurement added to the scientific credibility of the electrical devices. What could be more real or scientific than a numerical reading on a dial? Even though the physics of electricity and magnetism was not well understood, anyone could see their almost magical and mysterious properties. Magnetism could penetrate the thickest iron (at least that's how it was perceived) and electricity in a lightening bolt was surely awesome and powerful.

A scientist named W. R. Wells wrote in 1869 that all disease was caused by a loss of balance of the two forces of electricity—he was referring to the positive and negative charges. The brain, he wrote, was "the great electrical reservoir of the physical system" that "furnishes electricity to it." The brain carried electro-nervous fluid to all parts of the body and was the source of health and disease. Wells believed that venous blood was negatively charged and arterial blood positively charged, and that the application of electricity restored imbalance to diseased organs.[11] Another scientist writing in 1873 claimed that all illness was the result of a deficiency of electricity that could be remedied by the application of external electricity. One wonders if he happened to sell electrical devices. As we'll see in the next chapter, at that time that would not have been surprising.

Textbooks of Medicine and the Use of Electricity

Ever since John Wesley first suggested using electricity for angina, numerous heart-related conditions such as congestive heart failure, carditis (inflammation of the heart), and other conditions were touted as being responsive to electric current. The credibility of using electrotherapy for cardiac conditions was enhanced by textbooks of medicine recommending such therapy. Poore's 1876 *Textbook of Electricity in Medicine and Surgery* gave specific techniques for treating cardiac diseases. Enough anatomy was then known to appreciate how important nerves entered the heart from the vagus nerve and cervical nerves in the neck. Poole recommended the direct electrical stimulation of these neck nerves. He cited several case reports in which patients received relief from such treatment.

Others preferred stimulation directly over the left nipple. George M. Beard and Alphonse Rockwell in their 1891 textbook *On the Medical and Surgical Uses of Electricity* described a patient with angina who responded to electricity: "In the midst of the pain the positive pole was suddenly applied over the nipple, and a very intense current sent through the body. . . . The pain left him and . . . he found it impossible, by any effort he could make, to bring on another attack."[12] Beard and Rockwell had published their first textbook on the subject of medical electricity in 1871, *A Practical Treatise on the Medical and Surgical Uses of Electricity*. Extensive directions, including what garments the patient should remove, are given for general *faradization* (stimulation by electricity from an induction coil). In this procedure the patient's feet rested on a metal plate and the therapist rested his hand or a sponge on the head or ailing part of the body.[13] That same year the two authors asked to read a paper before the New York Medical Society, but were turned down on the grounds that electrotherapy was quackery. Six years later, however, the Society had apparently found enough credible evidence to accept them as members.[14]

By today's standards, it seems silly to argue which route of electricity—chest, neck, or total body stimulation—is best for treating heart conditions. All are dubious, at least for the conditions in which they were advocated, yet such debates were common in the nineteenth century. Perhaps when true physiology is not known, peripheral and irrelevant issues take center stage. Many scientists and physicians claimed that total body electrification was most beneficial for cardiovascular disease. The names given to these types of therapy sounded more scientific than they were. "Electrohydriatics" or "electrobalneotherapy" referred to immersion in a tub of electrified water. A "static bath with cephalic douche" was really sitting in a dry tub with sparks applied to the head. "Autoconduction," also known as "inductothermic," involved standing inside a large circular solenoid cage. The cage used high-frequency electricity of several hundred thousand oscillations per second. According to its inventor, "These currents can be very powerful. They produce no pain or conscious phenomenon in the person treated. The current, nevertheless, acts very energetically on the tissues." This treatment was similar in principle to microwaving the entire body. High-frequency treatments were especially popular in France from about 1890 to 1930 and were used to treat diabetes, gout, obesity, and many other conditions.[15]

Did any of these newfangled methods work? It is doubtful, although perhaps the patient may have felt some relief because of a placebo effect or the increased circulation that allowed improved kidney function to excrete excess fluid. One medical author recognized this possibility: "The treatment consists of a course of baths with sinusoidal or faradic currents. The action of these electric baths, if properly given, is to improve the general circulation, especially the peripheral, diminish visceral congestion, and increase diuresis."[16]

It's easy to assume that such therapies were relegated to the historical dustbin. However, in 1989 *Vanity Fair* reported that then-British Prime Minister Margaret Thatcher took electrically charged baths as part of a health and beauty regimen. As one might imagine, the London tabloids had a field day.

FIGURE 29. *Treatment for constipation using a large static electricity generator. One electrode was placed on the abdomen and the other in the rectum. (Courtesy A.L. Chatterton and Co.)*

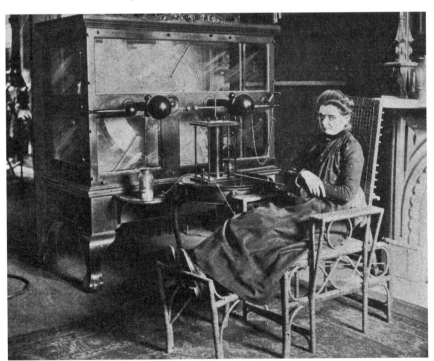

One headline proclaimed "The Switched-On Prime Minister's Amazing Secret" and another tantalized, "Shock Revelation on the Source of Mrs. T's Vigor."[17]

Electrotherapy as legitimate medical practice was widespread enough in the United States and Europe that it spawned numerous specialty journals. In 1894 one physician wrote, "About 10,000 physicians within the borders of the United States use electricity as a therapeutic agent daily. Many others find occasional use for it."[18] Physicians who used electrotherapy in their offices had devices ranging in size from portable battery-operated generators to massive machines involving large capital investments. The bigger the device and the more elaborate the polished brass, the more powerful it must be. The only means to recoup such investments would be to use, and charge (no pun intended) for its use, frequently. Along with the machines came a proliferation of training institutes offering special courses and fancy diplomas in electrotherapy.[19]

Enough anecdotal reports of benefit—and more than enough material interests—kept the electrotherapy industry alive and well. Reputable scientists occasionally demonstrated a "benefit" that stimulated belief in the healing properties of electricity. For example, Nicolai Tesla showed that tuberculosis bacteria could be killed by passing a high-frequency electric current through a test tube. Shortly thereafter, sensational banner headlines proclaimed the curative property of electricity for tuberculosis.[20] It is not unlike today when we read about breakthrough "cures" for AIDS or cancer. Unfortunately, a wide gulf exists between an isolated observation and practical widespread therapy.

The line between the quack and the scientist is a thin one indeed.
—Anonymous

ELECTROQUACKERY

« »

Electrotherapy and electroquackery were variations on the same theme. And although electroquackery never cured a disease, it served a different role—it kept alive the belief, and hope, that electricity had powerful curative properties. It is sometimes difficult to draw the distinction between quackery and mistaken medical science. A mistaken scientist or doctor sincerely believes the device offers some benefit, but simply doesn't have enough information to know he or she is in error. A quack, however, is someone who knows a device or nostrum will not work and only hopes for payment before the device kills the customer. In the nineteenth century both laypeople and scientists rarely applied the rigorous scientific method of proof as it is used today. "Proof" consisted more of anecdote and testimonial rather than reproducible observations or controlled and randomized clinical trials.

Between the quack and the mistaken scientist lay the business opportunist. He wanted to sell a product and make a profit and was interested more in marketing than scientific validity. But let us at least give him ethical credit: the seller of medical electrical devices in the nineteenth and early twentieth century did not want to *harm* anyone. He simply took advantage of the then-popular craze in medical electricity and tried to outmarket his competitor. Advertisements for home electrical devices, backed by copious endorsements and testimonials, filled popular magazines and newspapers. It wasn't until the Food and Drug Administration received authorization from Congress in 1940 to prosecute fraudulent medical devices that the advertisements and claims diminished. Prior to then the only avenue of restraint was prosecution for mail fraud, a laborious but sometimes effective deterrent.

Electricity was often the stuff that quackery was made of.[1] It is a mysterious, powerful, and unseen force; its strength covers the spectrum of the natural world extending from inanimate metals to living tissue. Ever since electricity was deemed beneficial for human ailments, it has been difficult to know who was in the majority: the scientist, the mistaken scientist, or the quack. For every legitimate study and proposal an equally illegitimate, specious, and economic self-serving claim would arise. Science progressed slowly in the face of fraud, and fraud was omnipresent in the field of electric therapy.[2]

Abrams' Ohm Cocktail

Perhaps the most successful charlatan to use electricity for medical treatment—at least from the viewpoint of amassing wealth—was Dr. Albert Abrams. When he died the American Medical Association's obituary gave him the dubious honor of being "the dean of all twentieth century charlatans." He was born in San Francisco in 1863, and at age nineteen received a medical degree from the University of Heidelberg, Germany. He was a successful psychiatrist practicing in San Francisco and became professor of pathology at Cooper Medical College. He was vice president of the California State Medical Society in 1889 and president of the San Francisco Society in 1893. He wrote profusely on medical topics and in 1910 published a thousand-page mainstream book, titled *Diagnostic Therapeutics.*[3]

Six years later he was in somewhat less traditional territory. None of Abrams's writings reveal why he departed from standard medical practice. Whatever the reason, his new career led him down the murky path of pseudoscience and exploitation. Abrams's quack theory, announced in a 1916 book, *New Concepts on Diagnosis and Treatment,* rested on the belief that all disease was a result of disharmony in the body's electrical oscillations. He believed each disease had its own characteristic pattern of oscillations. Electrons, not cells, formed the basis of life and disease. Abrams claimed the ability to both diagnose and treat. Diagnosis was simply the measurement of the vibrations associated with each disease and therapy became a matter of restoring the vibrations to their natural equilibrium.

His diagnosis machine was called the Pathoclast and the therapy machine the Oscilloclast. Abrams used a drop of blood to make the diagnosis—but the patient's signature would do if blood were lacking. The patient's blood would first be passed over a horseshoe magnet to cleanse it of unwanted electronic artifacts. Apparently the electrons in the blood cells were representative of the body writ large: "A single drop of blood with its billions of electrons is a condensation of the multitudinous vibrations of the human body." According to Abrams, "It is necessary to place a healthy control subject in the electrical circuit and test his skin reactions, which conform to the vibratory rate of the disease." This healthy subject stood on grounded metal plates with a wire connected from the machine to the forehead.[4]

Once Abrams had diagnosed the disease and determined the vibratory rate, he advised the patient to receive treatment from (surprise!) an Oscilloclast. The cure was carried out by dialing in the same vibratory rate. The machine would thus duplicate and neutralize the disease's specific vibrations. Invariably the patient would require multiple sessions with the Oscilloclast— diagnosis was quick and simple, but the cure apparently took a little longer.

Abrams's popularity peaked just after World War I. By then he had established societies, journals, and even a dozen schools—all designed to promote his "scientific" theories. Abrams even tried to use his theories to capitalize on Prohibition. He claimed that he could duplicate the vibrational frequency of alcohol and thus produce an electric "jag." A San Francisco newspaper wrote in 1920, "Hail the Ohm cocktail! The highball hilarious—Turn on the switches, and fill me with jolts!"[5]

It is impossible to determine exactly why something was so successful. Was it the dials, meters, levers, and readouts that gave the device its credibility? Was it the promise of a painless cure for all diseases? In a time studded with discoveries of invisible and insensible phenomena,[6] one more did not seem to stretch credulity. Whatever the reasons, the device became a raging success. By 1923 more than 3500 practitioners were using the Pathoclast and the Oscilloclast in their offices. Most were osteopaths who, according to one estimate, took in $1500 to $2000 a week using the machine. All the machines manufactured by Abrams were leased; the Oscilloclast rented for $200 plus a monthly payment of $5. Each machine was sealed and the practitioner leasing it had to sign a contract not to open the machine. No wonder—the machine was a total hoax; much of its wiring connected to nothing. In fact, it contained not a single complete electrical circuit.[7]

The *Journal of the American Medical Association* published articles demonstrating the quackery of Abrams's machines. One blood sample submitted by the AMA came from a sheep. The diagnosis came back that the "patient" was suffering from hereditary syphilis. (This is particularly hard to believe since the sheep had virgin wool.) Nevertheless, the practitioner stated that a cure could be guaranteed for $2500. In a series of 12 monthly articles *Scientific American* investigated the Electronic Reactions of Abrams and concluded, "At best it is an illusion; at worse it is a colossal fraud." Newspapers loved to report the fraud for what it was. The *Dearborn Independent* noted on May 19, 1923, "Various reports have appeared from time to time in the Journal of the American Medical Association of the results furnished to doctors when they sent samples of blood to Abrams' disciples for diagnosis. One guinea-pig was found to have congenital syphilis, and a sheep was found to be suffering from gonorrhea; but these animals were lucky compared to the rooster who was found to be suffering from congenital syphilis, gonorrhea, carcinoma, sarcoma, epithelioma, chronic malaria, and diabetes."[8] Scientific condemnations began to mount. Nobel laureate Robert A. Millikan characterized the machine as something a ten-year-old boy who knew a little about electricity would construct to fool an eight year old who knew nothing.[9]

Professional opinion alone could not stem the public's interest. It wasn't until Abrams's unexpected death from pneumonia on January 3, 1924, at the age of sixty-one that the ardor for his theories began to cool. Pneumonia was one of the diseases the Oscilloclast was supposed to treat. Abrams died two days before he was scheduled to give testimony at a fraud trial in Arkansas involving one of his practitioners who was caught making a diagnosis from chicken blood. The *San Francisco Examiner* ran a front-page obituary and wrote, "Worry over attacks launched on his theories in all parts of the civilized world by the medical profession led to a breakdown in his health."[10] At his death Abrams had amassed a fortune valued at two to five million dollars. The final irony is that Abrams earmarked his estate for a school of electronic medicine. His relatives contested the will and the school was never started.[11]

Violet Ray Machines and the Spark of Healing

Extremely popular as both home and medical office treatments were violet ray machines, which were sold by the millions and came in various models. Invented around 1900, they were most popular from 1910 to 1930 and were

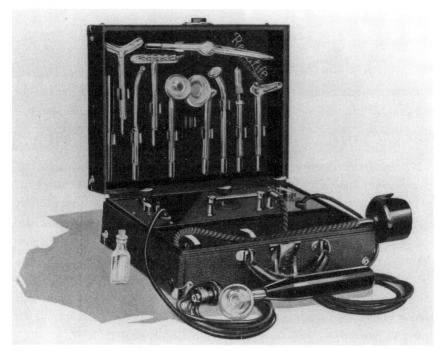

FIGURE 30. *Renulife Violet Ray machine with attachments. Electricity was supplied by a wall or light socket. Multiple models were available from a variety of manufacturers. This model cost $75 in 1920. The purple light emitted by the glass tube and the high-pitched buzzing sound added to the device's "healing properties."*

still used in reputable medical clinics as late as 1937.[12] The simplest model consisted of a single glass vacuum tube that glowed blue or purple after being electrified with a high-frequency current and emitted sparks when touched to the skin. The more elaborate models contained multiple attachments and each tube was designed to be inserted into a different body orifice or rubbed on a specific body part.

Violet ray machines were not totally innocuous. When using the glass comb-like attachment "guaranteed" to eliminate greying or reduce balding, the user was cautioned to avoid hair tonic containing alcohol—sparks from the glass comb could light the hair on fire. Yet violet rays were the perfect medical machine. They glowed, they emitted sparks, they were painful but not unbearable, and the sound caused by the high-frequency current served to enhance their therapeutic power. Furthermore, the device came with a pseudoscientific explanation and was endorsed by scientists and physicians.

The FDA Takes Action

The 1920s and 1930s were the heyday of electric quackery in America. Medicine had not quite solidified its position as a science-based discipline and the era of antibiotics and technological procedures was still distant. Another reason for the proliferation of these devices was lack of governmental regulation. The Food and Drug Administration's ability to regulate medical devices was not authorized by Congress until it passed legislation that became effective on New Year's Day 1940. The landmark 1906 Pure Food and Drug Laws did not cover medical devices.[13] Although the Post Office was occasionally successful in prosecuting quacks for mail fraud, there were too many con artists and too few government resources—changing a post office box or leaving town was far too easy.

The first device to be seized by the FDA under its new authority was the Electreat invented, marketed, and sold beginning in 1918 by Willie Kent. The device resembled a flashlight with a rolling pin attached to the end; numerous attachments could be inserted into the handle to increase its potential uses. It was operated by two standard D-size batteries and had a sliding controller that functioned both as a switch and a means of increasing energy. The flashlight-like handle contained a few turns of insulated wire wound around an iron core. A person felt a strong jolt of electricity in the hand holding the device and a strong tingle as the rolling pin or attachments were applied to parts of the body. An audible buzzing contributed to the device's potency.

An accompanying booklet told of the many ailments the device could treat: chest pain, dandruff, goiter, small bust, sweaty feet, weak eyes, and piles (hemorrhoids)—to name a few. The theory put forth to explain its healing properties alleged that electric current added "protectones" and took away "irritones." It also stimulated and relaxed muscles and served as a surrogate for physical exercise. The pamphlet cited testimonials from satisfied customers who described cures of appendicitis, paralysis, and other diseases.

The brochure cover highlighted a statement of irrefutable logic. "Two things cannot occupy the same space at the same time. Shooting Electricity in forces the pain out." Kent called his device a mechanical heart and explained: "Applying Electreat . . . causes rhythmic contractions of the arteries and veins and is like priming a pump. That is why we call it the Mechanical Heart." Kent sold the device at the wholesale price of $7—enough to earn him over $100,000 per year, a sizable sum in those days. They retailed in drugstores throughout the nation for $15.

The FDA didn't believe a word about the Electreat and its extravagant claims caused it to be seized as misbranded. Kent contested the seizure and the case came to trial in Kansas City on January 27, 1941. This was the first court case under the new legislation, and the FDA spared no effort. An expert witness for the FDA, professor Anton Carlson of the University of Chicago, testified that the device was a "blooming fake." Carlson said that the case involved "a difference in mental attitude between the scientific mind prepared to seek . . . scientific truths contrasted with those unthinking 'peculiar people" who blindly adhere possibly in faith to weird unproven scientific tenets of their so-called schools." Kent's defense was unscientific and weak. The judge agreed with the FDA, and the devices were ordered destroyed. Undaunted, Kent began manufacturing the Electreat again shortly after the war ended. This time he removed any therapeutic promises, though the testimonials remained. The FDA again seized the device and again the case went to trial. By this time Kent was seventy-six and too old to testify. Instead, testimony was given by a dozen witnesses who swore by the Electreat's benefit for their aches, pains, headaches, and stomach pains. No one doubts the placebo effect of a buzzing, electric-shocking device. The FDA came down hard on Kent because of the unknown number of people who believed the Electreat worked for appendicitis and other life-threatening conditions. Again, the judge agreed with the FDA and Kent was found guilty. He was fined $1000, the maximum under the law, and was not sent to jail because of his age.[14]

Ruth Drown and Mrs. Rice

One of the most dramatic legal battles against electroquackery involved Ruth Drown and her Radio Therapeutic Instrument—the latest in a series of gadgets she had concocted and claimed could cure all kinds of diseases. Drown's rise as a practitioner of electroquackery began in 1929 when she studied at the Los Angeles Chiropractic College and shortly after organized Drown Laboratories, Inc., in Hollywood—a combination school, manufacturing plant, "research" company, and treatment facility.[15]

World War II had put a temporary halt to the FDA's enforcement actions.

By 1948, however, the agency was back in the quack-busting business. Television and radar had captured the public's interest, and the quacks had moved in. Anything with the words "radio" or "radar" sounded scientific, important, *powerful*. People with serious illnesses grasped at the "hope" offered by quacks armed with these devices. Ruth Drown was one such quack; the Radio Therapeutic Instrument was her gadget; and Marguerite Rice of Blue Island, Illinois, was desperate.

In April, Rice was told by her doctor that a small lump in her right breast might be cancerous. Her doctor urged her to go to the hospital at once and get a biopsy, but Rice did not. First she called her husband, who was in California on business. A few days later he called her back to say, "Don't worry about hospitals and doctors; I've found a miracle."

The "miracle" was Ruth Drown and her Radio Therapeutic Instrument, which Mr. Rice had heard about from a friend. According to Drown, this gadget used radio waves to both diagnose and cure various illnesses. Her brochures claimed that the Radio Therapeutic Instrument would eliminate lumps from the breast and prevent cancer from forming in them. It would also cure heart trouble, loss of speech and memory, a tipped uterus, and low testicular function. The list of curable ailments was actually not noticeably different from those claimed by every other medical quack over the years.

Nor did the theories Ruth Drown offered for her device's remarkable performance sound all that different from those of other electrical quacks. The Radio Therapeutic Instrument, Drown had written, "tune[d] into the human body on the same principle as the commercial radio tunes into sound." Everything in the universe had its own unique and "individual rate of vibration."[16] What made her instrument unique was its ability to tap into the "animating Life Force," as she termed it, a quasi-religious concept that was all powerful but conveniently all unprovable. Drown combined the techno-speak of her generation with the evangelical language of a faith healer. Her writings are filled with such phrases as: Great Key to Life, Mighty Force, One Life, One Substance, One Energy, the Trinity is Wisdom (nucleus), Love (magnetism), Power (electron).[17]

Drown was in Chicago at about the time Mr. Rice returned home and the Rices went to visit her at her hotel. Drown took a blood sample from Mrs. Rice, put it in a black box (the Radio Therapeutic Instrument, of course), and twiddled some knobs. Out came the diagnosis, and Mrs. Drown gave her the news. No, the lump wasn't cancer—it was a fungal growth. However, Mrs. Rice was afflicted with several other maladies that she had not known about and a course of treatment with her wondrous Radio Therapeutic Instrument would take care of everything. A doctor in Chicago just happened to have one of Mrs. Drown's Radio Therapeutic Instruments, and Mrs. Rice could visit his office for treatment. Mr. Rice, concerned about the high bills from the Chicago therapist, contacted Drown. She suggested he purchase a Radio Therapeutic Instrument and sold him a home treatment model for $423, along with instructions on how to set the dials. Mrs. Rice meticulously followed directions, setting the nine dials and placing her feet on a metal electrode plate with another electrode on her stomach. The beauty of the treatment was that it worked twenty-four hours a day. When not attached to the machine directly, all Mrs. Rice had to do was place a blotter with a drop of her blood between the two electrodes.

Weeks went by, then months. Mrs. Rice felt worse. Finally, in response to Rice's anguished letter, Drown suggested she have her breast removed "if she feels she is not getting hold of the trouble with our treatment." We can treat the underlying condition later, Drown added. At about the same time she received Drown's reply, Mrs. Rice noticed an article in the *Chicago Tribune* condemning the Radio Therapeutic Instrument as quackery.

Upset and frightened, Mrs. Rice finally sought medical attention in New York City. She also got in touch with the FDA, who moved into action. The AMA was also involved, and worked to oust doctors in Illinois using Drown's electric gadgets. The FDA filed a libel action against Drown; she didn't contest it and lost. The agency continued to push, hoping to file outright criminal charges against her.

Ruth Drown agreed to a "trial by ordeal" for her Radio Therapeutic Instrument, demonstrating its power before a group of medical experts from the University of Chicago. In one test she attempted to show how her device could take X-rays of a patient's fractured femur. The patient was across town. Only a drop of the patient's blood on a blotter was used to take the X-rays. Everyone saw only simple fog patterns on the films, but Drown mumbled something about her equipment not being properly aligned. In another test, blood samples from ten patients were given to Drown for her diagnoses. She spent all afternoon on three samples and failed miserably. In fact, she wasn't even close. One sample was diagnosed as cancer of the prostate with metastatic spread to bones and organs. The specimen came from a healthy male physician (at least he thought he was healthy). The third test challenged Drown's claim that her device could stop hemorrhage. Two anesthetized dogs had their femoral arteries cut. One dog served as the control and had its cut artery tied off. The test dog was "treated" by the hemorrhage-control device located in an adjoining room. According to the final report, "Mrs. Drown stood in the doorway watching her animal bleed. From time to time we asked whether she thought her experiment was working." Drown must have taken pity on the poor dog for she finally asked for the artery to be tied. Under strict scientific controls, Drown's Radio Therapeutic Instrument failed every test. On the surface it is amazing that the University of Chicago had agreed to test Drown's instruments—how could such a prestigious institution lend its name to such a ridiculous study? The answer is simple: an avid and wealthy supporter of Drown was on the University's cancer board.[18]

Twenty months after the University of Chicago report, the FDA brought Drown into court in Los Angeles, charging her with criminal violation of the 1938 Food, Drug, and Cosmetic Act. The trial was spectacular, with ardent witnesses for both sides. Defense witnesses included the mother of actor Tyrone Power and the chairwoman of the Los Angeles School Board. Mrs. Patia Power testified that she had given remote treatment to her Marine son during World War II and he never once had to go to sick bay. The chair of the school board stated that she had been successfully treated from Los Angeles for a pneumonia she developed in Atlantic City. In response to the prosecuting attorney's question, she also claimed that she would be healed even if she had an automobile accident in Moscow and were hemorrhaging to death. She was certain that not even the Iron Curtain could stop the vibratory waves. Another defense witness gave enthusiastic support of Drown's admonition to preserve body magnetism. From this it logically followed that one should not take showers—he explained that water is a conductor that would connect him to the vibrations in the sewer and if he took a shower his body magnetism and energy would flow down the drain. The minutes of the trial contain no mention of the judge's expression during this testimony.

The government's witnesses included numerous eminent doctors and medical experts—and the husband of Marguerite Rice. By now Mrs. Rice, whose breast cancer had metastasized and become incurable, was too weak to travel. Drown took the stand in her own defense, but did her cause more harm than good. "To call this a radio," assistant district attorney Tobias Klinger said in his summary to the jury, "well, you might as well call it a cat." It took the jury only seven hours to find Ruth Drown guilty on September 24, 1951, of violating the Food, Drug and Cosmetic Act.

It cost the government $50,000 to take Drown to trial. The guilty verdict cost Ruth Drown $1000 in fines and the loss of her ability to sell her device interstate. It cost Marguerite Rice her life; she died of cancer on November 17, 1952.[19]

Drown continued to use her Radio Therapeutic Instrument on patients in her own office. In 1963 the state of California filed grand theft charges against her and a trial was scheduled for 1965. But Ruth Drown died three weeks before the case went to trial. It wasn't the last quackery case involving electricity that the FDA would prosecute. But it was certainly one of the most dramatic—and tragic.

Electroquackery and Legitimate Therapy

Electroquackery, with all its flashy devices and self-serving promoters, did not directly lead to an effective cure for heart disease or sudden death. But it did have an impact. Electroquackery made electrotherapy part of mainstream medicine. The public could recognize the outrageous quack—at least most of the public most of the time. What the public could not evaluate were claims made by seemingly credible individuals or institutions. If an electric therapy device were sold in the Sears and Roebuck Catalog, how quackish could it be? Electroquackery is easy for us to define in retrospect. That electricity was powerful was never in doubt; how to unlock its magic was the challenge.

Death may usurp on Nature many hours,
And yet the fire of life kindle again
The o'erpress'd spirits.
—William Shakespeare, *Pericles*

DEFIBRILLATION IS THE SPARK OF LIFE

« »

Electricity was used in many medical situations, both fraudulent and inexplicable. But not until researchers uncovered the connection between it and ventricular fibrillation would electricity make headway as a mainstream treatment. Ventricular fibrillation—chaotic contractions of the heart resulting in no pulse or blood pressure—can only be treated with electricity.

Before worrying about how to control and correct the heart's rhythm, physicians needed to study and then recognize fibrillation as a key event in cardiac arrest. Over the centuries, based solely on their finely tuned tactile and auditory senses to feel the pulse with their fingertips or hear the rhythm with their stethoscope, physicians described hundreds of different pulses and cardiac rhythms and coined many colorful names and descriptions. However, there are several logical reasons why fibrillation was not recognized until relatively recently. For example, ventricular fibrillation has no associated pulse and the heart makes no sound. The rhythm lasts for only minutes following death, so a doctor would have to begin observing the heart immediately to detect the rhythm. Also, ventricular fibrillation is usually not seen in traumatic deaths. Galen and other early observers of the death of gladiators and people in other traumatic situations probably did not encounter fibrillation. Moreover, ventricular fibrillation is not a common rhythm in animals. Though a common cause of death in humans, it is primarily seen in animals only when the animal's heart is electrically stimulated. Thus, it was-n't until electric experiments on animals became commonplace and there was a means to record the pattern of the rhythm that researchers began describing ventricular fibrillation.

In 1850 the German researchers Carl Friedrich Wilhelm Ludwig and Moritz Hoffa were the first to depict ventricular fibrillation, having demonstrated that strong electric currents applied directly to the ventricles of a dog's heart caused fibrillation. Researchers used a variety of terms for these early descriptions of fibrillation in animal hearts—"tremulations fibrillaires," "delirium cordis," "intervermiform [worm-like] movements," "fibrillar contractions," "herz-delirium," "undulatory movements," and "intervermicular actions."[1] It is not completely clear why ventricular fibrillation predominated, but the term is very apt since the irregularity only occurs in the two ventricles (the atria are not involved) and seems to weave in and out of groups of muscle fibers (fibrillation refers to the clusters of fibers).

Ludwig was also known for his development of the kymograph, a device consisting of a rotating smoked drum and stylus used to record physiological data graphically from the body, such as blood pressure or heart rhythm. Ludwig's invention was the direct precursor of the electrocardiogram. Though he did not specifically use his kymograph for ventricular fibrillation, such a procedure would one day become crucial in the treatment of this fatal rhythm.[2]

For many years ventricular fibrillation was mostly considered a curiosity with little relevance to humans. For example, the 300-page *Textbook of Electricity in Medicine and Surgery,* published in 1876, devotes one paragraph, almost a *non sequitur,* to electricity and its ability to induce fibrillation in the heart of a dog. There is no mention of how or why this is relevant to humans. Another textbook notes that the heart is sensitive to electricity but cannot recover once spasmodic contractions begin. In the late nineteenth century, paralysis was the main indication for electric therapy, not heart attacks.[3]

John McWilliam

John McWilliam (1857–1937), in a series of articles from 1887 to 1889 published in the *British Medical Journal,* made the first detailed descriptions of ventricular fibrillation. His writings were also the first to postulate its importance in humans.[4] There had been one or two earlier clinical accounts in which patients with very fast heart rates had been successfully treated with electricity—one case involved a twenty-one-year-old woman with diphtheria-associated heart inflammation. Her heart began to race uncontrollably and was returned to a normal heart rate with repeated electric shocks to her chest. This woman, however, did not have ventricular fibrillation since she would have died instantly. She probably suffered from intermittent atrial tachycardia (fast heart rate, often up to 180 beats per minute, which can lead to symptoms of dizziness but is rarely fatal), a condition that is responsive to electricity. Even today, the administration of small electric shocks is one form of therapy. Nevertheless, it is probably one of the first instances in which a fast heart rate was successfully treated with electricity.

In McWilliam's day it was assumed that sudden cardiac failure took the form of a sudden standstill—in other words, no electrical activity. The heart just stops. Doctors postulated a variety of causes for such a standstill. According to McWilliam, these causes included "over-distension or strain of the organ due to sudden exertion or excitement, pressure on the heart or rupture of its walls, inhibitory influences transmitted by the vagus nerve . . . or exhausting influences of a more obscure character."[5]

McWilliam performed experiments on dogs that laid to rest this idea of cardiac standstill. He wrote that the heart "assumes, on the contrary, the form of violent, though irregular and uncoordinated, manifestation of ventricular energy. Instead of quiescence, there is tumultuous activity, irregular in its character and wholly ineffective as regards its results." In fact, McWilliam's descriptions of ventricular fibrillation, written over a hundred years ago, are classic:

> The normal beat is at once abolished, and the ventricles are thrown into a tumultuous state of quick, irregular, twitching action; at the same time there is a great fall of blood pressure. Ventricles become distended with blood, as the rapid quivering movement of their walls is wholly insufficient to expel their contents. The muscular action partakes of the nature of an arrhythmic, uncoordinated, and rapidly-repeated contraction of the various muscular bundles . . . instead of a coordinated contraction leading to a definite narrowing of the ventricular cavity, there occurs an irregular and complicated arrhythmic oscillation of the ventricular walls. . . . This condition is very persistent, and it is easy to kill a dog by applying a faradic current to the ventricles.

It seems to me in the highest degree probable that a similar phenomenon occurs in the human heart, and that is the mode of cardiac failure and the direct and immediate cause of death in many cases of sudden dissolution. It is strange indeed if the phenomenon of fibrillar contraction is never manifested in the human heart. . . . For this phenomenon has been observed in all warm-blooded animals examined; it is, as far as I am aware, a universal feature in the behaviour of the mammalian heart; and at the same time it is much more readily induced and much more persistent in the higher mammals than in the lower forms.[6]

In addition to studying dogs, McWilliam performed experiments on cats, rabbits, rats, mice, hedgehogs, eels and chickens, both in young and adult animals. His work on animals provided him with ample observation of many real events, which led to several notable facts. He used those facts to reach two important general conclusions: (1) All mammal hearts can fibrillate; (2) the hearts of larger mammals can sustain ventricular fibrillation. Then he combined those two conclusions with a third known observation—(3) humans are large mammals—to deduce still another, new conclusion: (4) therefore, humans experience ventricular fibrillation, and the rhythm does not spontaneously revert to normal rhythm. McWilliam described sudden cardiac arrest even though his terminology was different than that used today: "a sudden, unexpected, and irretrievable cardiac failure may, even in the absence of any prominent exciting cause, present itself in the form of an abrupt onset of fibrillar contraction (ventricular delirium). The cardiac pump is thrown out of gear, and the last of its vital energy is dissipated in a violent and prolonged turmoil of fruitless activity in the ventricular walls."

McWilliam never tried electricity to stop the fibrillations of a heart muscle. It is not certain that he even thought of this possibility. One would not intuitively assume that the electrical stimulation that caused the fibrillation could also be used to put an end to it. Though McWilliam did not suggest electricity as a means to end fibrillation, he was certainly interested in finding such a therapy. He describes a very early example of pacing a dog's heart after the heart was at a standstill by stimulation of the vagus nerve. The stimulated heart could maintain a blood pressure, though not as high as the dog's normal blood pressure. "In certain forms of cardiac arrest, there appears to be a possibility of restoring by artificial means the rhythmic beat, and tiding over a sudden and temporary danger," he wrote. "Such is especially the case in those instances where cardiac failure assumes the form of an inhibition of the heart beat by impulses reaching the organ along the vagus nerves." McWilliam proposed doing this in humans by placement of electrodes on the chest and back.[7]

Unfortunately, much of McWilliam's work was ignored, both during and after his lifetime. The world of human cardiology was simply too primitive during the years of his most productive work. There was no appreciation of ventricular fibrillation because there was no context in which that observation could be useful.

In 1887 McWilliam speculated that anesthetic-related deaths may be associated with ventricular fibrillation, yet no one picked up on this comment until 1911 when Alfred Goodman Levy and Thomas Lewis convincingly showed the relationship between chloroform and fibrillation.[8]

It would not be anesthesia, however, that would provide the necessary clues but electrocutions. In the last two decades of the nineteenth century as Western nations went electric, accidental deaths from electrocution entered the consciousness of both scientists and the public. In the 1880s investigators believed that death from electrocution was caused by respiratory paralysis resulting from an overwhelming trauma to the central nervous system: "the condition after the shock is merely one of suspended animation in which respiratory function is suspended."[9]

Prevost and Battelli

Electrocution was finally proven a cause of ventricular fibrillation at the turn of the century. Jean Louis Prevost and Frederic Battelli, both physiologists, reported in the March 1899 issue of the *Journal de Physiologie et de Pathologie Generale* that a weak current passed through the heart, or through the intact chest, could fibrillate the heart. In a footnote they make what turned out to be a crucial discovery for the eventual development of defibrillation: a stronger shock was capable of terminating fibrillation. They wrote that 40 volts was sufficient to induce fibrillation, and that prompt application of a current of 240 to 4800 volts could terminate it—a rather staggering amount of current! Prevost and Battelli thus became the first scientists to show that electricity is an effective treatment for ventricular fibrillation; they were the first to defibrillate.

R. H. Cunningham

The same year that Prevost and Battelli made their discovery, R. H. Cunningham, writing in the October issue of *The New York Medical Journal*, graphically described the effect of electricity: "If the thorax of an animal is opened immediately after a strong continuous electric current . . . and the heart is exposed . . . the various minute bundles of muscle fibres are alternatively contracting and relaxing with considerable vigor in various parts of the ventricles." He also alluded to defibrillating a dog's heart using electric current, noting that "the application of such a current to the fibrillating dog's heart . . . materially hastens the restoration of the coordinated heart beat."[10] Though his article was published six months after the French article, Cunningham made his observations completely independently of Prevost and Battelli. Sensitive to the issue of plagiarism as well as the matter of who was the first to do the work, Cunningham wrote in a footnote that he became aware of the French physiologists' work only after his research was completed in February 1899. The publication of Cunningham's article was delayed because it was under consideration for a prize by the Alumni Association of the College of Physicians and Surgeons of New York.

Louise Robinovitch

Dr. Louise Robinovitch provided another paving brick on the road to defibrillation. During the years 1906 to 1909 she conducted a series of experiments published in *The Journal of Mental Pathology* in which she described cases of respiratory and cardiac collapse that required more than just artificial respiration. She cited the Sylvester method of artificial respiration. In instances of chloroform-related deaths and severe morphine poisoning with profound respiratory paralysis, she wrote that "the ordinary means of resuscitation are useless." She mentioned that extraordinary means of resuscitation such as open-chest cardiac massage were also useless, primarily because of the loss of time that occurred in setting up for the surgery. She proposed instead "various electric currents that produce respiratory movements of required amplitude accompanied by cardiac beats." The cardiac beats strengthen as the ventilation improves and, over several minutes, the electrical stimulation can be withdrawn. The benefit of this method is that it can be applied quickly. She essentially proposed a device to cause respirations by stimulating the phrenic (diaphragmatic) nerve, which simultaneously paced the heart. Her therapy would be effective for those cases in which the heart is not in actual ventricular fibrillation but still has a faint heartbeat, even if too feeble to feel. The device consisted of two metal plates applied to the mid-back; the operator regulated the rate and intensity of electricity.

Although most of her experiments were conducted on dogs, Robinovitch did provide one interesting case report of a young woman who arrived at the hospital suffering from a morphine overdose with respiratory depression—a respiratory rate of four per minute. The usual Sylvester technique did not improve the patient's deeply blue cyanotic color, and Robinovitch was called to the case and agreed to try the new device. After twenty minutes, it was retrieved and applied to the patient. Within thirty seconds of stimulation the patient's color improved. The woman opened her eyes and said, "Oh, I feel so cold in my back." The cold she felt was the wetness of the metal electrodes. The woman lived, probably because the device stimulated her breathing.

Severe respiratory depression and asphyxia from any cause lead to an initial speeding up of the heart and then, if the respiratory problem continues, a slowing and weakening until the heart stops completely. Respiratory depression generally does not cause ventricular fibrillation. Nevertheless, Louise Robinovitch came close to inventing an external defibrillator. Had she focused on fibrillation instead of respiratory depression, her technique might have been successful in supplying enough energy across the chest wall. Robinovitch was aware of the work of Prevost, Battelli, and Cunningham, and knew about electrocution-associated ventricular fibrillation. She believed, however, that Battelli's recommended energies were too damaging to the body. In other words, the cure would kill the patient. Other investigators had utilized a pathway of head to abdomen to attempt defibrillation. When Robinovitch tried to duplicate such experiments, she succeeded only in losing a whole series of dogs. According to her, such a pathway merely fried the brain.[11]

Robinovitch believed her device would be useful in cases of electrocution, especially since her electric pathway avoided the brain completely. She adapted her device for use in ambulances, presumably to attach to patients with respiratory difficulty. She wrote: "The method of resuscitation consists in causing artificial blood-pressure and respirations by means of rhythmic electric excitations until normal function is restored." While it may have been

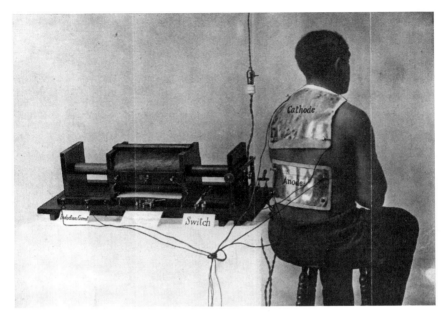

FIGURE 31. *"Portable" device developed by Louise Robinovitch to stimulate breathing in a nonbreathing person. Electricity was supplied by line current.* (*Courtesy* Journal of Mental Pathology)

useful in cases of stunned patients or those with respiratory arrest, it is doubtful it would have defibrillated a fibrillating heart. Robinovitch recognized this difficulty and wrote that resuscitation from "ventricular tremulation" is especially difficult. The ambulance device required household current to operate.[12] She did not give any details about the device's weight or its intended use in homes. Nevertheless, it bears an uncanny resemblance to modern-day defibrillators.

Robinovitch almost got it right. Her device could assist in selected cases of respiratory arrest—according to her, it caused artificial breathing "superior to all other forms of artificial respiration known to us to-day." But it would not work for the far more common condition of ventricular fibrillation. The ideal device, she said, would be "the invention of a simple, always ready, quickly applicable, and infallible method of resuscitation."

It is unclear why none of Robinovitch's scientific colleagues followed the thread of electrical defibrillation. Apparently no one appreciated the significance of the work done by Prevost, Battelli, and Cunningham, or its relevance to humans. The bottom line appears to be that no one believed anything could be done. In 1913 the Electric Light Association commissioned a report addressing resuscitation from electric shock that acknowledges fibrillation as a cause of death in linemen, but also states that "a solution of the problem in a manner permitting the life of the individual to continue may be impracticable."[13]

During this detour, researchers pursued nonelectrical interests, particularly chemical defibrillation. In the first two decades of the twentieth century, chemical defibrillation was used to stop fibrillation in the hope that a regular heartbeat would resume or could be started with another chemical. Salts of potassium chloride were the most common agents used, and calcium chloride was occasionally successful in starting a stilled heart.[14] Potassium chloride was particularly potent in stopping fibrillation, though it worked by totally wiping out all heart activity. Once the chemical induced asystole, it had to be flushed out and efforts undertaken to restart the quiet heart. Turning ventricular fibrillation into asystole is a little like treating a severe migraine with decapitation.

Enter William Kouwenhoven

The connection between electricity and defibrillation was picked up again in the 1920s. In 1926 the Consolidated Electric Company of New York City turned to the Rockefeller Institute for advice on how to respond to and deal with the alarming number of fatal electric accidents. The Institute in turn funded research at several universities, including Johns Hopkins, and wanted a research team that included both medical doctors and electrical engineers. The M.D.s were Orthello Langworthy and Donald Hooker, from the university's School of Hygiene and Public Health. The engineer was William Kouwenhoven.

Throughout the early 1930s, the three researchers carried out many studies on the effects of electrical currents on the heart. Kouwenhoven was also exploring the damage caused by electrical shock to the nervous system, and the possibility of using potassium salts for defibrillation. In 1930 Hooker, Kouwenhoven, and Langworthy began to study the effects of electricity directly on the heart and published their findings in the *American Journal of Physiology* in 1933.[15] They showed that electric shocks, even small ones, could induce ventricular fibrillation in the heart and more powerful shocks could erase the fibrillation. They induced ventricular fibrillation in dogs and were then able to defibrillate the heart without opening the chest.[16] But their closed-chest defibrillation was successful only if the fibrillatory contractions were vigorous and the period of no circulation or breathing did not exceed several minutes. If it lasted longer, open-heart massage was necessary before the electric shock could defibrillate the heart. The term "countershock" was derived from their research. Since an initial shock was required to place the heart in ventricular fibrillation, it was only logical to call the subsequent shock, which defibrillated the heart, the countershock. For many years the term was used synonymously to mean defibrillation.

The research of Hooker, Kouwenhoven, and Langworthy was well on its way toward developing effective defibrillation in humans; unfortunately their work had to be halted because of World War II. It was resumed under the sponsorship of the department of surgery at Johns Hopkins[17] and the studies were again funded by the Edison Electric Institute.

Claude Beck, "Dr. Heart"

Claude Beck, professor of surgery at Western Reserve University (later to become Case Western Reserve) in Cleveland worked for years on a technique for defibrillation of the human heart. Born in 1894 in a small town in the mining country of eastern Pennsylvania and educated at Johns Hopkins University Medical School, Beck probably witnessed his first cardiac arrest during his internship in 1922 while on surgery service. During a urologic operation, the anesthetist announced that the patient's heart had stopped. To Beck's amazement, the surgical resident removed his gloves, went to a telephone in a corner of the room, and called the fire department. Beck remained in total bewilderment as the fire department rescue squad rushed into the operating room fifteen minutes later and applied oxygen-powered resuscitators to the patient's face. The patient died, but the episode left an indelible impression. Twenty years later he wrote, "surgeons should not turn these emergencies over to the care of the fire department." Recalling the same event, he remarked to medical students in typically understated fashion, "The experience left me with a conviction that we were not doing our best for the patient."[18]

Based on the work of Hooker and Kouwenhoven, Beck constructed an alternating current internal defibrillator.[19] He realized that ventricular fibrillation often occurred in hearts that were basically sound and coined the phrase "Hearts Too Good to Die."[20] Beck believed that for heart surgery to have a future a surgeon must learn how to handle the emergency of ventricular fibrillation. "And so," he said, "I prepared myself to handle it." In 1939 he recommended that every hospital should have a "resuscitation squad" to respond to patients. Such a system was established at University Hospital in Cleveland, although as his colleague David Leighninger notes, he and Beck were the only "squad" the hospital ever had. The squad was summoned by paging "Dr. Heart" over the speaker system.[21]

By 1941 Beck was closing in on his goal of restarting a fibrillating heart. In an issue of the *American Journal of Surgery*, Beck described his technique of getting air into the lungs and red blood to the brain by hand-pumping the heart. He also explained open-chest electrical defibrillation of the heart and wrote about two patients who were defibrillated during surgery and lived two and four hours, respectively.[22] Beck was getting close.

During the early 1940s surgeons had reported a handful of cases of ventricular fibrillation that spontaneously changed to a normal rhythm in response to cardiac massage or injection of potent medications. These cases involved only temporary success and the patient invariably died several hours later. It was obvious that time was of the essence. A thoracic surgeon writing in the August 29, 1942, issue of *JAMA* noted, "In cardiac cessation the odds in favor of resuscitation decrease with each minute that passes before proper measures are applied. The stakes are high—a human life. The half-hearted attempts at resuscitation should be replaced by early and bold attempts at resuscitation. . . . The feeling that once the heart has stopped the patient is gone and nothing will help should be replaced by the knowledge that a human life can and may be saved, and any attempt is justifiable."[23] It became obvious that electric defibrillation was the bold immediate therapy required.

In 1947, Beck accomplished his first successful resuscitation of a fourteen-year-old boy using open-chest massage and internal defibrillation with alternating current. The boy was being operated on for a severe congenital funnel chest. The boy's sternum was only one inch away from his backbone, and this limited his lung expansion and caused him to become short of breath when he was physically active. The surgery would correct the deformity and totally eliminate the breathing problem. In all other respects the boy was normal. He received nitrous oxide and ether anesthesia, and the three-hour operation was uneventful except for a forty-five-minute period of rapid heart rate of 160 beats per minute for which digitalis was used. (Digitalis, derived from the foxglove plant, was described as a therapy for dropsy—heart failure—in 1785, and came to be used for fast heart rates as well as heart failure.)[24]

During closure of the large incision in the chest, the boy's pulse suddenly stopped and his blood pressure fell to zero—he was in cardiac arrest. Dr. Beck immediately reopened the chest and began manual heart massage. As he looked at and felt the heart, he realized that ventricular fibrillation was present. He continued massage for thirty-five minutes and then took an electrocardiogram that confirmed ventricular fibrillation. Another ten minutes passed before the defibrillator was brought to the operating room. The first shock using electrode paddles placed directly on the sides of the heart was unsuccessful. Beck administered procaine—medicine designed to raise the threshold for fibrillation and thus allow the next shock to work. Beck gave a second shock that wiped out the fibrillation. In a very few seconds a feeble, regular, and fast contraction of the heart occurred. The boy's blood pressure rose from zero to fifty millimeters of mercury and the heartbeat remained normal. Twenty minutes after the successful defibrillation, the chest wound

FIGURE 32. *Electrocardiogram from the first human successfully defibrillated by Claude Beck, MD, in 1947. The top two panels, taken immediately before the defibrillatory shock, show ventricular fibrillation. The bottom panel, taken after the shock, depicts a near normal heart pattern. (Courtesy of the* Journal of the American Medical Association, *Vol. 135: 985–986, Copyright 1947, American Medical Association, Chicago)*

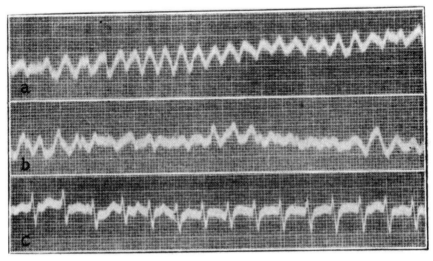

was closed. By three hours, the blood pressure rose to a normal level, and the child awoke and was able to answer questions.

The boy made a full recovery, with no neurologic damage, and reported that his exercise tolerance had considerably improved. It's not clear from Beck's report if the child ever realized how amazing his survival was. What started as a straightforward surgery led to forty-five minutes of death before resuscitation with the first successful human defibrillation took place.[25]

Beck is honored for his breakthrough in resuscitation but was criticized by Dr. Barnett Green, who in a letter to *JAMA* suggested that Beck actually caused the ventricular fibrillation by using digitalis. When the heart sped up to 160 beats per minute, Beck ordered digitalis to try to slow the rate. Green points out that the fast heart rate may have been due to the ether anesthesia or a relative lack of oxygen. Digitalis, he claimed, was not the correct drug to use since it would have been worthless in this situation, and in fact, the large dose may have triggered the episode of ventricular fibrillation. The onset of ventricular fibrillation two hours after the administration of the digitalis coincided with the time the medicine was likely to have its maximum toxic effect.[26] So who knows? Perhaps the first save was the result of an inadvertent medication error.

The defibrillators Beck used were individually made. Ever the scientist, Beck kept experimenting with different models to improve the machine's efficiency. Since these models were intended for open-heart defibrillation, he designed a model that would both shock and perform heart massage. Suction cups were attached to the walls of the heart and alternating suction would expand and allow the heart to relax. According to Beck, the machine could massage at the rate of 120 beats per minute, which he considered considerably better than the fifty to sixty beats achieved by surgeons. The device also relieved the surgeon of performing cardiac massage. The suction cups doubled as defibrillatory electrodes. Beck offered to "furnish this apparatus to anyone who would like to have it for the cost of the various parts."[27] It was an ingenious device, but ultimately an historical curiosity. Closed-chest compression and defibrillation turned Beck's defibrillatory machine into surplus dials, gauges, and wires.

Beck's interest in resuscitation remained paramount throughout his career. In 1961, shortly after the introduction of modern CPR, he learned of training manikins and the early reports demonstrating that laypeople could perform CPR. He established an organization called "Resuscitators of America" and over the next five years trained 5000 people.[28] The course, the first of its kind to train the public in CPR, occurred in a two-hour evening session. Instructors supervised each student's performance with Resusci-Anne, and a written test ensured competence. On January 28, 1966, the coordinator of Resuscitators of America described the program to members of the AHA Committee on Cardiopulmonary Resuscitation meeting in Miami Beach, Florida. James Jude was chairman of the committee and in attendance were Elam, Safar, and Gordon. Here was a golden opportunity for the AHA to endorse CPR for laypeople. The committee "gave serious thought as to whether or not the American Heart Association should reconsider its policy regarding the teaching of the laity the cardiopulmonary resuscitation procedures" and felt that further study was needed. In a bridge-building effort, the coordinator invited members of the AHA to serve on the Resuscitators' advisory committee, but the invitation was declined.[29] Caution ruled and the opportunity was dodged. The Resuscitators of America quietly faded into obscurity (mostly for lack of funds) over the next several years. Such a program would not surface again until 1972 in Seattle.

Kouwenhoven Redux

As we saw earlier, the Edison Electric Institute had funded research with the Electrical Engineering Department of Johns Hopkins to develop a portable device for closed-chest defibrillation. The major problem was providing enough energy through the chest and heart to bring all the muscle fibers to rest without damaging the nervous system or other organs. In other words, just enough energy was needed to defibrillate the heart, but not enough to irreparably damage other body parts. William Kouwenhoven's experiments were performed on anesthetized dogs, and he and his colleagues faced many questions: What type of energy should be used? Was alternating current more effective than direct? Which was safer? Where should the electrodes be placed on the chest? What size and shape should the electrodes be? Would the electrodes burn the skin? How long could the heart fibrillate before it could be defibrillated? Is there any danger to the machine operator? What if a shock were accidentally given to a heart not in ventricular fibrillation? In 1951 there were no answers to these questions.

Kouwenhoven initially experimented with DC discharges, but, after little success, focused his attention on alternating current.[30] Not surprisingly, Kouwenhoven found that considerably higher energy levels were required for closed-chest defibrillation compared to open chest. And, as other investigators had shown, if the heart remained in fibrillation for more than several minutes, the chances of survival fell. In experiments on 400 dogs, Kouwenhoven achieved a survival rate of 99 percent when the heart was in fibrillation for thirty seconds. When it was in fibrillation for one minute, two minutes, and four minutes, these rates fell to 90, 27, and 0 percent, respectively.

The optimal-size electrode for the dog's chest was a nine-square-inch circular shape. A plastic handle and plastic guard mounted an inch above the electrode protected the operator from accidental shock. Kouwenhoven found that 480 volts for one-quarter second was the optimal strength and duration. He also demonstrated that repeated shocks did not cause damage to the heart muscle and that a normally beating heart was not harmed by a 480-volt shock. Based on his dog experiments, Kouwenhoven created a prototype for use in humans. In 1957 the first closed-chest defibrillator Kouwenhoven developed weighed 270 pounds, but because it had wheels, it was portable (well, sort of). It used alternating line current—480 volts for adults and 240 volts for children. A foot switch delivered the shock. A timer could be set to alter the recommended duration if initial shocks were not successful.

Kouwenhoven's closed-chest defibrillator was used on two humans that year. One was a seventy-two-year-old man, who was defibrillated ten times over a four-day period, but did not survive resuscitation. The other was an eighteen-year-old girl who was in the hospital for repair of a congenital heart problem. While undergoing a diagnostic test, her heart fibrillated. Within seventy seconds, a defibrillatory shock was given and was successful. She regained consciousness within moments and remarked that she "must have fallen asleep." She was discharged three days later with no ill effects.[31]

Kouwenhoven invested decades studying defibrillation, yet his enduring fame came from his discovery of chest compression. Though he succeeded in developing an external defibrillator, in science glory goes to the first to publish. That honor would belong to a cardiologist in Boston, Paul Zoll, who scooped Kouwenhoven by a year.

Paul Zoll

For over forty years, Paul Zoll had been a recognized leader in cardiac pacing, defibrillation, and monitoring. His early research provided the foundation from which many of today's cardiac care technologies and instruments have evolved. Pacemakers, defibrillators, and cardiac monitors are just some of the revolutionary devices and procedures Zoll invented or nursed to maturity.

Paul Maurice Zoll was born in Boston on July 15, 1911. He received his A.B. from Harvard in 1932, graduating summa cum laude, and his M.D. in 1936. Zoll interned at Beth Israel Hospital in Boston and then at Bellevue Hospital in New York City from 1936 to 1939. After completing his internship, he returned to Boston to practice medicine. He decided to specialize in cardiology, and began doing medical research both at Beth Israel and Harvard Medical School.

When World War II broke out, Zoll joined the Army as a first lieutenant, and later rose to the rank of major. He was stationed at an army hospital in England, working with another doctor on techniques for removing shell fragments from the hearts of wounded soldiers.

Zoll went back to Boston after the war, and to both private practice and research. In 1948 he had an experience with a patient that would make a deep impression. "I was seeing this lady—a private patient—who was about sixty years old. She was having Stokes-Adams attacks that lasted on and off for three weeks. And she died. I was terribly frustrated at that," he said. "Here was a woman who was otherwise entirely well with an otherwise normal heart. It was just wrong." Stokes-Adams attacks were fatal in the 1940s. It is a cardiac condition in which the inherent pacemaker of the heart malfunctions and leads to a very slow heart rate. The condition comes on suddenly, without warning, hence the name "attacks." These attacks can occur repeatedly over days or weeks and may last for minutes or hours. Usually the patient has a very low blood pressure, due to the slow heart rate, and may become faint or lose consciousness. In 1948 there was no treatment for this condition, except to prescribe bedrest and hope the attacks would spontaneously cease.

Zoll was not willing to sit still and hope. Recalling his patient, he said, "And that made me remember those experiences in surgery in England during the war. I'd had the idea in the back of my head, I guess, for some time. But this experience with this patient activated me to do something." What Zoll did was build a wire with an electrode that he could run down the esophagus. In 1950 he tested his idea in animals and found that it was indeed possible to stimulate the heart with an electrical current running through the esophagus. Although he soon abandoned this method of stimulating the heart, it was a first step. Between 1950 and 1952, he and his colleagues worked out the details of external cardiac pacing in the laboratory. First used on human patients in 1952, the external pacer employed an electrical current to "encourage" a heart with a faulty beat to return to a regular rhythm.

Zoll realized that if externally applied alternating currents could help pace the heart, they might also jolt a fibrillating heart back into normal rhythm. He was in a minority with this opinion, however, and later recalled, "The general idea at the time [the early 1950s] was that external defibrillation would not work. It was too large an electric current." This negative opinion among most cardiologists was mainly based on the pronouncements of a prominent researcher who had worked on heart defibrillation for nearly thirty years. He had reached the conclusion that external defibrillation could never work because it would not be possible to supply enough current across the chest wall to reach the heart. The only place for defibrillation, he declared, was in the operating room. Only paddles placed directly on the heart muscle were effective. This opinion flew in the face of data from dog experiments that only three times the voltage used in open-chest defibrillation was needed for closed-chest defibrillation. The 160 volts on average was sufficient to achieve closed-chest defibrillation in dogs.[32]

This "authoritative" pronouncement sounded remarkably like the infamous "man will never fly" statements before 1903. Researchers since 1933, however, had successfully stopped ventricular fibrillation in animals with external alternating current across the closed chest. Now Paul Zoll wanted to take the next step—nor was he alone. "There were a number of people all over the country who were making efforts at external defibrillation," Zoll said. "I think there were at least a half a dozen. But I didn't know about them, so I had gone ahead and done the same things that others were doing."

The decision to develop an external defibrillator that used alternating current rather than direct current was a practical one. Alternating current derives its name from the back-and-forth motion of electrons carrying the current. Households in the United States have alternating current that changes directions sixty times per second. With direct current, electron flow goes in one direction. In contrast to household current, batteries produce direct current. "Direct current was not easily obtainable" at that time at the proper voltage, Zoll recalled. DC batteries both powerful enough to do the job and portable enough for practical use simply didn't exist in the early 1950s. "I talked to an electrical engineer I was working with at the time about why we couldn't use direct current," said Zoll. "He explained that it would take a room full of capacitors."

Like other researchers in the field, Zoll had spent several years perfecting his procedure in a series of animal experiments. He then turned to a small company in Norwood, Massachusetts, Electrodyne, to develop an external AC defibrillator that could be used on human beings. Zoll borrowed a transformer from Cambridge Power and Light Company. The transformer stepped up the AC current from a wall plug to a high enough voltage to cause defibrillation. The Electrodyne machine included the borrowed transformer, along with two copper electrodes mounted on heavily insulated handles.

The next dramatic step took place in 1955. On August 22, a sixty-four-year-old woman hospitalized five days earlier for a serious heart attack suddenly collapsed from ventricular fibrillation. Zoll and his colleagues applied a single 360-volt "countershock" using electrodes across the woman's chest. The ventricular fibrillation stopped at once, but her heart did not start beating normally and she died. The next two patients also died following successful external defibrillation. Zoll remained undaunted. Then, on November 17, the kind of success every doctor dreams about finally came. A sixty-seven-year-old man survived several episodes of ventricular fibrillation, thanks to Zoll's external defibrillator, and went home from the hospital fully recovered a month later. Over a period of four months, Zoll had successfully stopped ventricular fibrillation eleven times in four different patients. The energy required for defibrillation ranged from 240 to 720 volts and Zoll was worried about the potential damage such high energy might cause. He was gratified to write, "The complete recovery in Case 4 after repeated countershock indicates that external defibrillation can be accomplished without ill effect to the patient." Zoll's findings were published in the prestigious *New England Journal of Medicine* on April 19, 1956. His article was titled "Termination of ventricular fibrillation in man by externally applied electric countershock."[33]

The defibrillator designed by Zoll, as well as earlier versions invented by Kouwenhoven and Beck, were very large and heavy, primarily because they contained a transformer to step up the AC line current from 110 volts to approximately 1000. The larger voltage was required to do the job of defibrillating the heart; 110 volts was just not enough. Because of their size and weight, not many lives would be saved unless their inherent nonportability could be addressed.

Bernard Lown

The portability problem was solved by Bernard Lown. He devised a defibrillator that utilized direct current instead of alternating current. It was now possible to use power, supplied by a battery, to charge a capacitor over a few seconds. The capacitor stored the energy until it was released in one massive jolt to the chest wall. No longer would defibrillators require bulky transformers nor did they need to be tied to line current. The cord was cut—the defibrillator could travel to the patient.

Bernard Lown was born in Utena, Lithuania, on June 7, 1921. His family was Jewish, and, driven by anti-Semitic persecution, his father brought him to the United States in 1935 when Lown was forteen. He graduated summa cum laude from the University of Maine in 1942, receiving his B.A. in the classics. The same anti-Semitism that had driven his family from Lithuania was now ironically blocking his entrance into medical school. He was finally accepted at Johns Hopkins and received his M.D. in 1945.

As Lown would later recount, the story began in 1959. He had become concerned about the issue of sudden cardiac death, largely through the influence of his mentor, the cardiologist Samuel Levine. Like Levine, Lown was becoming convinced that sudden cardiac death was a serious problem that no one was working on. At about the same time, he had a patient with ischemic heart disease who was plagued with frequently recurring ventricular tachycardia. When the heart beats this fast, it loses the ability to pump adequate blood (it doesn't have enough time to fill between contractions) and blood pressure falls. If the ventricular tachycardia continues long enough, the patient will go into shock and die. How long the patient can tolerate ventricular tachycardia is a function of the heart's underlying condition. This rhythm in a young, healthy person can be tolerated for hours or days; in an older person with significant heart disease, it may be minutes. The only available treatment was injections of the drug Procainamide. Invariably, Lown's patient suffered these attacks at around 2 A.M., and Lown would have to rouse himself to give the man an injection. Lown was beginning to resent the loss of sleep from the resulting ten- to twenty-hour work day. "After about seven or eight bouts of this," Lown recalled, "the man's system became completely resistant to the Procainamide. But there was a lot of excitement at that time about Paul Zoll's AC external heart defibrillator. I thought perhaps we ought to utilize alternating current for this patient's tachycardia condition."

Lown decided to go ahead and try it on his patient. "I didn't know the first thing about how to use AC on a patient," he confessed later, "what type of current settings, amperage, and whatnot." But it worked—spectacularly, at first. The patient's tachycardia stopped at once, his blood pressure returned, and he was quickly discharged from the hospital. Within two weeks, though, he was back with a severe tachycardia. By this time Lown had discovered that low voltages with an AC defibrillator could actually cause ventricular fibrillation instead of stop it. He used 400 volts to shock the man's heart back to normal. Instead, the heart went into ventricular fibrillation.

Lown set out to discover just what alternating current did to the heart. In a series of experiments with dogs he found that alternating current will induce fibrillation in a normal heart about one in four times. AC is also quite likely to cause a worse arrhythmic heart beat in a heart already beating abnormally. Finally, AC could cause other injuries to the heart. "Obviously, we had a technology that was very hazardous," he observed.[34]

He decided to look into other ways of delivering a lifesaving shock to the heart. DC current seemed the simplest, but little was known about its effects. Lown divided the problem into two parts: What is safe? What is effective? A series of animal experiments on dogs in 1960 and 1961 established that DC shocks were extremely effective in shocking the heart. It was also clear that DC would be many times safer than AC when applied through the chest wall.

These initial studies exclusively approached the issue of how to stop a fast heart rate using electricity. The treatment of ventricular fibrillation—namely, defibrillation—was not on the early agenda. The treatment for fast heart rates is known as cardioversion. Cardioversion is similar to defibrillation in that electricity is used to change an abnormal rhythm to a normal one. It is different, however, in the urgency of the treatment. Generally, cardioversion is used as an alternate or adjunct to drug therapy, primarily for heart rates that are dangerously fast. Defibrillation, on the other hand, is the only effective therapy for the fatal rhythm of ventricular fibrillation and must be applied within minutes. Modern defibrillators are usually combined with cardioverters. Lown initially developed the DC cardioverter, but it soon became evident that DC electricity was superior both for cardioversion and defibrillation. The fact that the same type of current was effective for both uses allowed one machine to serve a dual role. This is important because occasionally cardioversion, instead of leading to a normal heart rhythm, could result in the critical condition of ventricular fibrillation. In such a situation the physician must immediately change from the cardioversion mode of the machine to the defibrillator mode and give a defibrillatory shock. Having both modes in one machine is more than a matter of convenience—it can be lifesaving.

In a 1962 article in the *American Journal of Cardiology,* Lown noted that the incidence of ventricular fibrillation was ten times more frequent after AC than DC cardioversion. Lown did discover one short period during the procedure when a DC shock could induce ventricular fibrillation. Thus, the trick was simply to build a device that would shock the heart while avoiding this so called "vulnerable period" of a few milliseconds. An electrical engineer at the American Optical Company in Buffalo hand-built several different types of DC machines for Lown to test.

The first chance to use the newly developed DC device came in 1961 at the Peter Bent Brigham Hospital in Boston. An elderly Irish woman suffering an acute myocardial infarction developed a serious case of ventricular tachycardia. Drug treatment slowed the condition but sent her into shock. The resident treating the woman contacted Lown, who was then doing some work at the Harvard School of Public Health across the street. It was about 2:00 A.M., but Lown and another doctor "carried the device to the Brigham and set it up," Lown recalled. The patient was muttering that she was dying—"with adequate reason," Lown would later write. Lown gave her a single jolt from his new DC cardioverter. Though she was not in ventricular fibrillation her rhythm was so fast (200 beats per minute) that he reasoned it would respond to the synchronized electric shock. "She came right out of the tachycardia rhythm," said Lown. "It was so remarkable." The woman's heart failure improved at once, and her blood pressure went back to normal. "The funny story about her," recalled Lown, "was that she felt so good that she thought she'd died and we were angels! It took me about an hour to persuade her that I wasn't the angel Gabriel." Lown's report of this case and several others was published in the November 3, 1962, issue of *JAMA*. It was reprinted in the same journal twenty-four years later and honored as a Landmark Article, a distinction given to only a handful of scientific reports.

Lown's work to perfect a DC defibrillator takes on greater significance because its development coincided with that of modern mouth-to-mouth ventilation and chest compression. Prior to CPR, the opportunity to defibrillate was a rare event. It had to happen in a hospital with a defibrillator immediately at hand. In such a case it would not have mattered much whether the defibrillator was AC or DC. The ability to prolong the dying process with CPR suddenly gave an urgency to find the best type of defibrillatory shock.[35] Now the machine could be rushed to the patient because CPR bought a few precious minutes. The real significance of DC defibrillation is that small and portable defibrillators were now possible. Lown envisioned his machines primarily in hospitals, but in moments of unbridled imagination he hoped they would be used to attack sudden death directly in the community.

Suppose John Colven suffered his cardiac arrest in the early 1960s, in his own city of Federal Way, Washington. June and John are having lunch at home with their next-door neighbor. John collapses. June recognizes what has happened and dials the local fire department. The universal 911 emergency number will not come into place until the 1970s, so June must dial the standard seven-digit number. The dispatcher she reaches cannot provide any instructions over the telephone. Their neighbor wants to help but doesn't know what to do, since CPR training of the public will not begin until the mid-1970s. The fire department rescue personnel soon arrive. They have been trained in CPR and they start it at once. But the rescue squad does not have a portable defibrillator, nor are they paramedics with the requisite medical training. So they load John into the aid vehicle and drive to the closest hospital, continuing CPR.

John's heart may have gone into ventricular fibrillation at the moment of his collapse. But by the time the aid car arrives at the hospital, thirty minutes have passed since his cardiac arrest. A moonlighting doctor (emergency medicine will not become a medical specialty until 1978) in the emergency room checks John's pulse and attaches an electrocardiograph machine: flatline. Even with ongoing CPR, it has taken too long for John to reach a defibrillator.

Rushing to the closest hospital with sirens wailing and CPR in progress makes for high drama, but not many lives were saved. Resuscitation required both the skill and the means to deliver it quickly. The way was found by a crusty cardiologist in the unlikely city of Belfast, Northern Ireland.

Part V

THE WAY
IS FOUND

« »

. . . they shall run and not be weary, and they shall walk, and not faint.
—Isaiah 40:21

BELFAST LEADS THE WAY

« »

A sudden cardiac arrest is not, of course, a scheduled or even predictable event. John Colven survived because emergency care and equipment reached him quickly enough. CPR was crucial; it kept his brain and heart oxygenated until more advanced care arrived. Defibrillation was equally critical because it treated his heart's fatal rhythm. And medications and placement of an airway tube also kept his heart in a normal rhythm. The function of emergency medical services is to deliver these advanced levels of care rapidly.

The system of emergency medical service involves multiple agencies and people working together to create a whole far greater than the sum of its individual parts. It is a system with a 200-year history that includes Napoleon's surgeon and a determined cardiologist in Belfast, Northern Ireland.

The First Ambulance

In 1792 Baron Dominique-Jean Larrey, Napoleon's chief army surgeon, devised the first ambulance service to bring aid directly to the injured soldier. When Larrey first entered the military, ambulances were required to be stationed two and a half miles to the rear of the army. After the fighting ended, the ambulances would pick up the fallen soldiers and take those still alive to field hospitals. The term "ambulance" itself denotes this age-old function. Originally a military term, the word probably derives from the Latin *ambulo*, meaning "move slowly," because a gentle motion was necessary in the transport of injured soldiers.

Larrey was shocked by the delays in providing even minimal care to soldiers. His indignation led him to design a lightweight, two-wheeled ambulance that allowed a surgeon to be mobile and work directly on the battlefield. These vehicles were called "flying ambulances" because they traveled with the "flying artillery" on the field of battle.[1]

Not all innovations in ambulance service involved the military. James Curry, a London physician, writing in his book *Observations on Apparent Death from Drowning, Hanging, Suffocation by Noxious Vapours, Fainting-fits, Intoxication, Lightning, Exposure to Cold, Etc, Etc.* (1815), proposed a vehicle to aid drowning victims after they have been removed from the water. His caravan was designed to heat the victim during the journey to the closest house where further resuscitation could be performed. It had a small stove that circulated heat and was designed so the exhaust vent could "enter a chimney in any ground floor room." The caravan was also "sufficiently narrow to enter the ground-floor apartment of any house where there is not a sharp turning." Curry recommended that a few shavings be lit in the small furnace, so that the bed would be warmed by the time it had been wheeled down to the riverside.[2] Though Curry wished that many of these "Resuscitation Apparatus," as he called them, would be stationed strategically throughout the country, there is no evidence that even one was constructed.

During the Crimean War (1854–1856), the British Army attempted to organize an ambulance corps (the Land Transport Corps) for the sick and injured. Florence Nightingale helped improve hospital care by introducing sanitary hospital practice during this war. By this action, she achieved a dramatic fall in mortality from infections. In 1859 Jean Dunaut of Switzerland proposed that every country should organize civilian relief societies to assist the wounded in time of war. This formed the basis for the International Committee of the Red Cross, founded in 1863.

In the United States, organized transport services for battle casualties first appeared in the Civil War. Although ambulance corps were proposed early on, none were used in the Union army until the Battle of Antietam in 1862. The effectiveness of care received by severely wounded soldiers transported to field hospitals was limited. Already suffering from shock and trauma, they often faced the additional trials of amputation, infectious shock, and gangrene.

During World War I, evacuation of the wounded to field hospitals still required twelve to eighteen hours. Among U.S. casualties, the mortality rate was 8.1 percent of those who received treatment. In World War II the time lag from injury to surgery was reduced to a maximum of twelve hours, and the mortality rate of the wounded fell to less than 5 percent.

Antibiotics helped play a role in this reduction in mortality. The Korean War (1950–1953) saw the introduction of Mobile Army Surgical Hospital (MASH) units. Helicopters and rapid ground transport carried the wounded to MASH units, and substantially reduced time intervals of two to four hours from injury to definitive care. The overall mortality rate dropped to 2.5 percent. During the Vietnam War rapid transport was further improved, decreasing transport time from injury to emergency care to seventy-five minutes, and the overall mortality rate was reduced to less than 2 percent.[3]

Urban ambulance services for civilians first appeared in Cincinnati in 1865 and New York City in 1869. The New York service began with two ambulances located at Bellevue Hospital. The initial rules required "two horses, one of which shall always be in harness, and ready to be attached to the ambulance." An experienced driver could hitch the horse and start rolling within thirty seconds. The ambulance was alerted either by a call to the hospital or telegraph signals from fire or police alarm boxes. Once the hospital was notified, "an electric switch is turned which communicates with the sta-

FIGURE 33. *Old ambulance from Bellevue Hospital, New York City, 1877 (Courtesy of the Society of the Alumni of Bellevue)*

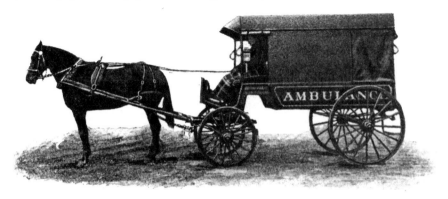

ble, ringing the gong, unhitching the horse, opening the door, stopping the clock, and turning up the gas (if the call be in the night). The trained horse, now unloosed, runs into place; the driver pulls down the shafts, and clasps the patent collar and hames, attaches the reins into the bit-rings, and drives out." A surgeon was simultaneously notified of the call and met the ambulance as it departed from the stable. Each ambulance was equipped with a medical box located under the driver's seat containing tourniquets, bandages, splints, and—most important—"one quart flask of brandy." Ambulance drivers received an annual salary of $500, which included room and board. The delivery of mail must have been a crucial undertaking in 1869, for hospital regulations stated that "an ambulance has the right of way over all other vehicles except the Fire Department apparatus and the United States mail wagons."[4]

During its first year of full operation, the New York City service responded to 1500 calls from one hospital (Bellevue). By 1883, nineteen ambulances operating out of seven hospitals handled more than 10,000 calls. Stationing the ambulances at hospitals provided convenient and ready access to a surgeon. The model of hospital-based ambulances predominated well into the 1930s and 1940s in the United States. In Europe hospital-based ambulances still remain the predominant mode. The response time in 1880 was reported as five to eight minutes per mile. These initial ambulances were purposely designed to be open and attractive, thereby instilling public confidence. It was important that they not resemble "Black Marias," the name given to vehicles used to transport those suffering from contagious diseases. Any attempt to conceal the contents would merely raise the suspicion of contagion and the public would never willingly enter such a vehicle. The vehicle's open nature also protected the driver and surgeon from acquiring an infection. A source from 1888 concluded, "Most ambulance surgeons have sat behind many contagious cases, but we have yet to hear of a single surgeon by whom the disease was contracted."[5]

For civilians, ambulance service was merely a means of bringing the patient to the hospital. In a few cities interns rode ambulances as part of their training, but provided no medical care. During the 1930s and 1940s, municipal fire departments in some cities (including Los Angeles, Columbus, Baltimore, and Seattle) began to offer rescue, first aid, and resuscitation care. In 1966, the U.S. National Academy of Sciences and the President's Commission on Highway Safety issued reports decrying the unevenness of ambulance personnel competency and lack of standard procedures. The Commis-

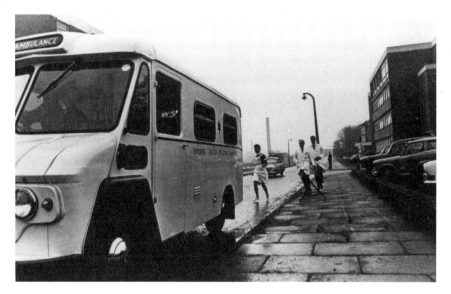

FIGURE 34. *Flying squad mobile intensive care unit (MICU) developed by J. Frank Pantridge, MD, and John S. Geddes, MD, in Belfast, Northern Ireland. The program began in 1966 and was staffed with doctors and nurses shown hurrying to the vehicle. (Courtesy of John S. Geddes)*

sion described the carnage resulting from traffic accidents as the "neglected disease of society." The subsequent National Highway Safety and Traffic Act of 1966 authorized the Department of Transportation to establish a national curriculum for prehospital personnel. Out of this came the birth of Emergency Medical Technicians.

Emergency Medical Technicians (also known as EMTs) did much to upgrade the general performance of ambulance services throughout the nation. Their eighty-hour course and certification ensured proper care for victims of motor vehicle accidents and other emergencies, and people suffering traumatic injuries. The training of EMTs included CPR. Thus, they could provide artificial ventilation and closed-chest massage at the scene as well as enroute to the hospital.

However, EMTs were not trained or authorized to perform definitive care for cardiac arrest. They could not provide defibrillation, endotracheal intubation, or administer intravenous medications. The sad reality was that EMTs saved few if any victims of sudden cardiac arrest. By the time EMTs arrived and transported the patient to the closest emergency department, too much time had elapsed for resuscitation to be successful. Not even letter-perfect CPR can save a life if defibrillation and other advanced procedures occur too late.

People with hearts too good to die were still dying. The breakthrough came in 1966, led by a forceful and somewhat irascible British physician working in Northern Ireland.

J. Frank Pantridge

Frank Pantridge was born in the small Northern Ireland plantation village of Hillsborough, a predominantly Protestant part of the province. He developed his fiercely independent streak quite early. In his autobiography, *An Unquiet Life*,[6] Pantridge recalls being sent as a child to a preparatory school in a small town about two miles from his home. "But [I] absconded so frequently that I was declared persona non grata and transferred to the Downshire School in the village." Pantridge was also fascinated with riding horses as a youngster, and frequently fell. "The numerous falls on my head may well have had something to do with my juvenile delinquency," he wrote (perhaps with tongue in cheek).

The doctor in Hillsborough during Pantridge's youth was a Dr. Boyd, who sported a long beard and did his rounds on horseback. Impressed, the young Pantridge decided he wanted to become a village doctor, somewhere in Northern Ireland.

Pantridge attended Friends' School (run by the Quakers) in the town of Lisburn. He claims that his academic performance was "less than average," and he did poorly in foreign languages and indifferently in mathematics and science subjects. He also encountered religious bigotry for the first time. While waiting for a bus, Pantridge recalled, he was attacked by a larger and older boy. Pantridge responded by kicking the fellow in the crotch and jumping onto the bus. He heard someone on board yell, "You should have killed the Catholic bastard!" Pantridge realized that the attacker had struck at him simply because his school blazer labeled him a Protestant. Things in Northern Ireland were such that virtually no Catholics went to Protestant schools, and vice versa.

In 1934 Pantridge entered Queen's University in Belfast and started his five-year medical course. One of his professors was T. Thompson Flynn, father of the famous movie star Errol Flynn and something of a character in his own right. Pantridge's first year was not a pleasant one, and he began to wonder if he had made the right decision. In 1935 he fell ill with diphtheria and missed many classes. After he recovered, Pantridge knew he might have to redo the whole year. He went to Flynn and asked for help. Flynn was most sympathetic and gave him permission to take an equivalency test for the zoology course, which he passed. His botany professor refused such an arrangement, but when Pantridge appealed this decision to the Dean of Faculty he won.

Pantridge began clinical work at the start of his third year of medical school in 1937 at the Royal Victoria Hospital. He would spend his entire professional life there, with the significant exception of World War II. Despite a self-proclaimed "undistinguished" undergraduate career, he graduated with honors in 1939.

In September, Britain declared war against Germany and its Axis allies Italy and Japan. Pantridge joined the Royal Army Medical Corps and shipped out to Singapore. He was assigned to a military hospital, and his ingrained resistance to incompetent authority soon asserted itself. He had several disagreeable tangles with his superior officer, was indirectly threatened with death for mutiny, and posted to another hospital.

Two years later the war came to Malaya. December 7, 1941, saw not only the Japanese attack on Pearl Harbor, but also their invasion of Hong Kong, Thailand, and Malaya. Pantridge served with the troops defending the British territory, helping the wounded during several attacks, ambushes, and retreats. For his courage on the field of battle he was awarded the Military Cross (an honor rarely won by doctors). In February 1942 Singapore fell. Not long after, Pantridge (along with other British troops) was captured by the Japanese and sent to the Changi prison camp. Pantridge continued to do his best to give medical treatment to others. All the while, he writes, he was "seething with rage" at both the Japanese and their brutal prison guards and at the British government for abandoning him and the other British troops.

Perhaps rage and hatred helped him survive. Perhaps it was an indomitable will to live, despite serious kidney problems, the danger of death from cardiac beriberi, starvation, the risk of cholera, brutal treatment by the Japanese, and later incarceration in the Tanbaya "death camp" in Burma. Perhaps it was a bit of both. One of his friends, Dr. Tom Milliken, was aboard the ship that picked up survivors of the Burmese camps after the war's end. He recalls asking several Australians if they knew of one of his colleagues, Dr. Pantridge. "'Ah!' they said, 'the doctor.' It was clear that the rough skeletons had acquired a considerable respect for 'the doctor,'" Milliken later wrote. "I found Pantridge in one of the many huts. . . . The upper half of his body was emaciated, skin and bones. The lower half was bloated with the dropsy of beriberi. The most striking thing were the blue eyes that blazed with defiance. He was a physical wreck, but his spirit was . . . unbroken."

Pantridge eventually returned to Belfast and the Royal Victoria Hospital. "He was withdrawn, usually monosyllabic, and appeared to know more about the world than those around him," his colleague Dr. Mary MacGeown later recalled. There is little doubt that his war experiences profoundly affected him—even though he apparently did not mention them often to others (his entry in *Who's Who* doesn't note his war experiences). Certainly it solidified his often ill-concealed contempt for authority figures—especially those with potential power over his own actions. And it may well have been the catalyst for Pantridge's willingness to challenge "conventional wisdom" and established medical practices.

Pantridge's personal medical problems during the war led him into research on the mechanism of sudden death from cardiac beriberi. That research won him a scholarship to the University of Michigan, where he worked with Frank Wilson, the world authority on electrocardiography. Pantridge returned to the Royal Victoria in 1949, with his course into the realm of cardiology and heart disease firmly established, and quickly introduced the surgical technique of opening up the narrowing of the heart's mitral valve. Later Pantridge established the Regional Medical Cardiology Centre at the Royal Victoria.

In 1965, Pantridge turned his attention to the vexing problem of heart attacks and sudden cardiac death. Publication on the lifesaving techniques of CPR and effective defibrillation had appeared only a few years earlier. His immediate sensitization to the problem came from two sources. First, personnel in the emergency department of the Royal Victoria Hospital repeatedly commented on the number of patients coming in DOA (dead on arrival). Second, a resident, John Geddes, showed him an article demonstrating that among middle-aged or younger men dying of acute myocardial infarction more that half died *within one hour* of the onset of symptoms.[7] Thus, the problem had to be solved outside the hospital, not in the emergency room or hospital ward. The emergency room was one stop too late for too many people. This was the era of coronary-care units and every hospital was jumping on the CCU bandwagon as a means of lowering mortality from acute myocardial infarctions. But Pantridge was not one to buy into the prevailing wisdom. He wanted to go right to the source of the problem. "The majority of deaths from coronary attacks were occurring," he wrote, "outside the hospital, and nothing whatever was being done about them. It became very clear to me that a coronary care unit confined to the hospital would have a minimal impact on mortality." He wanted his coronary care unit in the community.

His solution was simple—and revolutionary: the world's first mobile coronary care unit. Pantridge staffed it with an ambulance driver, a physician, and a nurse.

But Pantridge encountered several obstacles. "Of course, there was the problem of obtaining money," he recalled. "This we eventually did. We obtained a grant from the British Heart Foundation for, I think, 2100 pounds. In dollars at that time [1965] I would suppose it was something on the order of about $4000. That paid for the junior resident, John Geddes, and for the ambulance driver. We resuscitated an old disused ambulance from the depot." He also used money from this grant to purchase equipment—one defibrillator.

There were, of course, other obstacles. "My non-cardiological medical colleagues in the hospital were totally unconvinced and totally uncooperative," Pantridge said. "It was considered unorthodox, if not illegal, to send junior hospital personnel, doctors, and nurses outside the hospital."

Doctor in the Hot Seat

John Geddes was a resident in cardiology at the Royal Victoria Hospital and worked on Pantridge's service. Geddes shared this responsibility of riding in the ambulance with four other residents on the service. Ironically, Pantridge, the father of pre-hospital coronary care, rarely joined them. Said Geddes, "Pantridge was the sort of person who got other people to do things, but he tended not to do things like that himself. It was his way to have other people get involved in the action while he sat backstage directing operations. He is a genius, no question about it, and he was at his best looking at the data and thinking of the next idea. [But] he never had any enthusiasm for riding the ambulance."

Geddes recalled: "When I was an intern in the cardiology ward, the first [Bernard] Lown defibrillator arrived and was used for cardioversions of atrial fibrillation. Already we were attempting to treat cardiac arrests in the hospital with AC defibrillation, and it was uniformly unsuccessful. It so happened that during another part of my rotation, in the neurosurgical ward, we were all having coffee one morning around 11 o'clock. One of the hospital porters put his head around the door and said, 'Excuse me, there is a man who does not look very well out here.' The man turned out to be a patient who had been walking near the front door of that building and had collapsed. I and an anesthetist, who happened also to be present, ran out and found the man lying in a state of cardiac arrest. I started external cardiac massage, and the anesthetist gave him artificial respiration and then brought some anesthetic equipment and intubated him. He was moved to a nearby treatment room and defibrillation equipment was brought from the cardiology ward by Pantridge, which took about ten or fifteen minutes—it was on an enormous trolley—and we got the patient defibrillated. He was transferred to the CCU with a spontaneous circulation.

"That patient actually had a massive anterior infarct and died about eight hours later," Geddes continued. "But the point was that he regained consciousness for a time, and this event got us all fired up with the idea that you really could resuscitate people stricken with cardiac arrest. That was in April 1964." Pantridge at this time had already earmarked Geddes as one of the people who would work with him the following year, and he soon came as a junior resident. By then, there were patients having cardiac arrest once or twice a week in the hospital, and it fell to Geddes to arrive with the trolley and try to resuscitate them. The Royal Victoria Hospital in Belfast had an ideal layout for resuscitating patients in various wards. It consisted of a long horizontal corridor, with all the wards opening off it. A person could very quickly move from one point to another. Recalled Geddes, "From whatever ward it happened in, they would call the cardiology ward and say there was a cardiac arrest in ward 10, or whatever. Then the person at the telephone would push a button that set off the emergency pagers. The people on duty at the time would literally come running and go hurtling along the corridor with the trolley, which was quite heavy. During visiting hours we would have to shout at people to get out of the way, and of course some people are deaf so there were some near-misses.

"A physician and nurse always responded, and there was usually at least one medical student as well. There were very few people on the team, but the staff in the ward you went to helped continue with CPR. We were the paramedics, so to speak; we gave advanced life support while the other people continued to give basic life support."

Geddes and his colleagues were able to resuscitate quite a number of people—about one-third actually went home. Over a two-year period thirty-one of ninety-two patients with cardiac arrest were resuscitated and discharged alive.[8]

The creative spark that led to Pantridge's now-famous mobile intensive care unit (MICU) was struck by Geddes himself. "I was looking for a subject for a thesis to obtain a higher degree," Geddes recalled, "and it suddenly struck me, why not categorize these patients and look at the factors that helped them to survive. Not all had VF (ventricular fibrillation), and one thing that came out of my study was that, if they had asystole (a flat line on the ECG), they were very unlikely to survive for more than a few days. In the course of reading in preparation for handing in my thesis, I came across an article by Yater and his colleagues which described American servicemen in the Second World War, between the phenomenally young ages of eighteen and thirty-six, who had died of heart attacks. The most remarkable finding was that over 60 percent of those, in whom the interval between onset and death was known, died within the first hour. They were sudden deaths. The following Monday I showed the Yater paper to Pantridge and gave him a copy to read. When I discussed the high early mortality with him, he just immediately, like a flash, said, 'Well, if that is so, that is what is happening in Belfast; we are just seeing the tip of the iceberg. We must go out and get these people.' So that is what we set out to do."

Pantridge and Geddes had to jerry-rig a portable defibrillator since such technology did not exist in 1966. Geddes worked primarily with members of the hospital maintenance department to develop the means of powering the defibrillator. The problem they faced was to convert a low DC voltage (from batteries) to a high AC voltage with sufficient current output to operate the defibrillator. A maintenance engineer suggested a static invertor and a successful test of the idea took place in October 1965. The defibrillator they used in the first MICU was a standard American Optical machine, a large machine intended for hospital use that required electric line current to operate. It could, however, be operated from two twelve-volt car batteries connected through a static invertor. The defibrillator could be unplugged from batteries and taken into a house when needed, but if there was no electricity, it would be very cumbersome to lug the batteries. But if an electrical supply was present, which almost invariably it was, then the line-operated machine was easily connected to the wall supply. Today emergency medical service programs use small, lightweight battery-powered heart monitors and defibrillators. The heavy, clumsy defibrillators available in 1966 actually prompted Pantridge to develop his own portable defibrillator that was eventually manufactured and weighed a mere seven pounds.

Pantridge's new program began service on January 1, 1966. The first call was not received until January 6 at 5:30 in the afternoon. A general practitioner requested the unit for an elderly woman with chest tightness and shortness of breath. Geddes arrived to find her having a myocardial infarction complicated by a degree of heart failure. After appropriate treatment, no further complications occurred and the patient recovered. The only problem involved Geddes's irritation at the ambulance driver who wanted to go off duty and the nurse who wasn't there. Because of the time of day, a nurse could not be spared from the hospital. Ironically, this first call was the only time a nurse did not accompany the unit. Pantridge wanted the system to go full steam ahead and be widely publicized. Geddes, however, urged caution, since he didn't want it overwhelmed. To control the usage, Geddes insisted that he and Pantridge speak before small groups of family physicians. The service was designed to be activated by family physicians since patients with chest pain usually called their family doctor. The physician could then call an easy-to-remember number—2-44-44—that was a hot line direct to a phone in the nursing station of the hospital coronary-care unit. Usually a nurse, sometimes a doctor, answered and, if indicated, would call the ambulance quarters in the hospital grounds to request the MICU. "Send around the ambulance," was the usual order. They would then give the driver the address and other details after the team was enroute. The driver then picked up the doctor and nurse, often a senior medical student as well, and traveled with sirens blaring to the requested address. The nurses liked being assigned to the mobile ambulance since it was relatively light duty—having only one patient at a time was certainly easier than ward duty.

The program received much interest from newspapers and magazines. The *Sunday Telegraph* and *TV Times*, both national papers, ran glowing stories. For inexplicable reasons the mobile coronary-care unit received virtually no coverage in the Belfast newspapers until 1973 when funding cuts placed its future in jeopardy. Though the local media ignored the Belfast program, *Time* magazine appreciated its uniqueness. A story in its September 1, 1967, issue entitled "Medicine Immediate Countershock" stated:

> Top U.S. government physicians believe that in the case of at least one patient with a heart-attack history, namely Lyndon Johnson, the equip-

ment [a defibrillator] should be installed in his home—The White House. Since that is not practicable for Everyman, the alternative is to rush the equipment to the patient.

There is just one place in the world where that is being done consistently and effectively—Northern Ireland's dour capital city of Belfast . . . To Dr. Pantridge, it seemed silly to keep the intensive care unit in the hospital. The thing to do, he reasoned, was to take both equipment and expertise to the patient as fast as possible; he installed the gear in an ambulance. Now, a telephone call to the Royal Victoria gets the mobile intensive-care unit to the patient's door promptly—in four out of five cases, within 15 minutes. Out step a doctor and a nurse, usually with two medical students, armed with life-saving devices with which they give the most urgent emergency care.

Though the Belfast doctors make a fetish of avoiding "haste or fuss," the patient is soon on his way to the hospital in the mobile unit, with his heart monitored all the way. If it stops en route the doctors can restart it, just as they would in the hospital. The unit has proved so effective that in its first 15 months of operation not one of the 312 heart patients taken to the Royal Victoria has died in transit.[9]

The first successful resuscitation actually did not occur until ten months after the program began. Recalled Geddes: "I resuscitated the first survivor. He was a previously healthy male of about forty-five to fifty. At about 7:00 P.M. on an October evening I and the team, which included two medical students, arrived in a small second-floor bedroom to find the man with a pulse rate and blood pressure both around forty, with clear evidence of acute myocardial infarction on his ECG, which showed complete heart block. An infusion of isoproterenol increased his rate and blood pressure, but he developed an accelerating VT (ventricular tachycardia). At that point I sent the driver and nurse down to the ambulance to bring the defibrillator. When this had been unplugged from its socket and brought to the bedroom, the students tried to plug it in, since the patient was now in VF (ventricular fibrillation).

"There were then two sizes of wall sockets, fifteen and five amps. To overcome this potential source of delay, we had a so-called "Universal" adaptor on the defibrillator's cable. This was a flimsy piece of apparatus and it disintegrated when an attempt was made to plug it in. On my direction the students ripped the wires from what remained of the adaptor and each pushed a wire into the relevant hole in the wall (I don't think they connected the

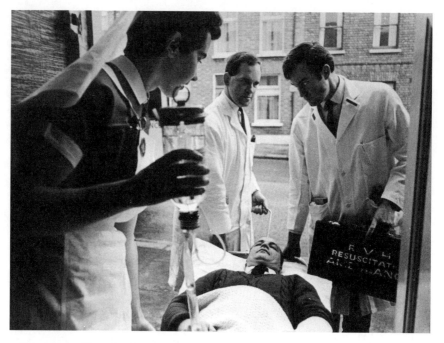

FIGURE 35. *Transferring patient from his home to the Belfast Mobile Intensive Care Unit (not pictured). Nurse Marlynne Kingston, Doctor John S. Geddes, and a medical student (left to right) (Courtesy of John S. Geddes)*

ground), making it possible to charge and operate the defibrillator successfully. The patient reverted to complete heart block. In order to stabilize him I inserted a bipolar pacing electrode via a left antecubital vein, succeeding in reaching the right ventricle blindly. This was no easy task. The enormous bed on which he was lying almost completely filled the small room, and I had to perform the procedure literally on my knees on the bed beside him. He was then transferred to hospital with pacing in progress, and later recovered normal conduction.

"He survived for only three weeks because of later rhythm problems. Still, it was our first resuscitation, and everybody was very excited."

We know today that sudden death resulting from ventricular fibrillation can be the end result of three conditions. One is myocardial infarction, another is ischemia or a temporary reduction in blood supply to a coronary artery, and the third is primary fibrillation without any symptoms. All three conditions exhibit the presence of an underlying coronary artery disease; in other words, there is atherosclerotic disease in the heart's arteries. But these conditions, especially the latter two, may give very little or no warning of impending fibrillation. The Belfast system was established to reach the first category of patients. The resuscitated patients were usually those whose hearts fibrillated after the ambulance was at the scene. The system reacted too slowly to resuscitate persons who fibrillated before the call was placed. It would require innovations in the system to reach the person who suddenly collapsed in cardiac arrest. That breakthrough took place not in Ireland but in North America.

What if John Colven's cardiac arrest had occurred in Belfast in 1967? Would he have survived? Certainly he would have had a better chance than in any other city, but because of the type of his arrest, the answer is most certainly "no." Colven's heart went into primary ventricular fibrillation with no symptoms of myocardial infarction or ischemia. There was no warning to trigger a call for help. The tiredness and fatigue he experienced were too vague to alert him or June of the impending danger. By the time June discovered that John had collapsed, called the MICU ambulance, and waited for it to arrive, too much time would have passed. And no CPR would have been performed at the scene. In 1967, few of the citizens of Belfast had been trained in CPR. Colven's brain would have been deprived of oxygen for too long. If Colven's ventricular fibrillation had been the result of an acute myocardial infarction, it is possible that help would have been summoned and the ambulance might have arrived at the moment of his collapse. Then he likely would have been counted as one of Pantridge's and Geddes's successes.

The team published the results of their program in the August 5, 1967, issue of *The Lancet* and reported their findings on 312 patients over a fifteen-month period. Half of the patients had a myocardial infarction and no deaths occurred during transportation. Of groundbreaking importance was the information on ten patients who had cardiac arrest. All had ventricular fibrillation and most arrests happened after the arrival of the MICU, though several took place prior to the ambulance's arrival. All ten patients were resuscitated and admitted to the hospital. Five were subsequently discharged alive. Pantridge and Geddes provide brief narratives of the ten resuscitations. The second resuscitation, typical of the others, reads: "A 55-year-old man developed chest pain while attending a meeting. He went home and summoned his doctor. The mobile unit was called. Ventricular fibrillation developed immediately after the patient was transferred to the ambulance. Defibrillation was achieved by a registrar (doctor). His period in hospital was uneventful and he was discharged on Dec. 6, 1966, and is now well."[10] The fifty-five-year-old man probably wasn't aware how historical his resuscitation was—he was simply happy to be alive.

Titled "A Mobile Intensive-Care Unit in the Management of Myocardial Infarction," the article assumed historical importance because it stimulated prehospital emergency cardiac-care programs throughout the world. August 1967 was exactly 200 years to the month from the founding of the Amsterdam Rescue Society. Both programs served as models for rescue efforts and each spawned dozens of similar programs. The rescue effort in 1767 in Amsterdam defined a collective will of society to attempt resuscitation for drowning victims, the prevalent form of sudden death in the eighteenth century. The rescue effort two centuries later in Belfast defined a successful way to achieve resuscitation for cardiac arrest, the sudden death of the twentieth century. It took 200 years for the way to be discovered and catch up with the will.

*Whatever America hopes to bring to pass in this world
must first come to pass in the heart of America.*
—Dwight D. Eisenhower

ACROSS THE ATLANTIC

« »

The *Lancet* has an extensive international readership, which helps explain why Pantridge's idea spread so fast to so many countries. Within two years similar programs began in Australia and Europe. Like the Belfast program, these also used physicians in the mobile intensive-care unit. William Grace started the first U.S. program in 1968, in New York City out of St. Vincent's Hospital in Greenwich Village. A program in Charlottesville, Virginia, begun by Richard Crampton soon followed. Both used specially equipped ambulances and placed physicians on board to provide advanced resuscitation care directly at the scene of cardiac emergencies.

William Grace

William Grace had visited Pantridge in Belfast, spent ten days learning about the program, and had actually gone out on emergency calls. John Geddes recalled Grace's visit, "He accompanied me on ward rounds in the CCU every morning and I was, as it turned out, quite needlessly in a state of some anxiety, as day after day this very senior individual listened intently but silently to the interpretations, opinions, and therapeutic decisions of a mere Registrar of less than two years' standing. Of course he did agree with what we were doing and set up his own mobile unit in New York along virtually identical lines."

Shortly after returning to New York City, Grace set about establishing an MICU patterned after the Belfast unit. Grace purchased some equipment with a small federal grant from the Regional Medical Program. This was one of Lyndon Johnson's "Great Society" efforts designed to attack heart disease, stroke, and cancer. The ambulance operated in the "catchment area" of St. Vincent's Hospital and Medical Center of New York, a radius running from 34th Street to Canal Street, and from Fifth Avenue to the Hudson River. Calls for medical emergencies in which chest pain was a complaint were passed on from the police 911 operator to the hospital. From there the ambulance would fight New York traffic to arrive at the scene. On board—besides the driver and his assistant—were an attending physician, resident physician, emergency room nurse, ECG technician, and a student nurse observer. A personal pager summoned each member of the team from throughout the hospital to the emergency department. Said Grace, "This team has four and one-half minutes to get to the emergency room, obtain their equipment and board the ambulance. Anyone who is not there within this time is left behind."[1]

Grace described the program's initial results in serving the first 161 patients. Only two instances occurred in which the doctor did not make the four-and-a-half minute deadline and the ambulance left without him. The ambulance usually reached the scene within fourteen minutes (plus of course the pre-response time). One call took twenty-five minutes because of heavy traffic. Among the first group of patients seen by the MICU were three people treated for ventricular fibrillation. One of the three survived.[2]

John Chadbourne, a cardiologist tapped by Dr. Grace to help run the program, vividly recalls one of his first saves. The call came in requesting the mobile unit for a forty-two-year-old man who had collapsed at home. When the unit arrived at the scene, Chadbourne and a nurse attached the monitor leads to the man's chest. Chadborne looked up at the monitor to see a disorganized wavering line. He asked the nurse to reattach the loose lead but she reassured him that they were all properly attached. If it wasn't a loose lead, then it had to be ventricular fibrillation. Chadbourne moved quickly to provide the defibrillatory shocks. The man was resuscitated and later returned home to his wife and seven children. Thirty-five years later, Chadbourne recalls the event as though it happened yesterday. Matter-of-factly he notes, "I guess you could say we saved his life."

Like the Belfast program, the St. Vincent's MICU was not established to provide primary response for sudden cardiac arrest. Its primary purpose was to treat the early period of acute myocardial infarction. Ventricular fibrillation, if it occurred after arrival, could be managed, but if it happened before arrival resuscitation seldom resulted. The forty-two-year-old man was one of the lucky ones.

Richard Crampton

In 1968, Richard Crampton was visiting Ireland with his family. "I went to Ireland almost annually," Crampton explained. "I have an Irish wife and half-Irish children. So we would go over and visit the family there." On this particular visit Crampton came across Pantridge's *Lancet* article. He was impressed, and concluded that resuscitation and defibrillation outside the hospital walls could and should be done. Crampton decided to check it out for himself. So he went to Belfast, met Pantridge, got the tour of the Royal Victoria Hospital, and rode with the MICU on a call.

Crampton was on the faculty at Columbia University and had two full-time hospital positions, at St. Luke's Roosevelt and at Lenox Hill, setting up their coronary-care units. Crampton had already had significant contact with William Grace—in fact, Crampton's superior, Robert Case, had urged Crampton to take Grace's course in coronary care. Crampton went to the course, met Grace and his colleagues—and ended up being invited to teach in the course. "I jumped from being a student one year to being on the faculty the next."

Meanwhile, Grace had moved ahead with his plans to begin a prehospital intensive-care unit in New York City. Crampton had liked what he had seen in Belfast; had been impressed by the work he had heard about; and was inspired by the efforts of Bill Grace. He began pressing the administors at Lenox Hill Hospital to consider establishing a mobile cardiac-care unit. The hospital, however, didn't buy into the mobile emergency care concept. "Lenox Hill already had its own private ambulance in those days," said Crampton, "which responded to emergency calls. And there were other specters hanging over it. One important one was costs. Another was simply that people didn't think it would work."

At about the same time his suggestions were falling on deaf ears at Lenox Hill, Crampton got a job offer he decided he couldn't refuse. The University of Virginia asked him to become the director of their coronary-care unit. Crampton accepted. "I realized," he said, "that in such a position I would have tremendous scope. I could do more" than what he'd been allowed at Lenox Hill.

When Crampton arrived at UV Hospital in 1969, he discovered a nearly ideal setup for a mobile intensive care unit. "The Charlottesville-Ablermoral Rescue Squad, which was our emergency medical service, was all volunteer," recalled Crampton. "It had been established in 1960, and there was no cost to the public. And they were open to try anything. They'd all learned Red Cross first aid, so the next step was to take them into CPR.

"We were able to get [our emergency response program] started in large part because of Bill Grace. He was aware of my interest in such a program, and he threw some grant money our way, through the Charles A. Fruealf Foundation," said Crampton. "The grant paid for the cost of a defibrillator and a bio-phone—the radio telemetry system."

By the end of 1970, Crampton's all-volunteer rescue squad was certified in CPR, and the new mobile cardiac response unit began operating in March 1971. Crampton staffed the unit with a resident physician and occasionally some nursing staff from the University of Virginia Hospital's emergency room. Though the Rescue Squad volunteers were enthusiastic, the "professionals" were not. "None of the cardiologists were enthusiastic. They sort of laughed at it. They felt it was impractical and that it wouldn't work."

The program started slowly, but not long after had its first important "save." "We had a prominent horse trainer undergo cardiac arrest at a horse show," Crampton recalled. "As you know, Virginia is a very prominent equestrian state. Anyway, the rescue squad defibrillated him, brought him to the hospital—and he became a long-term survivor." It was the first time such an event had happened in Charlottesville.

Crampton's setup used what he called "double teaming." "What that means," he said, "is that your rescue squad is at an ambulance depot. They get a call that Mr. Smith has collapsed at the shopping center or out at the farm. In those days," he added, "we didn't have '911.' Instead, everyone knew that if they dialed 295-1911, you'd get a pair of emergency service people there very quickly, in five minutes or less. So, they'd get the call and immediately send one ambulance straight out there with two people. Then they'd send a backup vehicle to the hospital emergency room and pick up the advanced life support equipment, and drive on out with it to the site. And if they thought it was a heart attack, the first ambulance would swing past the emergency room and pick up a physician."

Grace and Cramptom were innovators, but they were not revolutionaries. They imported a wonderful concept from overseas and made it work in their communities. The revolutionaries were Pantridge and Geddes. The New York and Charlottesville programs were pioneering efforts. Taking physicians and defibrillators and rushing through the city to reach a pulseless, non-breathing, comatose person was extremely unusual by 1969 standards. But these programs lacked a broader vision. They could work for some communities, but were not nationally applicable. For one thing, doctors were too expensive to be dedicated to standby status, waiting for an alarm to ring. This concept could conceivably work in cities with teaching hospitals where interns and residents in training form a potential, inexpensive pool for MICU staffing. Not every hospital or city had interns, and, more important, few hospitals could spare them. And since interns need supervision, who would watch the resuscitations? Would both an intern and supervising physician be required? It just wasn't practical. Nor was hiring fully trained physicians an economically realistic option.

What was needed was another conceptual breakthrough. Such a revolution in the management of sudden death happened almost simultaneously in five American cities.

RACING THE
ANGEL OF DEATH

《 》

Humanity's drive to cheat death took a giant step forward in 1969 and early 1970. That period witnessed a move from physician-staffed mobile intensive care units to paramedic-staffed units that took place independently and almost simultaneously in a handful of American cities. In each city the moving force for the change was a single person dedicated to saving lives: Eugene Nagel in Miami, Leonard Cobb in Seattle, Michael Criley in Los Angeles, Richard Lewis in Columbus, and Leonard Rose in Portland.

These men took a different approach to the problem of cardiac emergencies. Not only were paramedics used instead of physicians, but the programs were also established from the start to deal with the problem of sudden cardiac arrest. Pantridge's program was primarily established to reach the victim of myocardial infarction fast and thereby prevent mortality in the vulnerable early period. Thus, cardiac arrest was successfully treated only if it occurred as a complication of MI and only if the MICU was already at the scene or on its way. Because a physician had to be in attendance and was not standing by ready to jump in the ambulance, it was not possible to reach the scene in a few minutes. Patients with chest pain could not call the Royal Victoria Hospital and summon the special ambulance. First, they had to call their physician, who paid a house call and then requested the MICU. Occasionally, the emergency dispatcher could request the MICU for patients by calling 999 (similar to 911 in the United States) directly.

The programs in Miami, Seattle, Los Angeles, Columbus, and Portland were specifically designed not only to treat the early complications of MI but to attempt resuscitation for sudden cardiac arrest wherever and whenever it occurred. The U.S. paramedic programs thus carried Pantridge's concept one step further. Not only would medical technicians treat MIs in order to prevent cardiac arrest (and treat cardiac arrest should it occur after arrival), but reversal of death itself became a major purpose and goal. Because time was so crucial, patients or bystanders could summon the paramedics directly.

Several programs already had a strong base—their fire department ambulance service. In each city it was possible to build on that base and provide special training for firefighters and create paramedics. Using paramedical personnel took advantage of the strengths of the communities. This was not a conscious rejection of the Pantridge physician-based model, but an opportunity to take advantage of emergency services already in place and upgrade them.

Eugene Nagel: The First of Many

The Miami program was the first paramedic program in the United States. In addition to pioneering paramedical personnel, the program is noteworthy for using telemetry that allowed physicians to supervise care from a remote base-station hospital. The chain of events leading up to the service actually predates the Belfast program.

In 1962, when Eugene Nagel was a second-year resident in anesthesia at New York's Columbia-Presbyterian Hospital, one of the senior doctors suggested he look into something apparently new in the medical field that the doctor thought Nagel would find useful. It was called CPR.

Nagel's immediate reaction was a bit mixed. "I had not heard about it," he said. "Kouwenhoven and Jude's article had appeared in 1960, but I didn't know about it at the time. Well, this guy was prestigious and he was one of my bosses, so I said, 'Yes, sir.'"

Nagel wasn't sure where he was going to land after his residency at Columbia-Presbyterian. On the one hand, he had a hankering for a department head opening at Roosevelt Hospital in New York. It was a clinical position, and that appealed to him. On the other hand, he also was leaning toward another job in Florida at the University of Miami. It was an academic position, but "I had not really committed myself to academics," Nagel later commented. One thing Nagel did know: in either job, learning about the newly developed CPR technique would probably prove useful. "So off I went to learn it without really knowing what it was or why I was doing it."

Nagel took the Roosevelt position—and then quickly left it to go to Miami, despite his ambivalence about academia. "I figured I didn't want to be an academician because I thought I didn't want to do research," Nagel recalled. But there he was, at the University of Miami teaching anesthesia. It was all a bit baffling. "I had no clear picture," he said, "that I would stay or that I would enjoy it or that I would do well." In other words, Eugene Nagel was a newly married young man who, like many young people, still didn't have a good idea of What He Wanted To Do With His Life.

And as with so many other young people, the answer came looking for him. "I was invited to speak at a meeting of the International First Aid and Rescue Association," Nagel said, which was meeting in January 1964 at Miami Beach. He got the invitation because he was a member of the CPR Committee at Jackson Memorial Hospital. CPR was a hot topic, and Nagel was the local "expert." He shook his head at the memory of that meeting. "I don't even know what I talked about," he said. "And I was surrounded by a large number of equally befuddled doctors talking about bone injuries, this injury and that injury—talking to a group of largely laypeople who had absolutely no authority to do things like set splints and so on."

Later that year, James Jude became Chief of Cardiovascular Surgery at the University of Miami's Jackson Memorial Hospital. His arrival lit a fire under Nagel. "Suddenly I had the guru of CPR in my hospital," he recalled. Jude introduced some enthusiasm and organization to the CPR program at Jackson Memorial and made Nagel his de facto right-hand man. The CPR training he had done at Columbia-Presbyterian now became very important to Nagel and his career.

Shortly after the association meeting, Nagel visited Fire Station No. 1 and introduced himself. The Captain seemed genuinely interested in Nagel's proposal to teach CPR. Several men had years of experience at doing rescue— but practically no training. Nagel still had a lot to teach them about other aspects of resuscitation. "They were like eager sponges, willing to learn anything that made some sense to them. They knew almost as much as I did about the art of CPR. But there were facets of the resuscitation management, the airway particularly, that they were a little bit 'foggy' on, and we worked together very well," said Nagel. This connection with the fire department was one he thoroughly enjoyed—he loved to teach and be taught. Nagel later recalled his warm feeling toward his fire department students, "Their enthusiasm was infectious from the beginning. It was like a bonding. If they knew something from their experience that you did not know, they would share it, but it was not done in a 'I'll put you down' kind of way."

Because of Nagel's persistence and support, the fire department began to routinely initiate CPR in the field and bring patients to the emergency department. But this only created larger problems since the rescue personnel invariably faced a disinterested physician. Nagel observed, "We never seemed to save what we would call a true cardiac arrest. We'd bring them in in ventricular fibrillation and very often the doctor in the ER wouldn't even put the patient on the monitor (we didn't have quick look paddles in those days). The docs in the ER, I would say 75 percent, when you'd rush one in doing CPR, would tell you to quit and say he's dead. Disgustedly he would say this and ask 'Why are you bothering me?' This was very discouraging to the rescue guys." Just as stultifying was the lousy CPR on those cases in which the emergency department would take over. Nagel described these cases. "The firemen would come in trying to do 60 chest compressions a minute, interposed one breath every five—you'd come in under strict guidelines, depress the sternum one to two inches—you'd immediately get elbowed aside and somebody would be pushing with about as much compression as would dent a grape on the sternum and the ventilation would be abysmal." Nagel was determined to have some real saves. And if the ER docs wouldn't do it, he would have to look to his men in the community.

Nagel developed a camaraderie with the firefighters, rescue personnel, and their immediate superiors. However, his relationship with the Miami fire chief was not terribly simpatico. "When I conceived the idea of rescue personnel being able to do more than just CPR and first aid, and before I wrote a grant, I obviously had to discuss it with him," said Nagel. "His apprehensions were apparent from the beginning. It was clear he had deep reservations about going too far." The chief's greatest concern was that his department look good, that it excel and be a leader—and that it not fall flat on its face in some new experimental exercise and publicly disgrace itself. Nagel recalled one meeting: "I told the fire chief that I wanted to train the guys in defibrillation; they would not do it unless I was there. A big, tall, 6'3" Irishman by the name of Lawrence Kenny, he had been quite tolerant of me up to now. He took his finger and he punched me in the chest and drove me back about three feet with his one finger. He said, 'This is a fire department, not a hospital; these are firemen and not doctors. I don't want you to forget that.' Every time he would say something, he would punch me again in the chest with his finger which hurt a lot. I think that I probably got the idea."

For Nagel, that meant taking small steps instead of giant leaps. "So it was a selling job," Nagel explained. "We had to sell it to the medical community, to the medical school, to my department, to the fire department and especially the chief, and to the people he represented, which were the city commissioners."

In 1967, Nagel became aware of Pantridge's work. He believed that the Pantridge model of a doctor-staffed pre-hospital mobile intensive care unit was not going to work for the United States in general or Miami in particular. Nagel was focused on cardiac arrest and minutes were crucial. He became convinced that it was time to move away from a doctor-staffed setup to a paramedic one.

Nagel did not think he could initially sell the idea of paramedics working alone, even if they had authorization to perform medical procedures signed by physicians. "I saw no hope of a standing operating procedure," he recalled. "That would have been a major jump, and I didn't think I could sell it to anybody. But the fact that I, or a doctor like me, could be on the radio and give specific verbal orders to a fireman to perform a specific maneuver he'd been trained to do—well, that seemed semi-OK to the medical school and the fire chief."

So Nagel's first step was radio and telemetry.[1] Refined in the space program, telemetry allowed mission control in Houston to monitor each astronaut's heart rate. With minor modifications, it was just the technology Nagel needed to make his case. Nagel was joined by Jim Hirschman, a cardiologist who was an experienced amateur radio expert and interested in Nagel's telemetry effort. But before he could sell the need for defibrillation and medications, Nagel had to prove the existence of ventricular fibrillation—and that the ECG signal could be sent from the field to the hospital. Telemetry was something the fire chief could accept because it seemed unlikely to hurt the patient or embarrass the department. The firefighters on the rescue squad couldn't do anything else, though—no drug administration, no defibrillation. "What we did in Miami was to gradually systematize a lot of situations. Eventually, we gave the paramedics permission to do a number of things without radio contact," explained Nagel. "That included IVs, obviously, and then certain drugs in certain sequences." But for the first couple of years, it was one tiny step at a time.

During the initial telemetry experiments, the signal from the rescue unit went through the fire department voice channel and by phone line to Nagel's office in Jackson Memorial Hospital. When the system's practicality was proven, the receiving terminal was transferred to the post-anesthesia recovery unit where residents were on call twenty-four hours a day. As supervisors Nagel and Hirschman alternated being on call every other night. The telemetry was an ECG-modulated voice channel, and Nagel became accomplished at the art of using his ear to interpret the sound signal coming over the phone so he could diagnose the patient's heart rhythm. According to Nagel, there was no mistaking the absolutely unique sound pattern of ventricular fibrillation—once likened by him to a mezzo-soprano being goosed with an icicle during an aria. Hirschman, a cardiologist, wanted to see exactly what the rhythm was, and converted the sound waves into ECG signals. He could then read and diagnose the rhythm on standard ECG paper. The telemetry documented the rhythm causing the cardiac arrest, but for the first year there was no means of defibrillating the patient. Nagel knew the consequences of not being able to electrically shock ventricular fibrillation, "As soon as we got telemetry, it didn't take us very long to see that if it was VF in the field, they were not going to be successful without further treatment."

By the beginning of 1968, the fire rescue squads had a year of experience using telemetry and radio contact with Nagel and other doctors. Nagel in turn had a solid year's worth of telemetry data to use for his ongoing sales pitches to the fire chief and his superiors. By now Nagel had ingratiated himself with the chief and he made his request again. "I wanted to go to the City of Miami and I wanted to go to the University of Miami, with his permission, and ask that the fire rescue guys be allowed to defibrillate in the street. Whereas in '66 I got punched in the chest; in '68 I got a lot of lecture and a lot of moaning and groaning, but he finally said OK, that we would go together in front of the City Commission and we would go together in front of the Research Committee at the University of Miami and see if we could get permission for the experimental—that's what it was—work." They approved.

Nagel then began training firefighters in the use of defibrillators. At about the same time, he received a grant from the Florida Heart Association and was able to purchase additional equipment. With the chief's permission, he moved forward and bought a Physio-Control Lifepak 33 defibrillator in late 1968. "It was probably the first one they produced," he recalled with a smile. "That Physico Control unit lasted about one week and every nut, bolt, and screw fell out of it. I sent this bag of nuts, bolts, and parts back to Seattle and

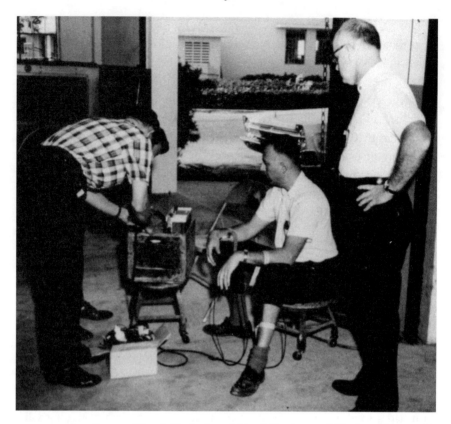

FIGURE 36. *Eugene Nagel (sitting) and Jim Hirschman MD (standing at his right), testing electrocardiogram telemetry equipment in 1967. Telemetry paved the way for Miami paramedics in 1969 to defibrillate patients without needing physicians at the scene. (Courtesy of Eugene Nagel)*

Hunter (Simpson), the head of Physio-Control, had one of his people come down and ride on the truck. We had only one rescue in the city of Miami. The truck was vintage World War II and it was the most rough riding thing I had ever been on, and it shook the hell out of all of our equipment. As a result of that, they went back and redesigned the Lifepak 33 and used lock washers and glyptol and other things so the unit wouldn't shake apart. They shock mounted certain delicate assemblies and whatever. It worked." It's fortunate that Physio-Control was able to improve their device because there wasn't much else on the market to choose from. The only other "portable" defibrillator weighed sixty-five pounds.

By 1969 Nagel and the fire rescue squads were going "full-bore" (as he phrased it). The City of Miami Rescue Unit quickly expanded to three trucks, and the annual number of rescue calls jumped from 8000 to 15,000. Nagel then asked the chief to authorize the paramedics to carry out IVs. This sales job involved a dramatic presentation, Nagel recalled. "I let a paramedic start an IV in me, lying on a table in front of the city commissioners at a public meeting," he said. "There were a lot of people in the audience including the chief. I told the commissioners that these men had been well trained, and that I had as much confidence in them as I did in most of the people at the hospital. And that did it. They accepted it." Once the struggle for intravenous lines had been won, Nagel surprisingly had no difficulty convincing the chief to allow medications.

Nagel had a more difficult job selling the chief on intubation (the placement of a tube down the throat and into the trachea). To Nagel, the need for intubation was obvious; someone in cardiac arrest does not breathe and the tube allows oxygen to reach the lungs. Without intubation, it was too easy for the tongue to block the air passage or vomit or saliva to clog up the trachea. Intubation was not without risk. If the tube was inserted down the esophagus instead of the trachea, it would make a critical situation even worse. But Nagel, confident in his skills as an anesthesiologist, knew he could teach the procedure. To overcome Chief Kenny's reluctance, Nagel trained nine paramedics using dummies and visited the morgue to practice on unclaimed bodies.

The chief had heard of the visits to the morgue and, according to Nagel, "made complaining sounds in his throat, much like a bear waking up in the spring." But since Nagel didn't hear a flat-out "no," he decided to proceed with training using live humans. As Nagel recalled, "Finally one memorable night I enlisted one of our residents, Harry Heinitsch. Harry was the perfect candidate for me to ask since he enjoyed scuba diving to extreme depths, jumping out of planes, and other ways to endanger his life. So why not cater to his obvious death wish? We sprayed each other with topical anesthetic. I then intubated Harry, awake, demonstrating the technique. All nine paramedics then intubated Harry successfully. Harry then intubated me and the paramedics followed his lead." Nagel describes himself as a prodigious gagger, claiming that "even looking at a tongue blade makes me gag." But liberal amounts of anesthetic got him through the evening, and neither Nagel nor the resident reported even so much as a sore throat. The following morning he presented the results of the evening's training; the chief remonstrated weakly, but finally conceded that the paramedics had demonstrated proficiency and allowed them to intubate.

It should not be surprising that the medical directors of the various paramedic programs would remember the first resuscitation in their city. Nagel vividly recalled Miami's first save. The collapse occurred near Station 1, on the fringe of the downtown area, where the tony part of town meets the underside. He reminisced: "There was a well-known alcoholic named Dan Jones who was then about sixty years old. He lived in a rooming house near our rescue unit. Dan Jones was familiar to the guys since they had hauled him to Jackson Memorial Hospital on several occasions. In June of '69 they got a call—man down. It was Dan Jones. They put the paddles on him, he was in VF, started CPR, zapped him, he came back to a regular rhythm, brought him in to ER and three days later he was out and walking around. In gratitude, about a week later, he came down to Station 1, which he had never done before, and he said he would like to talk to the man who saved his life. They told me they had never seen Dan Jones in a clean shirt and sober, both of which he was that day. He would periodically come to the fire house and just say hello and he seemed to be sober. In my talks in those days I said this was the new cure for alcoholism. That was our first true save."

Nagel recalls that there was much exchange of information among the pioneers of prehospital cardiac-care programs. "There was a lot of movement in this country. People came to Miami, Criley came to Miami—I'm not sure if Leonard [Cobb] did or one of his people. And we went to Columbus, Ohio, to see Warren's system. . . . We were talking with Grace. It was like a small town. If you have ever lived in a very small town—everything they did, we knew; everything we did, they knew. It was a very close community. There was obviously competition, no question about it, but there was, I think, very free passage of information."

Leonard Cobb and "Medic 1"

Draw a diagonal across the country from Miami and you come to Seattle. Nagel's program began in early 1969, and Leonard Cobb's effort in Seattle hit the streets a year later. The two cities thus anchored the national move to paramedic-staffed emergency medical services. Seattle's program is renowned for the use of a tiered response system (sending the closest aid unit simultaneously with the paramedic unit) and the training of its citizens in CPR. Numerous articles and news shows (including *60 Minutes*) refer to Seattle as the best place in the nation to have a heart attack—the published survival rates following out-of-hospital cardiac arrest in Seattle, and surrounding

King County, Washington, are consistently the highest in the world. The Seattle program was also one of the first in the nation and its preeminence is due to the determination of a cardiologist, Leonard Cobb, working in tandem with a fire chief, Gordon Vickery.

Leonard Arthur Cobb was born on June 23, 1926, in St. Paul, Minnesota. At age seventeen, he enlisted in the Navy. Much of his naval service took place stateside, in "exotic locales" such as Chicago and Houston; he rose to the rank of Electronics Technician's Mate Third Class, and was honorably discharged in 1946.

Like many young returning veterans, Cobb plunged into college after the war. He entered the University of Minnesota in 1946 and then went on to medical school. He graduated in 1952, and after working as a medical resident at UC San Francisco and a cannery worker in Alaska, went to Switzerland in 1953, where he studied metabolism at the University of Zurich.

Cobb returned to the United States in 1954 and a series of medical positions in San Francisco, Boston, and Stanford. In 1957 the University of Washington in Seattle offered Cobb a teaching position at the then prestigious salary of $7000 a year. By 1964 Cobb had put down roots in Seattle and was head of cardiology at Harborview Hospital.

For Leonard Cobb, the immediate spur to move from dreams to action came in 1967 when he read the article by Belfast's Frank Pantridge in *The Lancet*. "I remember reading Pantridge's report," Cobb recalls, "and it was kind of interesting. I think it was the first time anyone had come forth with an organized effort to provide prehospital care for patients with cardiac disease."

Pantridge's article energized Cobb. He knew the Seattle Fire Department was already involved in first aid. Cobb looked up Fire Chief Gordon Vickery and discovered another helpful situation. The fire department already had effective systems for documenting first-aid runs. Cobb realized that they could provide scientific documentation for the efficacy (or lack thereof) of Pantridge's suggestions. Cobb suggested to Vickery that they pool their knowledge and resources. Vickery knew of Martin McMahon's work with the Baltimore Fire Department and felt it was time for Seattle to enter the world of resuscitation in a big way. A medical study recently completed in King County bolstered their resolve to change the way first aid was delivered to heart attack victims. The study had shown that deaths from coronary disease in King County in people under age fifty took place within an hour of the first symptoms in 63 percent of those fatalities. Less than a quarter of the victims lived long enough for a doctor to examine them.[2] The findings were similar to those that helped catalyze the Belfast program.

Armed with these statistics, Cobb and several medical colleagues first sought a grant in 1967 to fund a program in Seattle building on Pantridge's work in Belfast. It was turned down. They tried again, and succeeded. "In 1968 we got a grant from the Washington/Alaska Regional Medical Program," says Cobb. Cobb and his colleagues specifically requested funds to start a mobile intensive coronary care unit and were awarded $450,000 for a three-year period. The funding primarily paid the salaries for fifteen firefighters to be trained as paramedics. Salaries were then approximately $10,000 a year. The first goal was to save lives. Their second was to see if nonphysicians really could carry out resuscitation and management of cardiac arrest. If successful, this approach would be a major change in the role of a fire department. Their third goal was to try and learn more about sudden cardiac death.

Cobb ran into considerable skepticism from his own colleagues. Members of the King County Medical Society and the Red Cross thought his idea was a waste of time—the Red Cross was then still on record as opposed to teaching CPR to the general public.

Cobb and Vickery pressed ahead. With money from the grant, the fire department purchased a mobile intensive-care unit and one of the deputy fire chiefs personally drove it from the Midwest back to Seattle. The "mobile unit" they got was actually a motor home with rounded sides, an Oldsmobile Toronado engine, and front-wheel drive. It had a kitchen sink, hot and cold running water, a refrigerator and freezer, and a toilet. The mobile unit soon acquired several nicknames—Wonder Bread Van, The Red Van, and Moby Pig.

The toilet was soon replaced by other equipment. The conversion from motor home to mobile intensive-care unit was all done on intuition and inspiration. The unit ended up with a huge coronary-care console installed and carried then-state-of-the-art portable DC defibrillators and all the necessary tubes and medications. A patient stretcher sat in the center, surrounded by the technology to keep the person alive. The first group of trained medics helped construct the mobile unit. They also took part in devising protocols for treatment, copying much from then-current practices in hospital CCUs.

In mid-1969, Vickery began looking for firefighters to volunteer for the new mobile unit, and in October helped select Seattle's first fifteen medics. Cobb personally supervised their training. It wasn't exactly clear what to teach them since there was no precedent to follow. Cobb put together a com-monsense curriculum that included ECG rhythm interpretation, defibrilla-tion, emergency administration of medication , and IV use. The training lasted a few months, and took place mostly at Harborview Hospital.

In March 1970 the first class of paramedics—as they had begun calling themselves—took to the streets of Seattle. An official ceremony launching the vehicle took place at City Hall, but none of the first group of fifteen actu-ally received a "diploma"—they just started saving lives.

"We were like sponges," says Greg Brace, one of the first group trained by Cobb. "When we first started riding, we knew how to do CPR, but not really. I mean, it's one thing to know how to do it 'in your head,' and still another to actually have a real patient lying there."

The mobile unit—and there was only one at first—was stationed outside the Harborview Hospital emergency room. As Cobb himself points out, the mobile unit was not the real innovation—it was the concept of a "tiered response" to medical emergencies. The idea was "that we would get someone out there quickly"—via the fire department's already-existing mobile first aid units—"and then a secondary response would come from the mobile inten-sive coronary care unit." The beauty of the tiered response system was the efficient use of fire department personnel. The system allowed aid personnel to reach the scene quickly, on an average of three minutes, to start CPR. A few minutes later paramedics arrived to provide more definitive care such as defibrillation. In this way the brain could be kept alive until the electric shock converted the heart to a normal rhythm. After the patient was stabi-lized, the paramedics would transport the person to the hospital.

From the very start, Cobb was sensitive to the politics and economics of resuscitation. He wanted the support of the medical community and did nothing to jeopardize the doctor-patient relationship. The policy was to transport the patient to the hospital of his or her choice. Cobb considered the consequences if such a policy didn't exist. "If we had said we're going to take all these patients, resuscitated patients, to Harborview, the doctors for sure would be moaning and groaning. We've bent over backwards to be sure that we do not interfere with doctor-patient relationships. . . . The doctor would be resentful if people were out there trying to scoop up their patients, so to speak, and taking them somewhere else."

Today Cobb's mobile cardiac-care unit is known as Medic 1. In fact, that's the generic name used in many communities to identify such mobile emer-gency units. The name itself originated with Gordon Vickery. As Cobb recalls, "Vickery and I were talking one day, soon after the big rig had arrived. And we were wondering what to call this. The rig itself had this huge name on its side—Seattle Fire Department Mobile Intensive/Coronary Care Unit. We started pondering acronyms like 'MCCU.' Vickery said, 'Well, in our engine companies we all have number designations'—like Engine Company 34 and so on—'so why don't we call this one 'Medic 1'? And that sounded fine to me."

For the first nine months, the paramedics had a doctor aboard on their emergency runs. Cobb used the physicians as a kind of safety net and a reassurance to the medical community, but it was always his intent to run the program with paramedics. Before the year was out, the paramedics were on their own. The physician was miles away at the base-station hospital, though voice connection by radio or phone was always an option. One critical skill learned from working with the doctors was how to put in tracheal tubes. This was not on the initial training agenda, but it soon became apparent that tracheal tube insertion was a vital resuscitation skill. There were concerns, Cobb admits. "But it was obvious after about a day and a half that it worked just fine" without doctors on the runs.

During the first year Cobb's experiment resuscitated sixty-one patients; thirty-one survived long enough to leave the hospital. One of those made national news, on CBS's *60 Minutes*. The *60 Minutes* crew came to Seattle to film a segment on the burgeoning citizen CPR program and rode with the unit, filming several resuscitations. The one that made the program was a resuscitation of a woman with multiple sclerosis.

The word was starting to spread nationally. But within Seattle the program was in jeopardy—problems with funding occurred even before it celebrated its third anniversary. The initial funding grant had to absorb a 25-percent cut, leaving the total grant of $450,000 over $100,000 short. The city would not make up the difference and reminded Cobb that the grant had promised funding for a full three years. Cobb and Vickery decided to do their own fund-raising. It was not a big fancy corporate or institutional campaign and Cobb was initially skeptical. He later recalled, "Initially I said, oh my God, we've got to go out with a hat on the corner and beg people to allow us to stay in business. In retrospect it was okay, but at the time it sure didn't seem like that was a very good idea." The newspapers supported the effort with front-page thermometers showing the progress of the campaign. It was a real grass roots effort—barbers donated a day's earnings, car dealers gave money, teenagers put on walk-a-thons in the city, donation jars were set up in malls. Over $200,000 was raised, double the amount needed to keep the program in business.

The Seattle paramedic program did more than pioneer paramedics and develop a tiered-response system. It was the first program in the world to make citizens an active part of the emergency system. Cobb reasoned that the best way to ensure early initiation of CPR was to train bystanders. Along with the support of Vickery, Cobb began a program in 1972 called Medic 2 with the goal of training over 100,000 people. Cobb recalled how the idea was first proposed. "One day he [Vickery] said, 'Look, if it's so important to get CPR started quickly and if firemen come around to do it, it can't be that complicated that other folks couldn't also learn—firemen are not created by God to do CPR. You could train the public.' I said, 'That sounds like a very good idea.' Shortly afterwards the program started." Cobb decided to use an abbreviated course. He later described how the training was set up. "We weren't going to do it by traditional ways where they had to come for twenty hours or thereabouts. So they had to do it at one sitting—how long will people participate? Well, maybe three hours. And that's pretty much the way it was." Cobb cautiously did not state how long it would take to train 100,000 people—he had no idea. In fact it took only a few years. By the twentieth anniversary of the Medic 2 program, over 500,000 people in Seattle and its surrounding suburbs had received CPR training.

As with the paramedic program, Cobb's plan to train the public in CPR encountered skepticism. The critics were silenced thanks to some fortunate saves. Cobb recalled one resuscitation, involving a fifty-four-year-old man, soon after the Medic 2 program began. "In March '73 there were these kids playing golf at Jackson Park. They came across a victim a quarter of a mile from the clubhouse—so these kids had taken the CPR course over at the local high school. Two or three of them began doing CPR and the other kid ran off and phoned the fire department. Shortly they came with the aid car and Medic 1 screaming over the fairways." The man was in ventricular fibrillation and required three shocks to be converted to a regular heart rhythm. Cobb concluded the story, "They got him started up again. He survived; he's alive today [1990]. That was a very convincing story. I didn't mind it being written up in the *Reader's Digest.*"

"I think," Cobb said, "there were skeptics all along who didn't have much belief in CPR, resuscitation, or even CCUs. . . . Basically we took stuff that was on the shelves already and did some packaging of it and made some modifications. We didn't have to develop CPR—CPR was done in 1960; we didn't have to develop a portable defibrillator—it was already there. . . . We just put a good package together."

Michael Criley and the Hollywood Paramedics

Los Angeles was another pioneer in the use of paramedics. In 1969 nearly seven million people lived in Los Angeles County, more than 3.5 percent of the American population. A young doctor named J. Michael Criley was concerned about the way many of those people were going to die. Criley was thirty-eight, and on the faculty in the department of medicine at the University of California, Los Angeles. He was also head of the Cardiology Division at Harbor General Hospital in Torrance, a county hospital affiliated with the UCLA Department of Medicine. He had come to Harbor General in 1967 and set up their first Cardiac Care Unit. Criley knew that, based on prevailing medical statistics, some 20,000 people in L.A. County would likely die of cardiovascular disease that year. Probably over half would die outside a hospital. Worse, some 5000 to 10,000 would succumb despite having "a heart too good to die"—that is, as a result of potentially reversible cardiac conditions. Criley determined to do something about it.

He had been aware for a couple of years of the work in Belfast by Frank Pantridge. At first, however, Criley felt almost overwhelmed by the prospect of making it work in Los Angeles. "All I could think of," he recalled, "was how vast the Los Angeles base was compared to Belfast, and how difficult it would be to have that many doctors and nurses that could be geared up to respond. It seemed impossible." Of course, there were also possible political difficulties. "There are 80 cities within the boundaries of Los Angeles County, and all these different jurisdictions," noted Criley.

By early 1969 Criley felt a bit differently. He had heard of a similar program being tried in Florida that used specially trained firefighters, or paramedics, to administer emergency cardiac aid. He started wondering if the same system could be set up in the Los Angeles area. It would use the services of existing L.A. County Fire Department rescue squads, which were, as Criley put it, "busy doing things like rescuing cats from trees."

Criley discussed this idea with Les Smith, the Administrator at Harbor General Hospital. Smith was not only an ambitious young administrator, he also knew whom to talk to. He approached the hierarchy in the Los Angeles County Department of Health, and started gaining their interest and support.

At about the same time, someone else was attacking the problem. Walter Graf, president of the local chapter of the American Heart Association, was also the personal physician for Kenneth Hahn, chairman of the County Board of Supervisors and one of the most powerful politicians in California. Hahn got Graf the funds for a mobile coronary-care unit for the Inglewood area of L.A. County. Unfortunately, Graf's single mobile unit got broadsided in a traffic accident, severely damaging the van and a lot of expensive equipment.

Les Smith contacted Hahn, and briefed him on Criley's proposal. Hahn signed on. Two of his areas of responsibility on the Board of Supervisors were the County Fire Department and Harbor General Hospital, where Criley was head of the Cardiology Division and where the new mobile coronary-care system would be based. "Hahn was the key," said Criley later. "He had appropriated the funds to get Harbor General started in the first place, so he was kind of our patron. And we needed his help with the fire department. All the top brass in the fire department opposed our idea. They felt the training was too specialized for firefighters, that they'd lose out in promotions, that they didn't really need that kind of training anyway, or shouldn't have it. Hahn kind of browbeat them into it."

The first mobile unit began rolling in December 1969. It was a station wagon commandeered from the forestry service, with "Rescue Heart Unit" lettered on its side. In addition to residual grass seeds, the wagon carried a portable defibrillator. Their first save was sudden death from a "cafe coronary," recalled Criley. "It was at a place called the Alpine Village, a sort of year-round German Oktoberfest transplanted to Southern California. We got this call from the emergency 'Rescue Heart Unit' and there's the 'um-pa-pa' polka music in the background. This guy had slumped under a table. He had been talking, and the polka band was playing, and he was trying to talk too loud and swallow at the same time. This huge chunk of meat got stuck in his throat, and he was in defib arrest. They countershocked him, and alerted the emergency room to prepare for a tracheostomy. They did it and saved the guy's life. He came to our twentieth anniversary. He's still alive and well."

In 1970, the need to enable paramedic authority made the legislators' agenda in Sacramento. The extent of Kenneth Hahn's helpfulness became fully apparent during the battle to pass the Wedworth-Thompson Paramedic Act. As the final version was wending its way through the California legislature, medical special-interest groups were exerting enormous pressure to kill it. Kenneth Hahn stepped in. "It was June or July of 1970," recalled Criley. "Several of us had made repeated trips to Sacramento to lobby various legislators. And we were just getting a blank stare. So Hahn went directly to then-Governor Ronald Reagan. Right into his office. He lobbied Reagan into getting it passed." Because of the legislation, paramedics were "cut loose" in the July 1970 and began functioning without the presence of a nurse. From then on, all medical supervision was at the other end of a radio or telephone with ECG telemetry.

A Jack Webb TV show may have also helped. In 1970, Webb got interested in the mobile coronary-care units and thought they'd make the basis for a great television series. His producer, Robert Cinader, rode with paramedics from County Fire Station 36 and learned the ropes firsthand. The resulting series, *Emergency*, became a major hit. "It was a major force in not only legitimizing the paramedics in our county," recalled Criley, "but also for exporting the idea across the country. People would watch and hear the fire sirens, kids would watch and see all these marvelous things going on. That gave us tremendous impetus. It put the spotlight on L.A. County and its fire department." Added Criley, "And Kenneth Hahn had no trouble getting appropriations."

Warren and Lewis: Columbus's Dynamic Duo

The early paramedic programs did not begin in sequence nor did one catalyze another. It is almost as if five dormant seeds simultaneously sprouted. In the Midwestern city of Columbus, Ohio, the program began with the vision of James Warren and the energy of Richard Lewis. The unique contribution of the Columbus system lay in its extensive training of paramedics to handle all types of medical emergencies.

Lewis's involvement with mobile cardiac care units began almost with his first day as a junior faculty member working with Dr. James Warren, department chair at Ohio State. The year was 1969 and Lewis was fresh from a residency and two years of military duty as an Army physician. Warren had long been interested in the problem of sudden cardiac death, and had set up the region's first in-hospital cardiac-care unit in 1955. An inveterate traveler, Warren attended several meetings of the British Cardiac Society in the early and mid-1960s and met Frank Pantridge. By then Pantridge had already started his mobile cardiac-care system in the Northern Ireland capital city. Warren had been deeply impressed by Pantridge's work, and decided to adopt it for use in Columbus.

He and Lewis were fortunate: Columbus was a city already primed for such a revolutionary medical development. The city fire department had been in the rescue squad business since 1931. In that year an oxygen ventilator was donated to take care of firefighters overcome by smoke. Although it was not intended for the general public, it soon evolved into a community service. In 1934 the fire chief personally responded to a call to assist an electrocuted telephone linesman. The resuscitation was unsuccessful, but newspaper publicity resulted in citizens beginning to call the fire department for medical emergencies. That same year, using donated supplies from the Red Cross, the department established a rescue squad for public medical emergencies. So the precedent of responding to medical emergencies was there for decades before James Warren proposed his extension of the service.[3]

"Jim [Warren] started talking with the fire department about his idea around 1967 or 1968," Lewis recounted. "A local industrialist got interested, and Jim also got the Advanced Coronary Treatment Foundation involved." Along with the local chapter of the American Heart Association and the Regional Medical Programs, Warren forged a coalition to spearhead funding. In April 1969 they began putting the pieces together and grafting them onto the Columbus fire department's existing Emergency Medical System.

Lewis arrived at Ohio State three months later. "Jim Warren came up to me shortly after I arrived and asked me if I'd be interested in being involved with this," Lewis recalled. "Well, I had never given it any thought at all. But you don't turn down things for your new Chairman!"

Lewis was to be the de facto medical director for this revolutionary medical service. He had good human "material" to work with. The firefighters on the new cardiac "flying squad" had chosen to specialize in what they were doing and Lewis's Army experience had taught him that medical corpsmen could be excellent caregivers with proper direction and training. "We took fifteen of them," said Lewis, "and gave them training in what would essentially be an advanced life-support—much more than that, really." Lewis had great confidence in the expertise of his medics. "I didn't have any problems letting non-physicians do stuff," he said. Because of the fire department's decades-long experience in the rescue business, Lewis set out from day one to train his men in a full spectrum of emergencies. Though all the paramedic programs began with a cardiac focus, they quickly evolved into "full-service" programs.

The original "heartmobile," as it was called, was a converted lumbering mobile trailer, based at the University Hospital in special quarters. It resembled Seattle's Moby Pig. At least three trained medics were available twenty-four hours a day, and a medical resident accompanied the crew to provide cardiology assistance and supervise care. When a call came to the fire department's emergency rescue unit that sounded like a heart attack, the unit would send its standard squad and also roll the "heartmobile" with its paramedics and doctor. Having only one vehicle and needing to wait for the doctor, who may have been in the middle of rounds on the eleventh floor, created a less than rapid response system. But it was a breakthrough. Lewis and his associates collected all the data from every such "run."

The program officially began in October 1969 and it soon became clear that the mobile cardiac-care unit was saving lives. "People were getting defibrillated, given atropine for bradycardia [slow heart rates], and getting to a hospital more quickly," Lewis noted. "And the firemen were very good. They'd look at ECGs and be just as good as the medical resident at diagnosing the arrhythmia."

The residents at University Hospital were very enthusiastic about the program. They were seeing something rarely encountered in medical training—patients brought back from clinical death. And although their support never flagged, their time and energy did. Recalled Lewis, "It was the end of 1970. We needed to keep the system going. So I decided the best way to do it was to have the [paramedics] do it by themselves without direct supervision. We felt on the basis of our experience so far that they could." During the summer of 1971, Lewis convinced the Columbus Safety Director to expand the system to three medic vehicles instead of one.[4]

To help build momentum for the conversion to paramedic-only service, Leonard Cobb was invited to Columbus to share his experience. Cobb gave an emphatic endorsement of paramedic skills and urged the Columbus program to take the leap and leave the doctors in the hospital.

What was initially conceived by Warren as a clone of the Belfast program evolved under Lewis's leadership into a new direction. Paramedics, working alone in the community, were saving victims of sudden death.

Leonard Rose and the Rose City

Portland, Oregon, also pioneered paramedic services, but with a different model of staffing. Instead of building on and using fire department personnel and equipment, the Portland program was the first to train private ambulance personnel as paramedics. Privately operated paramedic programs have now become a common model throughout the nation.

Leonard Rose's interest in cardiac resuscitation began in the early 1950s when he published a report on external cardiac pacing in a Stokes Adams case. Stokes Adams is a critical condition in which the heart slows down so much that the patient loses consciousness. A year later, Rose came west to Portland, Oregon and went to work as a cardiologist at Good Samaritan Hospital. By 1961—"after dozens of committee meetings," as Rose wryly put it—he put together Good Samaritan's first mobile resuscitation cart. Defibrillation was still confined inside hospital doors, but at least it was on wheels. The cart had the latest version of monitor, pacemaker, and defibrillator, along with everything else necessary to deal with cardiac arrest.

Rose was well aware of what was happening in the world of mobile cardiac units. He knew about Pantridge's pioneering efforts in Northern Ireland and William Grace's work in New York City. He made a point of visiting several people on the front lines, including Nagel in Florida.

Rose took the next step forward: training ambulance drivers to use portable defibrillators. "We were trying to get the ambulance company [Buck Ambulance] to install one in one of their ambulances," said Rose, "and to train the men. We had an EMT program by this time. We had an active medical society, and they were interested in the emergency medical technician program. They wanted to upgrade the training of the ambulance attendants." Buck Ambulance, though, wasn't buying.

Oregon's state health officer, Dr. Edward Press, had become interested in Leonard Rose's work. Press convened a lunch meeting in September 1968 that included representatives of the Oregon Medical Association, Buck Ambulance Company, and Good Samaritan Hospital—namely, Leonard Rose. Everyone agreed with Rose's goal of a swift emergency response and adequate care for cardiac patients. The problems were a lack of equipment and trained people—and of course money. Rose offered to train several specially selected ambulance attendants, and try to obtain the needed equipment on loan from some manufacturer or distributor. Buck Ambulance, in turn, agreed to give its people time off to undergo training. The hospital offered to provide classroom space, lab space, and equipment for training. Another series of meetings with the Oregon Medical Association and Multnomah County Medical Society gained approval for the project.

Rose's setup differed from Pantridge's MICU in Belfast. "He hadn't felt it was logical to have the paramedics do the defibrillating," Rose explained. "We thought that the mobile coronary unit as described by Pantridge was wonderful but not practical for our society. Instead, we thought it more likely that the EMTs would be the first ones to encounter such emergencies."

"We also developed stages in training," Rose explained. "We gave them certificates as advanced emergency medical technicians. They weren't called paramedics yet. We didn't invent the term paramedic but we had a curriculum. We published our curriculum in *JAMA*."

Rose moved slowly but steadily, gradually expanding the program. "We started with a pilot program, with just one ambulance in a limited geographical area near the Good Samaritan Hospital," said Rose. "This way, we could supervise what they were doing even though we weren't riding with them then. We even had volunteer coronary care unit nurses who rode with them initially to assist and supervise in their training. They [the paramedics] became pretty adept at reading an ECG or rhythm strips." The service soon became recognized in the community, and grass-roots support began to build. Rose continued to expand. Within a couple of years, they had four or five ambulances fully equipped to deal with cardiac emergencies.

The Amazing Sixties

The decade of the sixties opened with the development of CPR—the elements of artificial ventilation and artificial circulation fused. Publicity and news accounts about the benefit of CPR spread throughout the world. By the mid-1960s, the first effort to rapidly reach patients with myocardial infarction in the community began in Belfast, Northern Ireland. Soon after, the concepts of the program were cloned in New York City. More important, however, was the creation of paramedic-staffed ambulances. By the end of the decade, programs operated in Seattle, Miami, Los Angeles, Portland, and other cities. EMS services grew exponentially and every major city in the United States soon had a paramedic program.

EPILOGUE

《　》

EPILOGUE

If a man die, shall he live again?
—Job 14:14

THE QUEST CONTINUES

« »

The journey recounted here from biblical to modern times is far more than a simple tale of people and events. Discovering the secret to reverse sudden death required four components—respiration, circulation, defibrillation, and emergency medical services—each with its own history. All four must integrate perfectly to succeed. And although it is easiest to relate these events in a chronological fashion, such a presentation can falsely represent reality. Resuscitation was not achieved through incremental pieces of scientific knowledge—it required both a change in mind set as well as proper skills and tools. One has to realize that the quest was both inconceivable as well as technically impossible until the Enlightenment, when the collective will to reverse sudden and unexpected death first appeared.

The world-view change engendered by the Enlightenment and the technical achievements of the last two centuries only partially explain the success of resuscitation. There is also the web of cultural context—a powerful force for shaping events and personalities and bringing them together. Understanding the context in which the actors lived makes their actions and motives more comprehensible. Perhaps the most important context is how humankind viewed death. Our quest to reverse sudden death is intimately connected to our perceptions of and attitudes toward death itself. The French historian Philippe Ariès postulated four historical eras to describe these changes in attitudes. His hypothesis may not be perfect or even entirely accurate, but it does give us a way of grasping this all-important context.

The first era, says Ariès, can be called "tamed death." It covered the period from ancient history to the late Middle Ages. During this era life was, as Thomas Hobbes wrote, "solitary, poor, nasty, brutish, and short." Death was ever-present, a concrete fact of life. Because of its dominance and familiarity, death was prepared for and accepted in a fashion we would likely find difficult to comprehend. Acceptance was made easier by a near-universal belief in an afterlife. Death was viewed as a grateful release from a life often unhappy and painful, and an opportunity for everlasting salvation.

Ariès's second era, termed "death of the self," lasted from the end of the Middle Ages (roughly the twelfth to the fifteenth century) to the Enlightenment (the eighteenth century). This period corresponds approximately to the Renaissance. The awareness of one's personal death now became prominent. During this era, manuals on how to die, called *Ars moriendi,* helped guide an individual's behavior when death was imminent. In both eras, sudden death would have presented a particular difficulty because it did not allow for proper religious or personal preparation. Ariès writes that sudden death "destroyed the order of the world in which everyone believed; it became the absurd instrument of chance, which was sometimes disguised as the wrath of God."[1] Sudden death had a distasteful taint to it. The only exception to this general feeling was sudden death on the battlefield. Knights and soldiers who died in the service of God were entitled to salvation. Not so for accidental death. A drowned body was, at worst, interpreted as a suicide and, at best, an accident invoked by God's judgment. In either case, such a death was shameful and ignominious. With such beliefs predominating, it is no wonder that resuscitation after sudden death was pretty much unthinkable.

Ariès describes his third era as "death of the other." During this period, roughly from the Enlightenment to the beginning of the twentieth century, the predominant attitude toward death was defined by the loss of relationships, of the companionship of a beloved. The historian John Morgan writes of this period, "The image of the beyond in the earlier periods, which had ranged from eternal sleep to a glorious heaven or damned hell, became in the nineteenth century the scene of the reunion of those whom death had separated."[2] Finally, resuscitation starts to become acceptable. Rescue societies begin to spring up in European and American cities. Scientists, doctors— and charlatans—proposed countless techniques of resuscitation, mostly centered on artificial respiration. Resuscitation prevented separation from a loved one, but people also began to question the certainty of an afterlife. The rise of science corresponded to a decline in the belief of an existence after death. Sudden, unexpected death becomes perceived for what it is: merely an accident of fate, not the terror of God's wrath.

Ariès calls the last era "death denied." This period corresponds to the twentieth century, and is the result of complex factors. They include decreased personal exposure to death (75 percent of all deaths now occur in hospitals); high expectations of positive results from medicine and technology; steadily increasing life expectancy; and a highly developed perception of the individual as unique and precious. Ernest Becker in *The Denial of Death* calls this last factor "the ache of cosmic specialness."[3] It may well be the most important aspect of Ariès's fourth era—but it is also the most speculative. Less speculative is the fact that we rarely encounter real death in our personal lives. Movie death and TV death are fictionalized versions of the real thing. And even real death as seen on the evening news or tabloid shows is somehow removed, held at arm's length by the numbing nature of television. After all, we're sitting in our living rooms or bedrooms as we watch the oftentimes horrific scenes. They can't be real. The medicalization of death—in a hospital room or ICU ward—also removes the process of death from the home and sanitizes ugly and unpleasant aspects of terminal disease. We create a technological barrier of monitors, respirators, and IV tubing between the dying person and his or her family, and also between the individual and the medical staff. Doctors and nurses themselves have been increasingly viewed in the twentieth century as wizards of technology instead of comforters to the dying. Ariès is not speaking of "death denied" in a cognitive sense—no one can really deny our century's ghastly dance with death, given two world wars, the Holocaust, famines, and AIDS. Rather, he is referring to a psychological denial.

The very words we use, our terminology surrounding death, help to strengthen that denial. The usual definitions of death no longer apply. Death is not absolute. We now speak of clinical death (lack of pulse and blood pressure) and biological death (irreversible death of cells). Furthermore, declaring a person dead isn't a simple process anymore. In past eras, death was defined by lack of pulse or the absence of breath fogging a mirror held to a person's mouth. Now, various levels of death exist: cardiac death, brain death, organ death. And these levels can only be certified by physicians who often require sophisticated equipment. It is true that the body dies in discrete phases (cardiac, respiratory, and brain death), but in most situations all three deaths are compressed into a matter of minutes. For most of human history, death appeared instantaneous. Not so today. Technology can intervene at each level to abort the dying process. For example, respirators can keep a person alive in the face of total respiratory failure. Respirators and intravenous feedings can do the same for a brain-dead person for long periods.

How does this denial of death relate to attitudes toward sudden death? Given all these forces, it is no wonder that its denial is even more extreme. If death is to be prevented at all costs, then premature death simply cannot be allowed to happen. When it does, we are jarred into disbelief. We therefore have the cultural imperative to act, to rob death of its premature visitation. Combined with today's technology, we have the both the will and the means to achieve successful resuscitation.

Is It Worthwhile?

Despite, or perhaps because of, the advances in rescuing people from the cold clutches of death, many of us are pondering a fundamental ethical question: Is resuscitation worth it? Or does it merely prolong a life already over? There is much validity to the concept of a completed life. A life lived fully, with satisfying personal accomplishments, an education, marriage, work, children, grandchildren—such a life need not be artificially prolonged. People express great concern about the dignity of death. Spending one's last days and hours ignominiously attached to respirators, monitors, intravenous lines, and bladder drainage strikes most people as nightmarish. Added to these indignities are tremendous hospital and doctor bills. Even more awful is the possibility of suffering mental or physical incapacitation and enduring a life whose remaining months or years are far less less than whole and dignified.

Many of those involved in the quest to reverse sudden death have also questioned whether resuscitation is worthwhile. Peter Safar asks if resuscitation is "socially, morally, and economically justified, or is it an antievolutionary undertaking?" He answers his own question: "Resuscitation applied without judgment and compassion is morally and economically unacceptable. The debilitated elderly patient or the otherwise terminally ill patient with incurable disease, particularly the one with irreversible coma or stupor, should be permitted to die without the imposition of costly and often dehumanizing efforts." On the other hand, those who die "from potentially reversible conditions imposed by the arbitrary mischances of Nature, before thay have had time to live full lives, should receive the benefits of emergency resuscitation . . . if there is a chance that life with human mentation can possibly be restored."[4]

To tell the story of resuscitation is not to argue for needless prolongation of life. Rather, it drives home the point that sudden death is often a premature death. Most men and women in their fifties, sixties, and seventies are hardly willing to call their life biologically or psychologically completed. Claude Beck wrote about "hearts too good to die." That phrase captures the essence of sudden cardiac death. A heart too good to die is one that is basically fine but unfortunately suddenly fibrillates. If the fibrillation can be reversed in time, the heart will have years left to beat. Sudden death occurs in hearts too good to die and in people with uncompleted lives. John Colven had such a life, and such a heart. Pulled back from death, he now relishes the second chance that resuscitation technology has given him. The golf course he lives next to never looked so good as it does now.

Of course, the opposite situation also occurs. Richard Cummins, Professor of Medicine at the University of Washington, refers to the dilemma when resuscitations occur in "hearts too sick to live." A team of EMTs and paramedics at the scene of a cardiac arrest cannot instantly determine who should be resuscitated or allowed to quietly die. Emergency medical personnel are trained to provide the full-court press on everyone they encounter in cardiac arrest. Occasionally, it is obvious that resuscitation is futile and perhaps cruel. A person with advanced terminal cancer perhaps should not be resuscitated. But it is not usually clear what the underlying situation is when the paramedics arrive at the scene. Their only option is to resuscitate, and sometimes hearts too sick to live are brought back to life. There may be extensive brain damage with long, expensive hospitalizations—we can hardly call this success.

The ideal situation would be to start all resuscitations with the belief that success will be total and full recovery will occur. And this is generally the case when care is provided rapidly. However, in "good hearts" with delayed care or with "sick hearts," the outcomes following resuscitation may not be optimal. This is a reality with a bright and dark side. The bright side is bright indeed—good lives brought back from the abyss of death. Two-thirds of survivors from ventricular fibrillation return to their previous life with no or minimal impairment from the cardiac arrest. The dark side ranges from shades of grey to black. The grey end of the spectrum is that one-quarter of survivors have moderate to severe impairments following the resuscitation. While these people can usually return home, memory and other cognitive problems are often present. The black end of the spectrum contains the worst outcomes. Approximately five percent of cardiac arrest survivors have significant problems and require extended nursing or medical care.

This is the current reality and we must not deny it. We still face the conundrum: Should we attempt to reverse sudden death? Ultimately the only answer must be personal. And it must be addressed before the event, since those in cardiac arrest cannot make their wishes known. Most of us, I believe, would want to be resuscitated from ventricular fibrillation (assuming a basically healthy heart), but would we decide to be defibrillated if there was an underlying terminal condition (such as Alzheimer's or advanced cancer)? That answer is less straightforward. The point is that I cannot know what you want. I cannot tell how you value a few extra days or months of life. I cannot tell how you judge quality of life. In the face of no information, my obligation is to call 911 and initiate CPR. I'm not sure I have an ethical obligation, though I know it is a societal expectation. Personally, I would do CPR for a friend or stranger simply because I would feel too guilty if I didn't. But how much better it would be if I did know what you wanted.

My mother died of Alzheimer's disease. I knew, even had she not confirmed it with a living will, that she did not want to be resuscitated. To call the paramedics when she stopped breathing, in order to buy a few more days or weeks of life, would have been cruel. My father died at age eighty-two of a cardiac arrest. I suspect (though I cannot know) that he was in ventricular fibrillation. Because his collapse was unwitnessed, there was no chance of resuscitation, even though paramedics were called to the scene. He was a vigorous and sharp eighty-two, but he also had early prostate cancer, fairly bothersome arthritis, and his short-term memory was starting to fail. Though I believe he had several more good years ahead, I don't know if he wanted to be resuscitated. I simply never asked. Though the point is moot, I wish I had. We should have no inhibition about discussing a person's wishes regarding resuscitation. There is widespread acceptance about the wisdom of living wills, but they generally involve hospital situations. There is too little discussion about prehospital events. The reality remains that sudden cardiac arrest is the leading cause of death among adults in Western countries. Let your spouse, or friend, or family know what you would want. I'd rather not decide for you.

There is another answer to the question of whether resuscitation is worth it. It is true that only a few will actually be resuscitated. But we must also acknowledge a greater truth: the effort of resuscitation is ennobling. It reveals much about our society's values. A primary one is that human life has value. As Peter Safar eloquently wrote about resuscitation, "Its moral impact and the commitment it represents may have a much broader influence in a world where life has too often been regarded as cheap." Resuscitation is ultimately a life-affirming act. "Medicine imposes compassion, reason, and decency on a random universe," says Safer. "Thus, an increasingly individual-oriented society makes resuscitation evolutionarily positive—it implies a commitment on the side of Life."[5]

Progress in Resuscitation

The quest to reverse sudden death is filled with many false starts, rediscoveries, and interesting anecdotes. Many who proposed useful techniques failed to recognize their importance, or the times could not accommodate the discovery into its existing science. Yet many managed to integrate the ideas of others into new medical systems, or helped publicize important techniques themselves. William Osler once said, "In science credit goes to the man who convinces the world, not to the man to whom the idea first occurred."[6] This history of resuscitation has identified many individuals. But to a real extent, the names are less crucial than the advances themselves. Peter Safar wrote, "Obviously, the question of who should get credit for an advance holds less importance for mankind than the fact that the advance occurred and was implemented."[7]

This account of the history of resuscitation stops in the early 1970s. By then CPR, defibrillation, and a rapid means to provide prehospital care were all in place. Both the will and a way to achieve reversal of sudden death had emerged and taken root. The quest took exactly 200 years. The structure to resuscitate victims of sudden death now existed and was proving successful. That most of the world in the 1970s did not have this structure in place had mainly to do with the time needed to spread the word and educate people.

But the story of resuscitation doesn't end in the early seventies. Major advances continued to occur. In 1980, the first program to train emergency medical technicians to defibrillate began in King County, Washington.[8] Similar programs started in Iowa and then throughout the country. This training required ten hours, and, in the first demonstration project, survival from ventricular fibrillation increased from 7 percent to 26 percent. In 1984, the first program to use automatic defibrillators also began in King County.[9] The use of automatic defibrillators simplified the training of emergency medical technicians and thus allowed the procedure to spread more rapidly. Automatic defibrillators require only three to four hours of training since the EMT does not have to interpret the cardiac rhythm—the machine does that and advises the operator whether to deliver an electric shock. John Colven was initially resuscitated by fire department EMT personnel using automatic defibrillators.

In 1981, a program to provide telephone instructions in CPR also began in King County. This program used emergency dispatchers to give instant directions while the fire department EMT personnel were enroute. This demonstration project increased the rate of bystander-initiated CPR by 50 percent.[10] Dispatcher-assisted CPR is now the accepted standard of care for dispatch centers throughout the United States, as well as in Israel, Scotland, England, and Norway.

All these programs are designed to provide lifesaving interventions more quickly. In 1973, 1979, 1986, and 1992, the American Heart Association convened national conferences to review and define the standards and guidelines for basic and advanced emergency cardiac care. They made minor adjustments in how to perform CPR and recommended new drug treatments for cardiac arrest. These national conferences affirmed the importance of rapid defibrillation. With each subsequent conference, doctors and other caregivers came to increasingly appreciate the critical role of rapid defibrillation, and stronger recommendations were made to provide defibrillation as quickly as possible. The 1992 guidelines call for CPR to be performed until a defibrillator arrives. Once ventricular fibrillation is determined to be present, electric shocks are to be provided in rapid sequence without even stopping to perform CPR between shocks. Clearly, electricity is the most important component of resuscitation therapy for cardiac arrest. The sooner it is provided, the higher the likelihood of successful resuscitation.

The Chain of Survival

John Colven's return from death happened because of a system. No single person saved Colven's life; many were responsible. Everyone involved with the resuscitation effort played a role. The dispatcher provided emergency telephone CPR instructions. And June Colven knew to call 911 immediately and then performed two full cycles of CPR before the EMTs arrived. The team of EMTs provided four defibrillatory shocks, resulting in vital minutes of blood circulation. The two paramedics administered intravenous medication to stabilize the heart and prevent its going back into fibrillation, and inserted a breathing tube to adequately oxygenate Colven's lungs. By the time Colven arrived at the hospital, he had a stable blood pressure and pulse and was breathing on his own.

Just as it is impossible to single out an individual, it is impossible to choose one procedure that saved his life. The American Heart Association speaks of a "Chain of Survival" in describing the sequence of interventions required for successful resuscitation. It is an apt metaphor, for it defines not only the interventions but the sequence as well. The four links in this chain of survival are: early access, early CPR, early defibrillation, and early advanced care.[11]

These links came together in just the right way for John Colven. June called 911 immediately, CPR was performed within two minutes of collapse, defibrillatory shocks were given within seven minutes of collapse, and advanced care (medications, airway tube) occurred within twelve minutes of collapse. Each link in this chain builds on the previous link, and a timely delivery of each link allows the next to be successful.[12]

It is a cliché to state that a chain is only as good as its weakest link, but in resuscitation the cliché is valid. If each link or step occurs rapidly, there is a good chance for successful resuscitation. Any delay in a step, however, means death is inevitable, regardless of how efficiently the other steps occur. The four steps or links in the Chain of Survival are simplified representations of what is actually a multitude of tiny links. Each link summarizes a series of small but vital actions, which must flow flawlessly. Again, any delay in any action can destroy the integrity of the entire chain.

The first, **early access**, involves these actions:
- The collapse must be witnessed.
- The person seeing or hearing the collapse must recognize the seriousness of the situation.
- The bystander must know what number to call—911 in most parts of the country—and must quickly give the needed information to the emergency operator.

During the second link or step, **early CPR,** the bystander:
- Must know CPR or live in a community where the dispatcher provides instant instruction over the telephone.
- Must be able to position the victim on his or her back, preferably on a hard surface.
- Must be able to tilt the head properly to open the victim's throat and airtube.
- Must be able to form a tight seal around the mouth in order to blow air into the victim's lungs.
- Must be able to find the correct position for chest compression.
- Must be able to compress the chest one and one-half to two inches at the proper rate and for the appropriate number of times. The correct ratio is two ventilations followed by fifteen chest compressions.
- Must be able to continue CPR without fatiguing until emergency personnel arrive.
- If the collapse has happened at home, must unlock the front door and tie up the dog.

Early defibrillation, the third link in the Chain of Survival, requires that:
- The first arriving emergency personnel must have a defibrillator and be trained in its use.
- The personnel must attach the electrodes properly.
- They must correctly operate the defibrillator, either an automatic or a manual type, so that the first shock is delivered within one minute of their arrival or as soon as possible.
- The emergency personnel must also take over CPR for the bystander and adequately ventilate the victim with 100 percent oxygen, preferably by mask.

The fourth link, **early advanced care,** requires that paramedical personnel:
- Continue defibrillation if not already successful.
- Begin an intravenous line.
- Perform an endotracheal intubation (placement of a plastic tube down the throat and into the airtube) and ventilate with 100 percent oxygen.
- Administer emergency medications such as epinephrine to stimulate the heart and lidocaine to stabilize its rhythm.

Technically, if a person received instant CPR, defibrillation, and advanced care, the chance of resuscitation would be near 100 percent. Communities with mature emergency medical service systems are able to achieve survival rates of 30 to 40 percent for patients with ventricular fibrillation. These are people who are discharged alive from the hospital with neurologically intact brains. Without the techniques of modern resuscitation, none of these cardiac arrest victims would survive.

The rate of 30 to 40 percent may strike many of us as not that impressive. But it isn't practical to expect much higher resuscitation rates given the logistics of supplying CPR and defibrillation within minutes. On the other hand, 30 percent is remarkable in the face of what would otherwise be certain death. Never before in the history of the world has it been possible to consistently and reliably reverse death at even this level. What is regretful is that such high resuscitation rates are found in only a few cities.

Cardiac Arrest and Resuscitation in the Cities

Several dozen communities have studied cardiac arrest and published their rates of resuscitation from ventricular fibrillation. By and large, these figures leave room for improvement and one can only assume that communities who have not published rates do so only because they are so awful. Cities and communities with documented resuscitation rates above 20 percent are King County (Washington), Milwaukee, New South Wales (New Zealand), Seattle, Tampa, Torrance (California), Vancouver (British Columbia). Cities and communities with survival rates of 10 to 20 percent include: Columbus (Ohio), Pittsburgh, Reykjavik (Iceland), Stockport (Great Britain), Tucson, and rural/suburban communities in Iowa, Minnesota, and Pennsylvania.[13]

The links in the Chain of Survival constitute the system of emergency medical services in any community. Ideally, these services, whether provided by fire departments, public emergency medical agencies, or private ambulance companies, should be able to resuscitate many victims of cardiac arrest. The reality is far from the ideal. In actuality, the success of emergency medical service programs in the United States and throughout the world is not very good. Only a few communities are able to consistently resuscitate over 25 percent of victims whose cardiac arrest is caused by ventricular fibrillation. This resuscitation rate refers to the percent resuscitated and discharged alive from the hospital. Most other communities achieve success rates of less than

5 percent. New York and Chicago have survival rates of 5 percent and 4 percent, respectively.[14]

Why this wide variability? Why are some communities so successful and others, to put it charitably, less so? What can be done to give people in every community a reasonable chance of surviving sudden cardiac death? The answers are straightforward, but the solution is difficult. The wide differences in survival rates among communities are explained by the variability in delivering rapid CPR, defibrillation, and advanced care.

A Community Survival Checklist

What can be done to improve the likelihood of successful resuscitation in a community? The first thing to realize is that there are usually good reasons for the type of emergency medical services in any given community. For example, the community's history, resources, political and medical leadership (or lack of it) all play a major role. Having said this, one then must ask, "What is the situation in my community?" The answers to the following "Community Survival Checklist" will not only define the likelihood of successful resuscitation, but will also suggest actions to take in order to treat "hearts too good to die."

Does my community have 911?	Yes	No
Does my community have basic and advanced EMS care?	Yes	No
Does my community have a dispatcher-assisted telephone CPR program?	Yes	No
Does every ambulance and emergency medical vehicle have a defibrillator on board, with personnel trained and authorized to use it?	Yes	No
Does my community have an EMS medical director?	Yes	No
Does the EMT unit with a defibrillator have a response time of four minutes or less?	Yes	No
Does the paramedic unit have a response time of ten minutes or less?	Yes	No

If you knew the answers, you could tell whether there would be a good or a poor chance of anyone surviving sudden cardiac death. Quite simply, if the answers are all "Yes," your community would be among the best dozen in the United States. If there is a "No" to any question, your community is likely to have a very poor resuscitation rate. More important, "No" answers suggest what can be changed or improved.

Being fortunate enough to live and work in a city with an excellent EMS system, I have seen firsthand the miracle of resuscitation. Shortly after starting my internship in 1971, I found myself treating survivors of sudden cardiac arrest. I was assigned to the CCU at Harborview Medical Center and Leonard Cobb was my attending. Patients would arrive comatose after being defibrillated by Seattle paramedics. Within hours (occasionally days), they would awaken. Though I was amazed at literally seeing patients come to life, I assumed such events were commonplace throughout America. Only later did I learn that few communities come even close to Seattle. And later still I have come to understand the reason. Cardiac arrest in Seattle is no different from arrest in New York or Chicago, and yet the likelihood of survival is 10 times higher in Seattle. The explanation: Seattle can delivery CPR, defibrillation, and advanced care quickly. There are no mysteries or secrets, any community can do the same.

I hope as you read this you will become both curious and indignant. Discover the situation in your community. Find out the answers to the Community Survival Checklist. Ask your mayor (or fire chief or EMS director) the likelihood of surviving ventricular fibrillation in your town. And if it's low (as I predict it will be), demand better—for your parents, your spouse, your neighbor, yourself.

In both 1767 and 1967 a skeptical world asked: Will it work? How much will it cost? Why should we do it? Who will care? And the answers have not consistently come down in support of EMS programs. In both years, the world did not greet the announcements with wild enthusiasm. Change and improvement come slowly, even when human life is at stake. Too many competing priorities in society and too many good ways to spend and use precious resources are always present. On the other hand, change can occur very quickly. In the brief span of two decades, paramedic programs have been accepted as a public responsibility. We have declared it a societal right to receive prompt emergency medical care. We have made it official policy to try to reverse sudden and unexpected death. We have found the way, but continue to need the will.

We have seen firsthand the success of modern CPR, defibrillation, and emergency care. Physicians, nurses, paramedics, emergency medical technicians, and countless others are committed to the belief that death is not irreversible. They have ceaselessly struggled to rob death of its premature visitations. And thanks to all their efforts, the miraculous is now commonplace.

Emergency Care Guide

Call 911 for immediate help in life-threatening situations.

CPR*

Place victim flat on back on a hard surface.

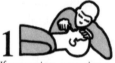

If unconscious, open airway.
Lift chin, tilt head.

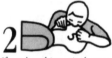

If not breathing, pinch nose, cover mouth with your mouth. Give 2 full breaths.

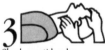

Check carotid pulse.
If pulse absent, begin chest compression.

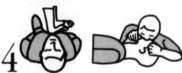

Depress sternum (breast bone between nipples) 1½" to 2". Give 15 rapid compressions, followed by 2 full breaths. Continue until emergency help arrives

First Aid for Choking

Conscious Victim

If the victim can speak, cough or breathe, do not interfere.

If the victim *cannot* speak, cough or breathe, give upward abdominal thrusts. Repeat until item is expelled or person can breathe.

If Victim Becomes Unconscious

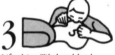

Lift chin. Tilt head back.
If not breathing, pinch nose, cover mouth with your mouth. Give 2 full breaths.

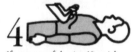

If unsuccessful, give 10 quick upward abdominal thrusts.

If unsuccessful, try finger sweep to remove object. Repeat steps 3 to 5 until emergency help arrives.

A CHRONOLOGY OF
RESUSCITATION

900 B.C.E.	Elijah the Prophet resuscitated the child of a widow.
850 B.C.E.	Elisha the Prophet resuscitated the son of a Shunamite woman.
35 C.E.	Jesus raised Lazarus from the tomb.
175 C.E.	Galen defined anatomy and physiology for the next millenium.
1543	Andreas Vesalius published *De Humani Corporis Fabrica*.
1600	William Gilbert published *De Magnete*.
1628	William Harvey published *De Motu Cordis* accurately depicting circulation.
1660	Otto von Guericke devised the first electrostatic machine.
1730	Stephen Gray demonstrated conductive nature of humans
1732	William Tossach resuscitated a coal miner using mouth-to-mouth technique.
1743	Johann Gottlob Kruger suggested electricity might have medical benefits.
1744	Christian Gottlieb Kratzenstein demonstrated the effect of electricity on paralysis.
1745	John Fothergill recommended mouth-to-mouth respiration as well as barrel roll technique of resuscitation for drowning.
1746	Pieter van Musschenbroek discovered the Leyden jar.

1752	Benjamin Franklin demonstrated the electrical nature of lightning.
1758	John Wesley opened an electric treatment dispensary for the poor.
1767	First rescue society formed in Amsterdam for the recovery of drowned persons.
1770	Nikolaj Abildgaard experimented with electric shocks to produce unconsciousness.
1774	Karl Wilhelm Scheele and Joseph Priestly discoved deflogisticated air (oxygen).
1774	Royal Humane Society founded by William Hawes and Thomas Cogan in London. The Society did much to promote rescue techniques for drowning and suffocations.
1774	Sophia Greenhill defibrillated(?) by Mr. Squires.
1776	John Hunter recommended deflogisticated air for resuscitation; also recommended electricity for resuscitation.
1780–1786	Humane societies formed in Philadelphia, New York, and Boston.
1782	The Royal Humane Society recommended inflation by bellows over mouth-to-mouth ventilation.
1787	Francis Lowndes opened facility specializing in electric medical treatments.
1788	Lavoisier experimented with and named oxygen.
1788	Charles Kite proposed that electric shocks be provided as a means of resuscitation and demonstrated a proto-defibrillator.
1791	Luigi Galvani published *De Viribus Electricitatis in Motu Musculari Commentarius* (*The Effects of Artificial Electricity on Muscular Motion*) and postulated the presence of animal electricity.
1792	David Hosack advocated rectal fumigation as a stimulant for drowning cases. This method had been periodically used in prior years.
1792	Baron Dominique-Jean Larrey develops the concept of using ambulances to bring aid directly to the victim.
1796	John Daniel Herholdt and Carl Gottlob Rafn published *Life-Saving Measures for Drowning Persons* summarizing thirty steps to be used in resuscitations.
1800	Alessandro Volta invented the chemical battery.
1803	Giovanni Aldini performed electric stimulation experiments on corpses of condemned criminals.

1811	Benjamin Brodie denounced rectal fumigation as danger-ous and the technique fell out of favor.
1820	Richard Reece published *The Medical Guide* containing a reanimation chair designed to electrically stimulate life.
1820	Hans Christian Oersted discovered the principle of electro-magnetism.
1821	Michael Faraday applied electromagnetism to make the first electromagnetic motor.
1828	J. Leroy found postmorten evidence of damage to the lungs that he attributed to the use of bellows. Shortly thereafter the Royal Humane Society withdrew its recom-mendation for bellows.
1850	Karl Fredrich Wilhelm Ludwig and Moritz Hoffa first described ventricular fibrillation in animals.
1855	Guillaume Benjamine Amand Duchenne published studies of electrotherapy in the treatment of nerve palsies.
1857	Marshall Hall advocated the "ready method" that consisted of rolling the drowning victim from stomach to side.
1858	Henry R. Silvester advocated arm-lift chest-pressure method of artificial respiration.
1858	Janos Balassa published the first report of external heart massage.
1862	The Royal Medical and Chirurgical Society recommended Silvester's method after performing experiments on cadav-ers. The technique was accepted as the preferred method by the Royal Humane Society and remained popular well into the first half of the twentieth century.
1865	Urban ambulance service began in Cincinnati.
1869	Ambulance service began in New York City.
1869	Benjamin Howard published his "direct method" of artifi-cial respiration.
1874	Moritz Schiff described open chest cardiac massage in ani-mals.
1878	R. Boehm discovered chest compression as "emergency circulation."
1887–1889	John A. McWilliam published a series of articles with the first detailed descriptions of ventricular fibrillation in ani-mals. He was the first to postulate the importance of ven-tricular fibrillation in humans.
1890	Edward A. Schafer developed a new method, called the "prone pressure" technique, that involved intermittent

	pressure on the back of the prone victim. The Schafer technique became popular in the United States and Europe.
1891	Friedrich Maass performed the first unequivocally documented chest compression in humans.
1894	J. V. Laborde offered his tongue-traction method of resuscitation.
1895	Howard Atwood Kelly advocated chest compression for chloroform associated respiratory arrests.
1899	H. B. Baker proposed his lift and drop method of resuscitation.
1899	Jean Louis Prevost and Frederic Battelli published a study demonstrating in animals the onset of ventricular fibrillation with an electric shock and the cessation of fibrillation with a stronger shock.
1899	R. H. Cunningham independently published similar findings as Prevost and Battelli.
1901	Kristian Igelsrud perfomed the first successful open-chest cardiac massage.
1904	George Crile performed the first American case of closed-chest cardiac massage.
1906	T. A. Green described forty cases of open-chest cardiac massage in humans.
1906–1909	Louise Robinovitch published a series of articles advocating electric stimulation to induce artificial respiration and cardiac pacing.
1932	Holger Louis Nielsen described the back-pressure arm-lift method of artificial ventilation. This method was considered superior to other methods and widely adopted in the United States and Europe.
1933	Orthello Langworth, Donald Hooker, and William Kouwenhoven published a study demonstrating the initiation and erasure of ventricular fibrillation with electric shocks. The investigators induced ventricular fibrillation in dogs and were able to defibrillate the heart without opening the chest. Their work rediscovers the findings of Prevost, Battelli, and Cunningham.
1936	Carl J. Wiggers demonstrated that open-heart massage could prolong the period in which an electric shock could terminate fibrillation.
1943	Frank C. Eve proposed the teeter-board method of artificial respiration.

1947	Claude Beck successfully defibrillated a fourteen-year-old boy using open-chest technique and an AC defibrillator. Beck coins the phrase "Hearts too good to die."
1946	James Elam performed mouth-to-nose ventilation on polio patients.
1951	Archer Gordon published a study demonstrating the superiority of Nielsen's back-pressure arm-lift method.
1954	Elam published a study demonstrating the effectiveness of exhaled air for artificial ventilation.
1955	Beck and David Leighninger save the first out-of-hospital cardiac arrest. The patient collapsed just outside the hospital entrance and was brought to the emergency department where his chest was opened and heart defibrillated.
1956	Paul Zoll demonstrated the effectiveness of closed chest defibrillation using AC defibrillators.
1956–1957	Peter Safar performed experiments demonstrating effectiveness of mouth-to-mouth ventilation in adults.
1957	Archer Gordon performed experiments demonstrating effectiveness of mouth-to-mouth ventilation in infants and children.
1957	The National Research Council/National Academy of Sciences endorsed mouth-to-mouth artificial respiration for infants and children.
1958	The American Medical Association Council on Medical Physics unequivocally endorsed mouth-to-mouth artificial respiration in children as well as adults.
1958	The National Research Council/National Academy of Sciences endorsed mouth-to-mouth artificial respiration for adults.
1959	First human saved with rediscovered chest compression.
1960	First prehospital cardiac arrest patient (Bertie Bish) saved with CPR and defibrillated in the emergency department.
1960	William Kouwenhoven, James Jude, and Guy Knickerbocker published a study demonstrating the effectiveness of closed-chest cardiac compression.
1960	Safar, Kouwenhoven, and Jude combine mouth-to-mouth ventilation with chest compression to create modern CPR. The first scientific presentation occurred at a Maryland Medical Society meeting in Ocean City.
1960	Asmund Laerdal developed and manufactured "Resusci-Anne" training manikins.

1961   Archer Gordon produced *The Pulse of Life* training film.
1961   International Symposium on Emergency Resuscitation in
            Stavanger, Norway, recommended training the public in
            mouth-to-mouth ventilation.
1961–1962   Bernard Lown demonstrated the superiority of DC over
            AC defibrillation.
1963   The term Cardiopulmonary Resuscitation (CPR) was first
            used to describe the combination of mouth-to-mouth res-
            piration with chest compression.
1966   The National Research Council/National Academy of
            Sciences endorsed CPR.
1966   National Highway Safety and Traffic Act authorized the
            Department of Transportation to establish a national cur-
            riculum for prehospital personnel, subsequently known as
            Emergency Medical Technicians.
1966   J. Frank Pantridge and John Geddes established the
            world's first mobile intensive-care unit program in Belfast,
            Northern Ireland.
1967   Pantridge and Geddes publish their findings in *The Lancet*.
1969   William Grace established a Belfast-like program in New
            York City.
1969–1970   Eugene Nagel in Miami, Leonard Cobb in Seattle,
            Leonard Rose in Portland, Michael Criley in Los Angeles,
            James Warren and Richard Lewis in Columbus established
            the first paramedic programs.
1971   Richard Crampton established Belfast-like program in
            Charlottesville.
1972   Leonard Cobb began a program to train 100,000 citizens
            of Seattle in CPR.

Since 1972 significant developments in cardiac resuscitation include defibrillation by emergency medical technicians, automatic external defibrillators,
widespread CPR training, and dispatcher-assisted telephone CPR.

GLOSSARY

« »

Alternating current (AC)   The flow of electric current that reverses at regular intervals. In the United States, AC current is 60 cycles per second. This is the type of current coming from wall outlets.

Angina   Chest pain caused by a temporary decrease in the blood supply to the heart muscle.

Atherosclerosis   A disease of the blood vessels, which become thickened and narrowed, reducing blood flow to body tissues.

Atrial fibrillation   An abnormal rhythm in which the atria are firing chaotically without contraction. The ventricles continue to beat in a coordinated fashion, maintaining blood pressure and pulse.

Atrio-ventricular (AV) node   A small bundle of conductive cells located between the atrium and the ventricles that directs the electrical impulse from the sino-atrial node down through the ventricles.

Automatic external defibrillator (AED)   A device used to identify ventricular fibrillation in a victim of sudden death, and automatically deliver an electric shock.

Automatic implantable cardioverter defibrillator (AICD)   A device surgically implanted into a patient's chest or abdomen that automatically delivers a shock when the heart goes into ventricular fibrillation or ventricular tachycardia. The device can also pace the heart if its rate becomes too slow. Patients who survive ventricular fibrillation are the primary candidates for AICDs. The newer term for this device is implantable cardioverter defibrillator (ICD).

Biological death   Irreversible brain death that results four to six minutes after the heartbeat and respirations stop.

Cardiac conduction system   A specialized network of electrical pathways along which electrical impulses move resulting in the coordinated contraction of the heart muscle and generation of a pulse.

Circulation   The movement of blood through the body with each heartbeat or, in the event of sudden death, the application of chest compressions.

Clinical death   Occurs immediately with the cessation of the heart beat and respirations.

Conduction   The transmission or movement of an electrical impulse.

Cardiopulmonary resuscitation or CPR   A technique of administering artifical ventilations and chest compressions to a victim of cardiac arrest to temporarily maintain circulation of oxygen and blood until more definitive care can be initiated.

Defibrillation   The delivery of an electric current through the chest wall and heart for the purpose of terminating ventricular fibrillation and restoring a perfusing rhythm.

Defibrillator   A device that delivers a predetermined flow of electricity to a heart in ventricular fibrillation.

Defibrillatory shock   The delivery of an electric current through the chest wall and heart for the purpose of terminating ventricular fibrillation.

Direct current (DC)   A constant flow of electric current in one direction only. This type of current comes from batteries.

Electrical therapy   The use of electricity over the ages in treating certain ailments or diseases.

Electrocardiogram (ECG)   A tracing of the electrical impulses traveling through the heart.

Emergency Medical Technician (EMT)   An individual who is trained in basic life-support services, such as CPR. This individual is often a firefighter or ambulance attendant.

Emergency Medical Technician defibrillation (EMT-D)   A specially trained emergency medical technician who can deliver an electric shock to a victim of sudden death in ventricular fibrillation.

Heart attack   The medical term is myocardial infarction; it is the death of a portion of heart muscle as a result of obstructed blood flow.

Implantable cardioverter defibrillator (ICD)   The newer term for devices surgically implanted in the chest or abdomen that automatically deliver a shock when the heart goes into ventricular fibrillation or ventricular tachycardia. The device can also automatically pace the heart if its rate becomes too slow.

Ischemia   A temporary decrease of blood flow to any part of the body.

Myocardial infarction   The death of a portion of heart muscle as a result of obstructed blood flow.

Paramedic   An individual who receives over 1100 hours of specialized medical training and can provide advanced life-support services.

Resuscitation   An attempt to revive a victim who has suffered respiratory and/or cardiovascular arrest or sudden death.

Seizure (or convulsion)   The involuntary, often violent, contractions or series of contractions of the voluntary muscles.

Sino-atrial (SA) node   A small bundle of conductive cells where an electrical impulse is generated. Sometimes referred to as the heart's internal pacemaker.

Sudden cardiac arrest (sudden death, cardiac death)   Occurs when the heart suddenly stops pumping blood, resulting in loss of consciousness and death unless rapid emergency care is provided to the body's tissues and organs.

Unstable angina   Chest pain that occurs at any time regardless of physical activity or emotional stress.

Ventilation   The artifical delivery of respirations to a victim of sudden death.

Ventricular fibrillation (VF)   A fatal arrhythmia in which there is a loss of coordinated contractions, resulting in sudden death.

NOTES

« »

PROLOGUE: APRIL 1991

1. The resuscitation described here occurred exactly as depicted. The EMT and Paramedic run report, transcripts of the 911 call, and interviews with the rescuers were used to make the account as accurate as possible. I interviewed John and June Colven (their names have been changed to protect their privacy) on March 10, 1992. The run reports and the tape recording of the call to the dispatch center were kindly provided (with the consent of the Colvens) by the King County Emergency Medical Services Division of the Seattle-King County Department of Health.

2. Paramedics operate manual defibrillators. In contrast to automatic defibrillators, used primarily by emergency medical technicians, manual defibrillators require human interpretation of the cardiac rhythm. Paramedics are trained to interpret normal and abnormal cardiac rhythms.

PROLOGUE: JUNE 1778

1. The resuscitation attempt described here is based on case number 351 found in *Reports of the Humane Society for the Recovery of Persons Apparently Drowned*, 1779–1780, London, pp. 108–109.

PART I: THE MOMENT OF DEATH

1. Sudden cardiac death is also known as sudden cardiac arrest. "Arrest" refers to the cessation of the heartbeat. A thorough discussion of sudden death can be found in Norman A. Paradis, Henry R. Halperin, Richard M. Nowak, eds., *Cardiac Arrest: The Science and Practice of Resuscitation Medicine* (Baltimore: Williams & Wilkins, 1995). A discussion centered more on the emergency medical services approach to sudden death is found in Mickey S. Eisenberg, Lawrence Bergner, Alfred P. Hallstrom, *Sudden Death in the Community* (Westport, Conn.: Praeger, 1984) and Mickey S. Eisenberg, Alfred P. Hallstrom, Lawrence Bergner, Richard O. Cummins, Sudden cardiac death, *Scientific American* 254 (1986):37–43.

2. Paul G. McGovern, James S. Pankow, Eyal Shahar, et al., Recent trends in acute coronary heart disease: mortality, morbidity, medical care, and risk factors, *New England Journal of Medicine* 334 (1966):884–890.

3. Lest one think that the heart is a time bomb ready to be destroyed at any minute, keep in mind that angina rarely leads to sudden death. Over six million Americans have coronary artery disease (atherosclerosis). Tens of millions of episodes of angina take place every year. Over a million episodes of myocardial infarction and approximately 400,000 sudden deaths occur annually in the United States (approximately one sudden death per minute). Still, while most of these deaths are caused by ventricular fibrillation, not every episode of angina or even every myocardial infarction leads to a fatal electric disturbance.

4. The discoverers of CPR in the fifties believed that direct compression over the heart squeezed blood out of the ventricles, and the heart valves allowed forward flow and prevented back flow. Pressure on the sternum pushed blood out of the heart. Releasing the pressure allowed the chest to return to its resting position and thus drew venous blood into the heart. With the next compression, more blood is expelled and the process is repeated. At the time, their explanation of how rhythmic chest compression worked seemed reasonable and convinced most physicians and scientists.

Investigators in the 1970s began to question this "squish theory" of forward flow. They provided evidence that pressure changes across the rib cage and small valves in the major veins caused forward flow of blood. Current opinion holds that not only changes in chest pressure but also squeezing blood out of the heart play a role.

PART I: THE FIRST RESUSCITATION

1. The first accounts shedding any light on attempted resuscitation come from the ancient civilizations of Egypt and Mesopotamia. Priests were clearly preoccupied with life after death, although there is no information about the acceptance of death. Boating accidents were undoubtedly common on the Nile and the Euphrates and Tigress rivers in Mesopotamia (modern Iraq). Thus, sudden accidental death would likely be encountered frequently. One Egyptian papyrus shows an inversion method of treating victims of drowning. This method, which allows the water to drain from the victim, is a commonsense action. No other drawings dealing with resuscitation exist from this period, but stories of resuscitation are present in Egyptian mythology. There is the story of the god Osiris who was dismembered by his brother; his sister

gathered the widely scattered pieces and reassembled them. So while it is impossible to look on myth and legend as proof of the impossible—namely, reversing the irreversibility of death—the idea was there in human imagination. There is little doubt, however, that the ancients would have agreed with the sixth century B.C.E. poet Ibycus: "You cannot find a medicine for life when once a man is dead." See also John Paraskos, Biblical accounts of resuscitation, *Journal of Medical History and Allied Sciences*, 47 (1992):310–320.

2. Peter V. Karpovich, *Adventures in Artifical Respiration* (New York: Assocation Press, 1953), p. 10.

3. Other accounts of resuscitation also appear in the Hebrew Bible. An account in Exodus describes the resuscitation of newborns. The Hebrew midwife Puah "breathed into the baby's mouth to induce the baby to cry" (Exodus 1:17). The Talmud, an interpretation of the Hebrew Bible, deals with the problem of "assisting in breathing in delivery." The following advice is given: "The newborn is held so that it should not fall on the earth and one blows into his nostrils" (Shabbath 128, b–4). Clearly the resuscitation of newborns involved intuitive actions. There were no recommendations for resuscitating adults—only God could do that.

PART I: BUILDING THE FOUNDATION

1. Galen's works constitute half of the existing ancient Greek medical literature. If one excludes the works of Hippocrates (460–370 B.C.E.), then Galen accounts for five-sixths of the ancient medical literature.

2. Lois N. Magner, *A History of Medicine* (New York: Marcel Dekker, 1992), p. 393.

3. Owsei Temkin, C. Lilian Temkin, *Ancient Medicine: The Selected Papers of Ludwig Edelstein* (Baltimore: Johns Hopkins Press, 1967), pp. 250–251.

4. A. B. Baker, Artificial respiration: The history of an idea, *Medical History* 15 (1971):336–346.

5. One of Galen's most significant accomplishments was to prove that arteries contain blood. It was previously believed that arteries were filled with air (more precisely, pneuma) and came from the lung via the left ventricle. Blood from a cut artery was explained by postulating connections between veins and arteries. The belief that arteries contained only air is not entirely far-fetched. In ancient Greece animals may have been strangled prior to vivisection. Such a mode of death would have pooled blood in the right heart and veins, leaving the arteries relatively void of blood. See Gene L. Colice, Historical perspectives on the development of mechanical ventilation, Martin J. Tobin, ed., *Principles and Practice of Mechanical Ventilation* (New York: McGraw-Hill, 1994), pp. 1–2. An excellent summary of Galen's contributions can be found in Sherwin B Nuland, *Doctors: The Biography of Medicine* (New York: Vintage Books, 1988), pp. 31–60.

6. Plato, Aristotle, and other Greek philosophers believed that the source of heat was the heart. For a discussion see E. Mendelsohn, *Heat and Life* (Cambridge: Harvard University Press, 1964), pp. 8–26.

7. Baker, pp. 336–346.

8. William Manchester, *A World Lit Only by Fire* (Boston: Little, Brown, 1992), p. 318.

9. Thomas Moore, *Care of the Soul* (New York: HarperCollins, 1992), pp. 3–25.

10. Edward Grant, *Physical Science in the Middle Ages* (Cambridge, England: Cambridge University Press, 1971), p. 88.

11. The book is generally known as *De Fabrica*.

12. Baker, pp. 336–346.

13. Vesalius equivocated about the right-to-left flow of blood through the heart. He stated that he could not find the pores in the heart's septum, though he did not go so far as to proclaim their absence. See Sherwin B. Nuland, *Doctors: The Biography of Medicine* (New York: Vintage, 1988), pp. 61–93 and C. D. O'Malley, Vesalius, Andreus, in *Dictionary of Scientific Biography,* ed. Charles C. Gillispie (New York: Scribner, 1970), Vol XIV, pp. 3–12.

14 Other versions explaining Vesalius's pilgrimage to Jerusalem are that he recovered from a serious illness and that he simply wanted to leave Spain and take a new job in Padua. See Nuland, p. 92.

15. William Harvey. *An Anatomical Disputation Concerning the Movement of the Heart and Blood in Living Creatures*, translated by Gweneth Whitteridge (London: Blackwell Scientific Publications, 1976), pp. 102–103.

16. *De Motu Cordis* had first been published in Latin—at that time the formal language of scientists and other intellectuals. The first English translation of *De Motu Cordis* appeared in London in 1653.

17. For a discussion of Harvey's works, see Frederick G. Kilgour, in *Scientific Genius and Creativity, Readings from Scientific American* (New York: W. H. Freeman, 1987), pp. 10–15 and Jeroome J. Bylebyl, in *Dictionary of Scientific Biography*, ed. Charles C. Gillispie (New York: Scribner, 1970), vol. VI, pp. 150–162.

18. J. T. Hughes, Miraculous deliverance of Anne Green: An Oxford case of resuscitation in the seventeenth century, *British Medical Journal* 285 (1982):1792–1793.

19. Martin H. son Holmdahl, Apparent death, current and historical medical explanations. Address at Gustav Adolf's Academy, November 6, 1990, pp. 1–9.

20. George Eliot, *Middlemarch* (London: Penguin Books, 1965), p. 482.

PART II: THE SEARCH FOR ARTIFICIAL RESPIRATION

1. The term scientist did not arise until the nineteenth century. During the Enlightenment, scientists were called natural philosophers.

2. William Tossach, A man dead in appearance, recovered by distending the lungs with air, *Medical Essays and Observations* (Edinburgh), 4th ed., 1752, vol. V, pt II, pp. 108–111.

3. John Fothergill, Observations on a case published in the last volume of the medical essays, etc. of recovering a man dead in appearance, by distending the lungs with air, *Philosophical Transactions*, No. 475, London, 1745.

4. Alexander Johnson, An account of some societies at Amsterdam and Hamburg for the recovery of drowned persons, 1773, London, p. 119.

5. Ralph H. Major, *Classic Descriptions of Disease*, 3rd ed. (Springfield, Ill.: Charles C. Thomas, 1945), p. 422.

6. William Buchan, *Domestic Medicine; or, the Family physician*, 8th ed. (London, 1784), pp. 672–673.

7. Fothergill.

8. Johnson, p. 4.

9. Richard V. Lee, Cardiopulmonary resuscitation in the eighteenth century, *Journal of the History of Medicine* (1972): October:418–433.

10. Johnson, p. 4.

11. Johnson, p. 8.

12. R. J. Cary, A brief history of the methods of resuscitation of the apparently drowned, *Journal of Johns Hopkins Hospital Bulletin* 270 (1918):243–251. See also Nora H. Schuster, The emperor of Russia and the Royal Humane Society, *Journal of the Royal College of General Practitioners*, 21(1971): 634–644; Elizabeth H. Thomson, The role of physicians in the humane societies of the eighteenth century, *Bulletin of the History of Medicine* 37 (1963):43–51; and Lee.

13. Johnson, p. 6.

14. Lee, p. 428.

15. "By a Physician"—A physical dissertation on drowning, London, 1766.

16. Johnson, pp. 27–30.

17. Lee, p. 428.

18. P. J. Bishop, *A short history of the Royal Humane Society* (London: Royal Humane Society, 1974).

19. Royal Humane Society, Annual Reports, 1787, 1788, 1789. London, p. 463.

20. William Meyler, Bath Human Society (London: Nichols and Son, 1806), p. 41.

21. Meyler, p. 12.

22. Bishop, p. 5.

23. Bishop, pp. 6–8.

24. Thompson, pp. 47–48.

25. Oxygen was independently discovered in the 1770s by Karl Wilhelm Scheele in Sweden and Joseph Priestley (1733–1804) in England. Schelle made his discovery using nitric acid, and Priestley heated mercuric oxide to prepare what he called "dephlogisticated air." Schelle's discovery occurred one year earlier than Priestley's, but because his report was published after Priestley's, most of the accolades go to the English scientist. Publishing is everything in science, as true in 1770 as today.

For additional information on Priestley and Lavoisier, see Royston M. Roberts, *Serendipity: Accidental Discoveries in Science* (New York: John Wiley & Sons, 1989), pp. 25–31; Robert E. Schofield, in *Dictionary of Scientific Biography* ed. Charles C. Gillispie (New York: Scribner, 1970), vol. XI, pp. 139–147; and Henry Guerlac, in *Dictionary of Scientific Biography*, ed. Charles C. Gillispie (New York: Scribner, 1970), vol. VII, pp. 66–93.

26. Lee, p. 424.

27. Stanton P. Nolan, John Hunter and cardiopulmonary resuscitation, *Surgery* 66 (1969):611–613.

28. B. A. Sellick, Cricoid pressure to control regurgitation of stomach contents during induction of anesthesia, *Lancet* ii (1961):404–405.

29. Nolan, pp. 611–613.

30. John Daniel Herholdt, Carl Gottlob Rafn, *An Attempt at an Historical Survey of Lifesaving Measures for Drowning Persons* (Copenhagen: H. Tikiob, 1796).

31. Royal Humane Society, *Case of Resuscitation by his Imperial Majesty the Emperor of Russia* (London: Nichols, Son, and Bentley, 1814).

32. M. Alexander, The rigid embrace of the narrow house: premature burial and the

signs of death, *Hastings Center Report* (1980) June:25–31.

33. Alford. E. Brown, H. A. Jeffcott, Jr., *Absolutely Mad Inventions* (New York: Dover Publications, 1970), pp. 118–119.

34. Royal Human Society, Annual Report, London, 1805.

35. Maria Trumper, The role of academic physicians in the German response to Galvani's discovery of animal electricity, 1791–1810 (Paper presented at the AAHM Conference, Seattle, April 1992.)

36. Alexander, pp. 25–31.

37. Charles Kite, *An Essay on the Recovery of the Apparently Dead,* London, 1788.

38. James Curry, *Observations on apparent death from drowning, hanging, suffocation by noxious vapours, etc.,* London, 1815, pp. 1–33.

PART II: A BETTER MOUSETRAP

1. Edwin Clarke, in *Dictionary of Scientific Biography*, ed. Charles C. Gillispie (New York: Scribner, 1970), vol. VI, pp. 58–61.

2. Peter V. Karpovich, *Adventures in Artifical Respiration* (New York: Assocation Press, 1953), p. 32. See also R. J. Cary, A brief history of the methods of resuscitation of the apparently drowned, *Journal of Johns Hopkins Hospital Bulletin* 270 (1918):243–251.

3. Arlo S. Hermreck, The history of cardiopulmonary resuscitation, *American Journal of Surgery* 156 (1988):430–436.

4. Henry R. Silvester, A new method of resuscitating still-born children, and of restoring persons apparently drowned or dead, *British Medicine Journal,* (1858) July 17:576–579.

5. Cary, p. 249.

6. Silvester, p. 579.

7. Karpovich, pp. 35–39.

8. Stewart. M. Brooks, *Our Murdered Presidents: The Medical Story* (New York: Frederick Fell, 1966), pp. 29–32.

9. Benjamin Howard, *Plain Rules for the Restoration of Persons Apparently Dead from Drowning* (New York: E. B. Treat and Co., 1869).

10. Benjamin Howard, The more usual methods of artificial respiration. With demonstrations of the "direct method" of the author, *Lancet* ii (1877):193–196.

11. R. H. Woods, On artificial respiration, *Transactions of the Royal Academy of Medicine, Ireland* (1906):136–142.

12. Karpovich, pp. 38–40.

13. P. Stroemback, *Redningen (The Rescue)*, Bra Boecker and the Swedish Red Cross, 1987.

14. A. S. Gordon, F. Raymon, M. Sadove, A. C. Ivy, Manual artificial respiration, *Journal of the American Medical Association* 14 (1950):1447–1452.

15. The Eve method involved strapping a victim on a long board that rocked back and forth like a teeter-totter. As the head tilted up, a small inspiration occurred; as the head rocked down, the abdominal contents fell against the diaphragm causing exhalation. This method was slightly better than the Silvester and Schafer methods, but was limited by the necessity of finding or improvising the proper rocking board.

16. A. S. Gordon, M. S. Sadove, et al., Critical survey of manual artificial respiration, *Journal of the American Medical Association*, 147 (1951):1444–1453.

17. Karpovich, pp. 162–181.

PART II: THE KISS OF LIFE

Interview with James Elam on August 6, 1990.

Interviews with Peter Safar on December, 23, 1988, and August 19, 1990.

Interview with Felicien Steichen on July 15, 1992.

1. Yandell Henderson, *Adventures in Respiration* (Baltimore: Williams & Wilkins, 1938), p. 184.

2. Jane S. Smith, *Patenting the Sun: Polio and the Salk Vaccine* (New York: Doubleday, 1990), pp. 27–88.

3. Hart Ellis Fisher, Resuscitation in *Medical Physics*, Otto Glasser, ed. (Chicago: Year Book Publishers, 1944), pp. 1241–1254.

4. Roderick E. McGrew, *Encyclopedia of Medical History* (New York: McGraw-Hill, 1985), p. 275.

5. James O. Elam, Rediscovery of expired air methods for emergency ventilation, in *Advances in Cardiopulmonary Resuscitation*, Peter Safar, ed. (New York: Springer-Verlag, 1977), pp. 263–265.

6. Ralph M. Waters, Simple methods for performng artificial respiration, *Journal of the American Medical Association* 123 (1943):559–561.

7. R. H. Woods, On artificial respiration, *Transactions of the Royal Academy of Medicine, Ireland* (1906):136–142.

8. James O. Elam, Elwyn S. Brown, John D. Elder, Artificial respiration by mouth-to-mask method: A study of the respiratory gas exchange of paralyzed patients ventilated by operator's expired air, *New England Journal of Medicine* 250 (1954):749–754.

9. Peter Safar. History of cardiopulmonary-cerebral resuscitation, in William Kaye and Nicholas Bircher, *Cardipulmonary Resuscitation* (New York: Churchill Livingston, 1989), pp. 1–53.

10. Elam, Rediscovery of expired air methods of emergency ventilation, pp. 263–265.

11. Ibid.

12. Peter Safar, Ventilatory efficacy of mouth-to-mouth artificial respiration, *Journal of the American Medical Association* 167 (1958):335–341.

13. Safar was not being figurative. The Army contracting officer called Lloyd's of London to explore the possibility of insurance for an accidental mishap during the experiments. Lloyd's turned the request down.

14. Safar, Ventilatory efficacy of mouth-to-mouth artificial respiration, pp. 335–341.

15. James E. Peppriell, Douglas R. Bacon, Mark J. Lema, et al., The development of academic anesthesiology at the Roswell Park Memorial Institute: James O. Elam, MD, and Elwyn S. Brown, MD, *Anesthesiology Analog* 72 (1991):538–545.

16. Mouth-to-mouth for children and infants had been recommended the previous year on March 8, 1957. The National Research Council/National Academy of Sciences had convened another ad hoc conference on artificial respiration since the Red Cross wanted new recommendations for resuscitation in infants and children. The meeting,

held in Washington, D. C., recommended the change from manual to mouth-to-mouth ventilation for children. Elam and Gordon were on the ad hoc panel chaired by David Dill. In addition, representatives from the Army, Navy, Air Force, Public Health Service, American Red Cross, and a liaison from the British Armed Forces attended the meeting. Peter Safar was listed as a guest. Gordon presented solid data in support of mouth-to-mouth respiration for children. With support from the U.S. Army Chemical Corps and the American Red Cross, Gordon carried out studies at the University of Illinois College of Medicine, and enlisted the help of parents whose children had been admitted to hospital for elective circumcision. The results were astounding. No manual method came close to the ventilation achieved with mouth-to-mouth respiration. Gordon wrote in a summary article of the conference, "Adequate ventilation is the *sine qua non* of resuscitation. As revealed by these studies, mouth-to-mouth breathing is unequivocally superior to all manual resuscitations methods in ensuring adequacy of pulmonary ventilation." These data convinced the panel to unequivocally recommend mouth-to-mouth ventilation for infants and children. The panel suggested training for "new mothers when discharged from maternity hospitals." Although the evidence for benefit was equally compelling for adults as well as children, the Council felt that the public would not accept and perform the method on adults. One member at the meeting stated, "People generally have great fear of the moribund and would probably hesitate to apply mouth-to-mouth resuscitation to persons who were cyanotic, vomiting, etc." Clearly it was assumed that people would disregard the aesthetic considerations in children but not in adults. (See Archer S. Gordon, Charles W. Frye, Lloyd Gittelson, Max S. Sadove, Edward J. Beattie, Mouth-to-mouth versus manual artificial respiration for children and adults, *Journal of the American Medical Association* 167(1958):320–328; National Academy of Sciences. National Research Council. Ad hoc conference on manual methods of artificial respiration. Tentative agenda, March 8, 1957; and National Academy of Sciences. National Research Council. Ad hoc conference on manual methods of artificial respiration. Minutes of second meeting, March 8, 1957).

17. David B. Dill, Symposium on mouth-to-mouth resuscitation (expired air inflation), Council on Medical Physics, *Journal of the American Medical Association* 167 (1958):317–319.

18. Nina Tjomsland, *From Stavanger with Care: Laerdal's First 50 years*. Printed by Aase Grafiske A/S, Stavanger, Norway.

19. Despite—or perhaps because of—personal tragedy, Safar seemed even more determined. He never flagged in his passion to defeat the Angel of Death. Nancy Caroline, an emergency and critical care colleague working at the University of Pittsburgh in 1975, later the medical director of Freedom House, recalls her first encounter with Safar. It was at a concert at the Jewish Community Center and Rudolph Serkin was performing a Beethoven sonata. Nancy was in the twenty-fifth row and midway through the concert saw someone slump over in his seat about ten rows ahead. "Before I could even register what I had seen, a figure leapt out of his seat like a jack-in-the-box, vaulted over five rows of concert-goers, dragged the unconscious man into the aisle, and started CPR. Someone else apparently called for an ambulance, for the Freedom House people arrived only minutes later and the whole group—Peter, the unconscious man, and the ambulance people—exited together with CPR in progress. Serkin, incidentally, didn't miss a beat." Caroline learned well from her mentor—she went on to establish the first nationwide paramedic service for Israel.

PART III: THE SEARCH FOR ARTIFICIAL CIRCULATION

Interview with James Jude November 1, 1990.

Interview with Guy Knickerbocker August 14, 1990.

1. Close reading reveals these early reports to be merely accounts of efforts to achieve ventilation.

2. Francis Robicsek, L. Littmann, The first reported case of external heart massage, *Clinical Cardiology* 6 (1983):569–571. See also Richard L. Taw Jr., Dr. Friedrich Maass: 100th anniversary of "New" CPR, *Clinical Cardiology* 11 (1991):1000–1002.

3. James R. Jude, William B. Kouwenhoven, Guy G. Knickerbocker, External cardiac resuscitation. *Monographs in Surgical Science* 1 (1964):59–117.

4. James R. Jude, Origins and development of cardiopulmonary resuscitation in Thomas B. Boulton, Richard S. Atkinsons, ed., *The History of Anesthesia*, International Congress and Symposium Series, Number 134 (New York: Parthenon, 1987), pp. 452–464.

5. Jean-Maurice Poitras, Pulmonary resuscitation—Howard Atwood Kelly, 1894. *Maryland State Medicine Journal* (1979) July:62–63.

6. Poitras, pp. 62–63.

7. Taw, pp. 1000–1002, and Jude, Origins and development of cardiopulmonary resuscitation, pp. 452–464.

8. Werner Overbeck, Historical views concerning cardiac arrest and resuscitaiton, in *Cardiac Arrest and Resuscitation*, Hugh E. Stephenson, ed. (Saint Louis: C.V. Mosby, 1969), pp. 27–40.

9. Peter Safar, History of cardiopulmonary-cerebral resuscitaiton, in *Cardiopulmonary Resuscitaiton*, William Kaye, Nicholas Bircher, eds. (New York: Churchill Livingston, 1989), pp. 1–53.

10. Safar, p. 17, Taw, pp. 1000–1002, and Jude, Origins and development of cardiopulmonary resuscitation, pp. 452–464.

11. Taw, pp. 1000–1002.

12. John W. Pearson, *Historical and Experimental Approaches to Modern Resuscitation* (Springfield, Ill.: Charles C. Thomas, 1965), p. 8.

13. Taw, pp. 1000–1002.

14. Jude, External cardiac compression, pp. 65. See also Pearson, p. 15.

15. Overbeck, pp. 35–36.

16. Jude, External cardiac resuscitation, p. 61.

17. T. A. Green, Heart massage as a means of restoration in cases of apparent sudden death, *Lancet* ii (1906):1707–1714.

18. Green, pp. 1707–1714.

19. Guy Knickerbocker, Contributions of William B. Kouwenhoven—reminiscences, in *Advances in Cardiopulmonary Resuscitation*, ed Peter Safar (New York: Springer-Verlag, 1970), pp. 255–258.

20. Vivien T. Thomas, *Pioneering Research in Surgical Shock and Cardiovascular Surgery* (Philadelphia: University of Pennsylvania Press, 1985), pp. 156–160.

21. Knickerbocker, pp. 255–258.

22. The first electocardiograph machine was commercially sold in 1908. By the 1950s electrocardiograms (ECGs) were routinely used in research and clinical practice.

23. Safar, p. 30.

24. Peter Safar, James O. Elam, James R. Jude, Robert J. Wilder, Paul M. Zoll.

Resuscitative principles for sudden cardiopulmonary collapse, *Diseases of the Chest* 43 (1963):34–49.

25. William B. Kouwenhoven, James R. Jude, Guy G. Knickerbocker, Closed-chest cardiac massage, *Journal of the American Medical Association* 173 (1960):94–97.

26. Kouwenhoven, pp. 94–97.

28. James R. Jude, William B. Kouwenhoven, Guy G. Knickerbocker, Cardiac arrest: Report of application of external cardiac massage on 118 patients, *Journal of the American Medical Association* 178 (1961):1063–1070.

28. Paul W. Kearney, If a heart stops beating—there's help at hand, *Readers Digest* (1960):Nov. 77:96–99.

PART III: THE BIRTH OF CPR

1. Recent advances in emergency resuscitation, *Maryland State Medical Journal* (1961) August:398–411.

2. The first version of *The Pulse of Life* was directed toward trained rescue workers since at the time no one advocated teaching chest compression to laypersons. Nevertheless, Adams and Gordon anticipated the need for general training. In a letter dated April 2, 1962, Adams wrote to an anesthesiology consultant, "If our film sifts down to a man on the street level, it would also be suitable for use as we have spelled out everything as simply as possible. We have tried to place heart compresseion in its true light—that is, as a last resort. We came up with what I think is a good gimmick—the ABC of resuscitation: A irpassage (open air passage), B reathing (restore breathing), C irculation (restore circulation) and always in this order for each step is dependent on the one that precedes it."

3. Jude, Kouwenhoven, and Knickerbocker produced a film, *External Cardiac Massage,* in 1961. It was funded by SmithKline French and circulated widely among physicians.

4. Los Angeles County Heart Association, Symposium on Cardiac Arrest, 11/3/59 (mimeo).

5. Closed Chest Cardiac Resuscitation AHA Statement, August, 1961, American Heart Association, Dallas, Texas (mimeo).

6. Efforts to spread the word about CPR were occurring internationally. In August 1961 Asmund Laerdal helped organize an international Symposium on Emergency Resuscitation in Stavanger, Norway. In attendance were the leading figures in CPR, including Jim Elam, Peter Safar, Archer Gordon, Bjorn Lind, and Ivar Lund. The conference's purpose was as much to educate as to develop international guidelines. Some attendees must have been shocked to learn of entrenched methods of artificial respiration. One anesthesiologist stated, "I am ashamed to say that in France only manual methods are taught." Similar comments came from British anesthesiologists. (See Proceedings of the Symposium on Mouth-to-Mouth Resuscitation and External Cardiac Resuscitation [Stavanger, Norway, August 21–25, 1961] *Acta Anaesthesiologica Scandinavica*: Supplement 9, 1961.) The recommendations from the conference, published in *Journal of the American Medical Association*, were the first to call for widespread training of the general public in mouth-to-mouth ventilation. Recommendation 4 stated, "First-aid workers of all categories, school children, and

the general public should be taught mouth-to-mouth and mouth-to-nose resuscitation." The conference unfortunately hedged a bit when it came to teaching chest compression to the general public. Recommendation 7 stated, "External cardiac resuscitation should be taught and used only in conjunction with artificial ventilation and, for the present, its use should be confined to medical personnel, nurses, and recognized life-savers." See Recommendations of the symposium on emergency resuscitation, Stavanger, Norway, *Journal of the American Medical Association* 178 (1961):748.

7. AHA Statement, August 1961.

8. Committee on CPR of the Division of Medical Sciences, National Academy of Sciences-National Research Council, Cardopulmonary resuscitation, *Journal of the American Medical Association* 198 (1966):372–379 and 138–145.

9. Peter Safar, History of cardipulmonary-cerebral resuscitation, in *Cardiopulmonary Resuscitation* by William Kaye and Nicholar Bircher, eds. (New York: Churchill, Livingston, 1989), pp. 1–53.

10. Ivar Lund, Bjorn Lind, eds., Aspects of Resuscitation, *Acta Anaesthesiologica Scandinavica,* Supplement 29, 1968.

PART IV: EARLY CURRENTS

1. David C. Schechter, *Exploring the Origins of Electrical Cardiac Stimulation* (Minneapolis: Medtronic, 1983), p. 15.

2. Ibid., p. 14.

3. Bern Dibner, *Doctor William Gilbert* (Norwalk, Conn.: Burndy Library, 1947), p. 5.

4. Richard S. Westfall, *The Construction of Modern Science: Mechanisms and Mechanics* (Cambridge: Cambridge University Press, 1977), p. 25.

5. Dibner, p. 11.

6. Robert Norman. *The Newe Attraction, Containing a Short Discourse of the Magnes or Lodestone.* London, 1581.

7. John L. Heilbron, in *Dictionary of Scientific Biography*, Charles C. Gillispie, ed. (New York: Scribner, 1970), Vol. V, pp. 515–517. See also Nancy Roth, A person not in the picture: Stephen Gray's conduction experiment, *Medtronic News,* vol. 20 (1):27 (no year given).

8. Nancy Roth, Early electromedicine and the Frankenstein myth, *Medical Instrumentation* 12 (1978):248.

9. Karl J. Fink, Johann Kruger on electricity "Cui bono," For whom to what good? Part I, *Electric Quarterly* (1990) 12 (3).

10. Licht, pp. 3–5.

11. Ibid., pp. 5–7.

12. Ibid., pp. 5–6.

13. D. J. Struik, in *Dictionary of Scientific Biography*, Charles C. Gillispie, ed. (New York: Scribner, 1970), Vol. IX, pp. 594–597.

14. Margaret Rowbottom, Charles Susskind. *Electricity and Medicine: History of their Interaction* (San Francisco: San Francisco Press, Inc, 1984), p. 9.

15. Nancy Roth, Electrical knowledge and the pursuit of happiness, *Medtronic News* 1989–90, p. 33.

16. Licht, p. 8.

17. Schechter, p. 33. Despite Franklin's skepticism about the benefits of electricity for paralysis, his negative opinion never reached Meriwether Lewis. During his famous expedition in 1806 Lewis described an unsuccessful effort to treat a paralyzed chief. He wrote in his journal that he wished he were in Philadelphia, where Franklin had experimented with electricity to treat paralysis, "I am confident that this [chief] would be an excellent subject for electricity." See Stephen E. Ambrose, *Undaunted Courage: Meriwether Lewis, Thomas Jefferson and the Opening of the American West* (New York: Simon & Schuster, 1996), p. 354.

18. Dennis Stillings, Benjamin Franklin's celebrated kite experiment, *Medical Instrumentation* (1973) 7:234.

19. John Wesley, *The Desideratum: or Electricity Made Plain and Useful, by a Lover of Mankind, and of Common Sense* (London, 1760).

20. Schechter, p. 48.

21. Dennis Stillings, The First Defibrillator? *Medical Progress and Technology* 2 (1974):205–206.

22. Schechter, Early experience with resuscitation by means of electricity, p. 364.

23. Charles Kite, *An Essay on the Recovery of the Apparently Dead* (London: C. Dilly, 1788), p. 166.

24. Kite, p. 125.

25. Schechter, Early experience with resuscitation by means of electricity, pp. 362–363.

26. Francis Lowndes, *Medical Electrician: Observations on Medical Electricity* (London, 1787).

27. Bern Dibner, *Luigi Galvani. An expanded version of a biography prepared for the Encyclopedia. Brittanica* (Norwalk, Conn.: Burndy Library, 1971), p. 10.

28. Hebbel E. Hoff, Galvani and the pre-Galvanian electrophysiologists, *Annals of Science* 1 (1977):157–172.

29. Bern Dibner, *Galvani-Volta. A Controversy that Led to the Discovery of Useful Electricity* (Norwalk, Conn.: Burndy Library, 1952), pp. 24–37. See also Bern Dibner, *Alessandro Volta and the Electric Battery* (New York: Franklin Watts, Inc., 1964).

30. Schechter, Early experience with resuscitation by means of electricity, p. 361.

31. These principles also explain the pain experienced when a person with silver or gold fillings bites down on a piece of aluminum. A miniature Volta pile is created because saliva serves as the medium that allows electric ions to flow between the metals. The resulting unpleasant sensation is actually a small electric current traveling through the filling to stimulate the root beneath.

PART IV: SEARCHING FOR THE SPARK OF LIFE

1. David C. Schechter, *Exploring the Origins of Electrical Cardiac Stimulation* (Minneapolis: Medtronic, Inc., 1983), p. 40.

2. Ibid., p. 42.

3. Ibid., p. 44.

4. Ibid., p. 45.

5. Bern Dibner, in *Dictionary of Scientific Biography*, ed. Charles C. Gillispie (New

York: Scribner, 1970), Vol. I, pp. 107–108.

6. David C. Schechter, Early experience with resuscitation by means of electricity, *Surgery* 69 (1971):360–372.

7. Alfred C. Garratt, Electro-physiology and electro-therapeutics; showing the best methods for the medical uses of electricity (Boston: Ticknor and Fields, 1861), second edition, p. 77.

8. Richard Reece, *The Medical Guide* (London, 1820).

9. Bern Dibner, *Oersted and the Discovery of Electromagnetism* (Norwalk, Conn.: Burndy Library, 1961), p. 16.

10. Harvey Green, *Fit for America. Health, Fitness, Sport, and American Society* (Baltimore: Johns Hopkins University Press, 1986), p. 168.

11. Green, pp. 168–169.

12. Schechter, *Exploring the Origins of Electrical Cardiac Stimulation*, p. 49.

13. G. M. Beard, A. D. Rockwell, *A Practical Treatise on the Medical and Surgical Uses of Electricity, Including Localized and General Electrization* (New York, William Wood & Co., 1871), pp. 190–193.

14. Sidney Licht, *Therapeutic Electricity and Ultraviolet Radiation* (New Haven, Conn.: Elizabeth Licht, Publisher, 1959), p. 20.

15. Ibid., pp. 22–23.

16. Schechter, *Exploring the Origins of Electrical Cardiac Stimulation*, p. 53.

17. David Armstrong, Elizabeth Metzer Armstrong, *The Great American Medicine Show* (New York: Prentice-Hall, 1991), p. 191.

18. Licht, p. 23.

19. Even reputable universities offered courses in electrotherapeutics. The University of Michigan, for example, established the Electro-therapeutical Laboratory in 1881 and charged $10 tuition for a six-week course. (See Bulletin of the Electro-therapeutical Laboratory of the University of Michigan, Jan, 1895 Vol 1, number 1, p. 1, Ann Arbor, Michigan.)

20. Licht, p. 23.

PART IV: ELECTROQUACKERY

1. The first electroquack was Elisha Perkins, born on January 16, 1741, in Norwich, Connecticut. No sooner had Galvini published his work on animal electricity than Perkins, an enterprising physician and sometime mule trader, capitalized on it to make a fortune. Apparently Perkins's "discovery" was the product of his observation during surgery that muscles would contract when touched by a scalpel. This observation led Perkins to read the experiments of Galvani and learn of bimetallic generation of electricity. According to correspondence to his son-in-law in October 1795, he happened to be treating a woman with ankle pain and, on impulse, drew his penknife downward from the calf to the painful ankle. Amazingly enough, the pain departed. His letter states, "If it was possible to monopolise the whole use or one hundredth part . . . it would make me and mine as rich as we ought to wish to be." Perkins patented his bimetallic rods in February 1796. Ironically, they were the first medical item patented by the U.S. government. See James Harvey Young, *The Toadstool Millionaires*

(Princton: Princeton University Press, 1961), pp 16–34; Roger M. Macklis, Magnetic healing, quackery, and the debate about the health effects of electromagnetic fields, *Annals of Internal Medicine* (1993) 118(5):376–383.

2. The late nineteenth century was a commercial paradise for purveyors of electric and magnetic therapeutic gadgetry. Traveling magnetic healers promoted magnetic salves and medications. They hawked numerous electric and magnetic pieces of apparel. Some of these products gained a certain commercial legitimacy. Electric health rings, electric linament, magnetic boot insoles (cost: eighteen cents a pair) were sold in the Sears Roebuck mail-order catalog. The special Sears Electric Rings were said to be "the first genuine electric rings introduced into the United States. All others are imitations." See Stewart H. Holbrook, *The Golden Age of Quackery* (New York: Macmillan, 1958), pp. 122–145.

3. Holbrook, pp. 122–145. Arther J. Cramp, *Nostrums and Quackery and Psuedo-Medicineicine* (Chicago: American Medical Association, 1936), Vol. III.

4. Nancy Roth, Good vibrations: Abrams's oscilloclast and the instrumental cure, *Medical Instrumentation* 15 (1981):383–384. See also David Armstrong, Elizabeth Metzger Armstrong, *The Great American Medicine Show* (New York: Prentice-Hall, 1991), pp. 192–193.

5. Armstrong and Armstrong, p. 192.

6. Roth, pp. 383–384.

7. Sidney Licht, *Therapeutic Electricity and Ultraviolet Radiation* (New Haven: Elizabeth Licht, 1959), p 21.

8. Roth, pp. 383–384.

9. Morris Fishbein, *Fads and Quackery in Healing* (New York: Blue Ribbon Books, 1932), p. 145.

10. Armstrong and Armstrong, p. 192.

11. Quackery doesn't love a vacuum. As Abrams's Pathoclast and Oscilloclast fell into disrepute, a new medical device took their place in 1926. Known as the I-ON-A-CO, it was not based on any pseudoscientific theories—it simply cured. The device was composed of two coils of insulated wire (worth $3.50, according to a critical report of the American Medical Association) worn around the waist or neck and plugged into household current. The smaller coil was attached to a flashlight bulb, and, when placed in close proximity to the large coil, would generate enough electricity (via induced current) to light the tiny bulb. Could there be better evidence of the magical property of the large coil? A detractor likened it to a "magic horse collar." (See Fishbein, p. 153.) It sold for $58.40 cash or $65 on the deferred-payment plan. According to inventor Gaylord Wilshire, the electric current was a "simple and effective method of using magnetism for the cure of human ailments." Any and all ailments. All one has to do, according to the directions is to "place over your shoulders the Wilshire Ring or I-ON-A-CO. That's all. You may then light a cigarette and read your newspaper for ten or fifteen minutes. Meanwhile its magnetic force is permeating your body, and effecting the cure. You see nothing, you feel nothing." (See Holbrook, p. 139.)

12. Licht, p. 23.

13. The 1938 Federal Food, Drug and Cosmetic Act changed the focus of the FDA from that of an agency primarily established to police adulteration of food and drugs to one concerned with regulating and evaluating new drugs and devices. (See P. M. Wax, Elixirs, diulents, and the passage of the 1938 Federal Food, Drug and Cosmetic

Act, *Annals of Internal Medicine* 122 (1955):456–461.) Wax argues that the major catalyst for the passage of the 1938 act was the 1937 mass poisoning involving 355 patients
treated with sulfanilamide that had been diluted with the poison diethylene glycol.
Over 100 people died. At the time there were no requirements for toxicity testing
prior to the release of a new drug.

14. James H. Young, *American Health Quackery* (Princeton: Princeton University
Press, 1992), pp. 187–198.

15. James H. Young, *The Medical Messiahs* (Princeton: Princeton University Press,
1967). See also W. Wagner, The Unreal World of Dr. Drown, in *Reader's Digest
Scoundrels & Scalawags: 51 Stories of the Most Fascinating Characters of Hoax and Fraud*
(Pleasantville, N.Y.: Reader's Digest Association , 1968), pp. 413–427.

16. Young, *The Medical Messiahs*, p. 249.

17. Ruth B. Drown, *The Theory and Technique of the Drown H.V.R. and Radio-Vision
Instruments* (London: Hatchard & Co., 1939); see also Ruth B. Drown, *The Science
and Philosophy of the Drown Radio Therapy* (Los Angeles: Ward Ritchie Press,1938).

18. Young, *The Medical Messiahs*, pp. 247–249.

19. Ibid., p. 257.

PART IV: DEFIBRILLATION IS THE SPARK OF LIFE

Interview with Bernard Lown June 2, 1992.

Interview with Paul Zoll March 8, 1990.

1. David C. Schechter, *Exploring the Origins of Electrical Cardiac Stimulation*
(Minneapolis: Medtronic, Inc., 1983), p. 68.

2. Nancy Roth, "First stammering of the heart": Ludwig's kymograph, *Medical
Instrumentation* 12 (1978):348.

3. George Vivian Poore, *Textbook of Electricity in Medicine and Surgery* (London:
Smith, Elder & Co., 1876). See also Wilhelm Erb, *Handbook of Electro-Therapeutics*
(New York: William Wood & Co., 1883), p. 108.

4. Hugh MacLean. John Alexander MacWilliam, *Aberdeen University Review* 24
(1937):127–132.

5. John A. McWilliam, Cardiac failure and sudden death, *British Medical Journal*
(1889) January 5:6–8.

6. Ibid., pp. 6–8.

7. John A. McWilliam, Electrical stimulation of the heart in man, *British Medical
Journal* (1889) February 16:348–350.

8. A. G. Levy, T. Lewis, Heart irregularities resulting from the inhalation of low per-
centages of chloroform vapour, and their relationship to ventricular fibrillation, *Heart*
3 (1911):99.

9. Schechter, p. 146.

10. R. H. Cunningham, The cause of death from industrial electric currents, *New
York Medicine Journal* (1899) October:681–622.

11. Louise G.Robinovitch, Methods of resuscitating electrocuted animals. Different
effects of various electric currents according to the method use. Importance of exclud-
ing from the circuit the central nervous system during resuscitation, *Journal Mental
Pathology* 8 (1909):129–145.

12. Louise G. Robinovitch, Induction coil specially constructed according to our indications for purposes of resuscitation of subjects in a condition of apparent death caused by chloroform, morphine, electrocution, etc., *Journal of Mental Pathology* 8 (1909):129–145.

13. Report of the Commission on Resuscitation from Electric Shock. Read before the National Electric Light Association, Chicago, June, 1913.

14. D. R. Hooker, On the recovery of the heart in electric shock, *American Journal of Physiology* 91 (1930):305–328. See also D. R. Hooker. Chemical factors in ventricular fibrillation, *American Journal of Physiology* 92 (1930):639–647.

15. D. R. Hooker, W. B. Kouwenhoven, O. R. Langworthy, The effect of alternating electrical currents on the heart, *American Journal of Physiology* 103 (1933):444–454.

16. William Kouwenhoven, Donald R. Hooker, Resuscitation by countershock, *Electrical Engineering* (1933):475–477.

17. James R. Jude, William B. Kouwenhoven, Guy G. Knickerbocker, External cardiac resuscitation, *Monograph in Surgical Science* 1 (1964):59–117.

18. John A. Meyer, Claude Beck and cardiac resuscitation, *Annals of Thoracic Surgery* 45 (1988):103–105.

19. Beck and Kouwenhoven probably never met. However, there was an indirect connection between the two. Apparently Beck's colleague Carl J. Wiggers visited Kouwenhoven's laboratory sometime during the 1930s, after Kouwenhoven's papers had been published, and discussed his work. It's possible that Wiggers's reports to Beck on Kouwenhoven's work influenced Beck's later work on external defibrillation.

Wiggers, a member of the department of physiology at the Western Reserve University in Cleveland, published the results of his studies on coronary circulation in animals in 1936. He showed that open-heart massage before rather than after application of countershock resulted in the resuscitation of hearts that had been in fibrillation for five to seven minutes, in most cases without use of drugs or chemicals. In a 1940 article, he wrote that the heart could remain in fibrillation for up to fifteen minutes and still be successfully defibrillated so long as one minute of open-heart massage preceded the shock. Wiggers advocated electric defibrillatory shocks and wrote that "the method should prove of value in revival of exposed human hearts that fibrillate accidentally during [the] course of cardiac operations." He realized that cardiac massage prior to the shock could buy time until the device was at hand. "Any procedure that extends the time for hopeful recovery by only few a minutes," he wrote, "becomes of practical importance." See C. J. Wiggers, Cardiac massage followed by counter shock in revival of mammalian ventricles from fibrillation due to coronary occlusion, *American Journal of Physiology* 116 (1937):161–162; and C. J. Wiggers, The physiologic basis for cardiac resuscitation from ventricular fibrillation-method for serial defibrillation, *American Heart Journal* 20 (1940):413–422.

20. Beck wrote other idioms attempting to communicate the idea of hearts too good to die, such as "The Heart Has Mileage Left In It" and "The Heart Needs a Second Chance to Beat." The latter two expressions never caught on.

21. David S. Leighninger, Contributions of Claude Beck, in Peter Safar, ed., *Advances in Cardiopulmonary Resuscitaiton* (New York: Springer-Verlag, 1975), pp. 259–262.

22. Leighninger, p. 260.

23. Samuel A. Thompson, George L. Birnbaum, Irving S. Shiner, Cardiac resus-

citation: With report of a case of successful resuscitation following auricular and ventricular fibrillation, *Journal of the American Medical Association* 119 (1942):18:1479–1485.

24. Louis J. Acierno, *The History of Cardiology* (London: Parthenon Publishing Group, 1994), p. 712.

25. C. S. Beck, W. H. Pritchard, H. S. Feil, Ventricular fibrillation of long duration abolished by electric shock, *Journal of the American Medical Association* 135 (1947):985–986.

26. Barnett A. Greene, Letter to editor re: article by Beck on ventricualr fibrillation abolished by electric shock, *Journal of the American Medical Association* 135 (1947):985.

27. C. S. Beck, H. J. Rand III, Cardiac arrest during anesthesia and surgery, *Journal of the American Medical Association* (1949) December 24:1230–1233.

28. Peter Safar, History of cardipulmonary-cerebral resuscitation, in *Cardiopulmonary Resuscitation,* William Kaye and Nicholas Bircher, eds. (New York: Churchill Livingston, 1989), p. 22.

29. Summary notes, Committee on Cardiopulmonary resuscitation, January 27–28, Miami Beach, Florida, American Heart Association, Dallas, Texas (mimeo).

30. W. B. Kouwenhoven, W. R. Milnor, Treatment of ventricular fibrillation using a capacitor discharge, *Journal Applied Physiology* 7 (1954):253–257.

31. W. B. Kouwenhoven, W. R. Milnor, G. G. Knickerbocker, William R. Chesnut, Closed chest defibrillation of the heart, *Surgery* 42 (1957):550–561.

32. Arthur C. Guyton, J. Satterfield, Factors concerned in electrical defibrillation of the heart, particularly through an unopened chest, *American Heart Journal* 167 (1951):81–87.

33. Paul M. Zoll, Arthur J. Linenthal, William Gibson, Milton H. Paul, Leona R. Norman. Termination of ventricular fibrillation in man by externally applied electric countershock, *New England Journal of Medicine* 254 (1956):727–732.

34. Bernard Lown, "Cardioversion" of arrhythmias (I), *Modern Concepts of Cardiovascular Diseases,* American Heart Association 33 (1964):863–868.

35. Lown, New method for terminating cardiac arrhythmias, pp. 548–555.

PART V: BELFAST LEADS THE WAY

Interview with John Geddes June 10, 1990.

Based on written reply from J Frank Pantridge to questions, September, 25, 1991.

Interview with Richard Crampton October 29, 1992.

1. Katherine Traver Barkley, *The Ambulance* (Kiamesha Lake, N.Y.: Load Go Press, 1978), p. 19.

2. James Curry, *Observations on apparent death from drowning, hanging, suffocation by noxious vapours, etc.* (London, 1815).

3. Thomas Hearne, The development of emergency medical services, Mickey S. Eisenberg, Lawrence Bergner, Alfred P. Hallstrom, eds., *Sudden Cardiac Death in the Community* (Bridgeport, Conn.: Praeger, 1984), pp. 29–43.

4. A. H. Buck, ed., *A Reference Handbook of the Medical Sciences* (New York: William Wood & Co., 1886), Vol. 1—Ambulances, pp. 128–133. See also Robert J. Carlisle, ed.,

An Account of Bellevue Hospital with a Catalogue of the Medical and Surgical Staff from 1736–1894 (New York: Society of the Alumni of Bellevue Hospital, 1893), pp. 65–76.

5. Buck, pp. 128–133.

6. J. F. Pantridge, *An Unquiet Life* (Northern Ireland: W & G Baird, 1989), p. xi. Most of the biographical material in this chapter comes from this book.

7. Wallace M. Yater, Arron H. Traum, Wilson G. Brown, Richard P. Fitzgerald, Murry A. Geisler, Blanche B. Wilcox, Coronary artery disease in men eighteen to thirty-nine years of age, *American Heart Journal* 36 (1948):334–372, 481–526, 683–722.

8. J. F. Pantridge, J. S. Geddes, Cardiac arrest after myocardial infarction, *Lancet* i (1966):807–808.

9 Twenty-five years later, during an award ceremony at a national meeting of the American Heart Association in Dallas, Pantridge remarked how he liked everything about the *Time* article except the reference to Belfast as dour.

10. J. F. Pantridge, J. S. Geddes, A mobile intensive-care unit in the management of myocardial infarction, *Lancet* ii (1967):271–273.

PART V: ACROSS THE ATLANTIC

1. William J. Grace, John A. Chadbourn, The first hour in acute myocardial infarction, *Heart Lung* 3 (1974):736–741.

2. William J. Grace, John A. Chadbourn, The mobile coronary care unit, *Diseases of the Chest* 55 (1969):452–455.

PART V: RACING THE ANGEL OF DEATH

Interview with Leonard Cobb March 27, 1989.
Interviews with Eugene Nagel July 2, 1989, and July 6, 1992.
Interview with Richard Lewis April 16, 1992.
Interview with Michael Criley April 27, 1992.
Interview with Leonard Rose February 2, 1993.

1. Eugene L. Nagel, Jim C. Hirschman, Sidney R. Nussenfeld, David Rankin, Edward Lundblad, Telemetry-medical command in coronary and other mobile emergency care systems, *Journal of the American Medical Association* 214 (1970):332–338. See also Eugene L. Nagel, Jim C. Hirschman, Paul W. Meyer, Frank Dennis, Telemetry of physiologic data: an aid to fire rescue personnel in a metropolitan area, *Southern Medical Journal* 61 (1968):598–601.

2. Cedric R. Bainton, Donald R. Peterson, Deaths from coronary heart disease in persons fifty years of age and younger: A community-wide study, *New England Journal of Medicine* 268 (1963):569–575.

3. John M. Stang, Martin D. Keller, Richard P. Lewis, Mobile pre-hospital coronary care, Columbus, Ohio, in A. A. J. Adgey, ed., *Acute Phase of Ischemic Heart Disease and Myocardial Infarction* (The Hague: Martinus Nijhoff, 1982), pp. 99–118.

4. J Michael Criley, A. James Lewis, Gaylord E. Ailshie, Mobile emergency care units, Implementation and justification, *Advances in Cardiology* 15 (1975):9–24.

EPILOGUE: THE QUEST CONTINUES

1. Philippe Ariès, *The Hour of Our Death* (New York: Alfred A. Knopf, 1981), p. 10.

2. John D. Morgan, Attitudes toward death in Warren Thomas Reich, ed., *Encyclopedia of Bioethics* (New York: Simon & Schuster, 1995), p. 524.

3. Ernest Becker, *The Denial of Death* (New York: Free Press, 1973), p. 4.

4. Peter Safar, Concluding statement in *Advances in Cardiopulmonary Resuscitation* (New York: Springer-Verlag, 1977), p. 297.

5. Ibid., p. 297.

6. William Osler, *The Evolution of Modern Medicine. Lecture Series of April 1913* (New Haven, Conn.: Yale University Press, 1921).

7. Peter Safar, History of cardiopulmonary-cerebral resuscitation, *Cardiopulmonary Resuscitation,* William Kaye and Nicholas Bircher, eds. (New York: Livingstone, 1989), p. 2.

8. Mickey Eisenberg, Michael Copass, Alfred Hallstrom, et al., Treatment of out-of-hospital cardiac arrest with rapid defibrillation by emergency medical technicians, *New England Journal of Medicine* 302 (1980):1379–1383.

9. Richard O. Cummins, Mickey S. Eisenberg, Paul E. Litwin, et al., Automatic external defibrillators used by emergency medical technicians: a controlled clinical trial. *Journal of the American Medical Association* 257 (1987):1605–1610.

10. William B. Carter, Mickey S. Eisenberg, Alfred Hallstrom, Sharon Schaeffer, Development and implementation of emergency CPR instruction via telephone, *Annals of Emergency Medicine* 13 (1984):695–700. See also Linda Culley, Jill Clark, Mickey S. Eisenberg, Mary P. Larsen, Dispatcher assisted telephone CPR: Standards and time requirements, *Annals of Emergency Medicine* 20 (1991):362–366.

11. Richard O. Cummins, Joseph P. Ornato, William Thies, Paul E. Pepe, et al., Improving survival from cardiac arrest: the chain of survival concept, *Circulation* 83 (1991):1832–1847.

12. Mickey S. Eisenberg, The perfect resuscitation, *Annals of Emergency Medicine* 21 (1992):1122–1123.

13. Mickey S. Eisenberg, Bruce T. Horwood, Richard O. Cummins, Robin Reynolds-Haertle, Thomas R. Hearne, Cardiac arrest and resuscitation: A tale of 29 cities, *Annals of Emergency Medicine* 19 (1990):179–186.

14. G. Lombardi, J. Gallagher, P. Gennis, Outcome of out-of-hospital cardiac arrest in New York City, *Journal of the American Medical Association* 271 (1994):678–683. See also Lance B. Becker, M. P. Ostrander, J. Barrett, G. T. Kondos, Outcomes of CPR in a large metropolitan area—where are the survivors? *Annals of Emergency Medicine* 22 (1993):1652–1658.

SELECTED READINGS

《 》

Adgey AAJ, Nelson PG, Scott ME, Geddes JS, Pantridge JF. Management of ventricular fibrillation outside hospital. *Lancet* 1969;i:1169–1171.

Albury WR. Ideas of Life and Death. Chapter in Bynum WF, Porter R (eds) *Companion Encyclopedia of the History of Medicine*, London: Routledge, 1993, pp. 249–280.

Alexander S, Kleiger R, Lown B. Use of external electric countershock in the treatment of ventricular fibrillation. *Journal of the American Medical Association* 1961;177:916–918.

Ariès P. *Western Attitudes Toward Death from the Middle Ages to the Present*. Baltimore: Johns Hopkins University Press, 1974.

Baum RS, Alvarez H, Cobb L. Survival after resuscitation from out-of-hospital ventricular fibrillation. *Circulation* 1974;50:1231–1235.

Beck CS, Leighninger DS. Reversal of death in good hearts. *Journal of Cardiovascular Surgery* 1962;3:357.

Beck CS, Weckesser EC, Barry FM. Fatal heart attack and successful defibrillation. *Journal of the American Medical Association* 1956;161:434–436.

Beck CS. Death after a clean bill of health. *Journal of American Medical Association* 1960;174:117–119.

Beck CS. Reminiscences of cardiac resuscitation. *Review of Surgery* 1970 (March-April):76–86.

Boyd DR. The history of EMS systems in the USA. Chapter in Boyd DR, Edlich RF, Micik SH (eds) *Systems Approach to Emergency Medical Care*. Norwalk, Conneticut: Appleton-Century-Crofts, 1983, pp. 1–82.

Cambridge NA. Electrical apparatus used in medicine before 1900. *Proceedings of the Royal Society of Medicine* 1977;70:635–641.

Cobb LA, Conn RD, Samson WE, Philbin JE. Early experiences in the management of sudden death with a mobile intensive coronary care unit. *Circulation* Supplement 1970 (Oct):III–144.

Cobb LA, Conn RD, Samson WE. Pre-hospital coronary care: The role of a rapid response mobile intensive coronary care system. *Circulation* Supplement 1971;II–45.

Cobb LA, Hallstrom AP. Community-based cardiopulmonary resuscitation: What have we learned? *Annuals of New York Academy of Science* 1982;382:330–342.

Crampton RS, Aldrich RF, Gascho JA, et al. Reduction of pre-hospital, ambulance and community coronary death rates by the community-wide emergency cardiac care system. *American Journal of Medicine* 1975;58:151–165.

Crile G, Dolley DH. An experimental research into the resuscitation of dogs killed by anesthetics and asphyxia. *Journal of Experimental Medicine* 1906;8:713–725.

Criley JM, Niemann JT, Rowborough JP. Cardiopulmonary resuscitation research 1960–1984: Discoveries and advances. *Annals of Emergency Medicine* 1984;13:756–758.

Cummins RO, Eisenberg MS, Hallstrom A, Litwin PE. Survival of out-of-hospital cardiac arrest with early initiation of cardiopulmonary resuscitation. *American Journal of Emergency Medicine* 1985;3:114–119.

Cummins RO, Chamberlain DA, Eisenberg MS, Bossaert L, Holmberg S, et al. The "Utstein Style": Recommended guidelines for uniform reporting of data from out-of-hospital cardiac arrest. *Circulation* 1991;84:960–975.

Cummins RO, Eisenberg MS. Prehospital cardiopulmonary resuscitation: Is it effective? *Journal of the American Medical Association* 1985;253:2408–2412.

Cummins RO, Eisenber MS, Litwin PE, et al. Automatic external defibrillators used by emergency medical technicians: A controlled clinical trial. *Journal of the American Medical Association* 1987;257:1605–1610.

DeBard ML. The history of cardiopulmonary resuscitation. *Annals of Emergency Medicine* 1980;9:273–275.

Driscoll TE, Ratnoff OD, Nygaard OF. The remarkable Dr. Abildgaard and countershock. *Annals of Internal Medicine* 1975;83:878–882.

Eisenberg MS. Improving out-of-hospital cardiac arrest. *Lancet* 1994;344:561–562.

Eisenberg MS. Charles Kite's essay on the recovery of the apparently dead: The first scientific study of sudden death. *Annals of Emergency Medicine.* 1994;23:1049–1053.

Eisenberg M, Bergner L, Hallstrom A. Paramedic programs and out-of-hospital cardiac arrest: I. Factors associated with successful resuscitation. *American Journal of Public Health* 1979;69:30–38.

Eisenberg M, Bergner L, Hallstrom A. Cardiac resuscitation in the community: The importance of rapid delivery of care and implications for program planning. *Journal of the American Medical Association* 1979;241:1905–1907.

Eisenberg M, Bergner L, Hallstrom A. Out-of-hospital cardiac arrest: Improved survival with paramedic services. *The Lancet* 1980;i:812–815.

Eisenberg M, Hallstrom A, Bergner L. Long-term survival after out-of-hospital cardiac arrest. *New England Journal of Medicine* 1982;306:1340–1343.

Eisenberg M, Hallstrom A, Copass M, Bergner L, Short F, Pierce J. Treatment of ventricular fibrillation: Emergency medical technician defibrillation and paramedic services. *Journal of the American Medical Association* 1984;251:1723–1726.

Eisenberg MS, Horwood BT, Cummins RO, Reynolds-Haertle R, Hearne TR. Cardiac arrest and resuscitation: A tale of 29 cities. *Annals of Emergency Medicine* 1990;19:179–186.

Elam JO, Green DG, Schneider M, Henning R, Archer G, Hustead R, Benson D, Clements J, Ruben A. Head-tilt method of oral resuscitation. *Journal of the American Medical Association* 1960;172:812–815.

Emergency Cardiac Care Committee and Subcommittees, American Heart Association, Guidelines for cardiopulmonary resuscitation and emergency cardiac care. *Journal of the American Medical Association*, 1992;268:2172–2302.

Ferris LP, King BG, Spence PW, Williams HB. Effect of electric shock on the heart. *Electrical Engineering* 1936;55:498–515.

Flagg PJ, Hosler RM. *The National Resuscitation Society's Respirocardiac Resuscitation Course*, New York: National Resuscitation Society, 1962.

Fleming D. Galen on the motions of the blood in the heart and lungs. *Isis* 1955;46:14–21.

France EM. Some eighteenth century authorities on the resuscitation of the apparently drowned. *Anaesthesia* 1975;30:530–538.

Fye WB. Ventricular fibrillation and defibrillation: Historical perspectives with emphasis on the contributions of John MacWilliam, Carl Wiggers, and William Kouwenhoven. *Circulation* 1985;71:858–865.

Garland TO. *Artificial Respiration*, New York, Macmillian, 1955.

Geddes JS, (ed). *The Management of the Acute Coronary Attack: The J. Frank Pantridge Festschrift*. London: Academic Press, 1986.

Geddes JS. Twenty years of pre-hospital coronary care. *Brain and Heart Journal* 1986;56:491–495.

Geddes JS, Adgey AAJ, Pantridge JF. Prognosis after recovery from ventricular fibrillation complicating ischemic heart disease. *The Lancet* 1967;ii:273–275.

Gordon AS, Fainer DC, Ivy AC. Artificial respiration: A new method and a comparative study of different methods in adults. *Journal of the American Medical Association* 1950;144:1455–1464.

Gordon AS, et al. Circulatory studies during artificial respiration of apneic normal adults. *Journal of Applied Physiology* 1951;4:421.

Gordon AS, Sandove MS, Raymon F, Ivy AC. Pole top and other resuscitation methods: A comparison study. *Industrial Medical Surgery* 1952;21:147–152.

Grace WJ. The mobile coronary care unit and the intermediate coronary care unit in the total systems approach to coronary care. *Chest* 1970;58:363–368.

Grace WJ, Chadbourne JA. The first hour in acute MI. *Heart and Lung* 1974;3:736–741.

Graf WS, Polin SS, Paegel BL. A community program for emergency cardiac care. *Journal of the American Medical Association* 1973;226:156–160.

Guildner CW. Resuscitation—Opening the airway: A comparative study of techniques for opening an airway obstructed by the tongue. *Journal of the American College of Emergency Physicians* 1976;5:588–590.

Gurvich NL, Yuniev GS. Restoration of the regular rhythm in the mammalian fibrillating heart. *American Review of Soviet Medicine* 1946;3:236–239.

Hawkins LH. The experimental development of modern resuscitation. *Resuscitation* 1972;1:9–24.

Howard B. The more usual methods of artificial respiration. With demonstrations of the "direct method" of the author. *The Lancet* 1877;ii:193–196.

Howard B. *Plain Rules for the Restoration of Persons Apparently Dead from Drowning*. New York: E. B. Treat and Company, 1869.

Iserson KV. *Death to Dust: What Happens to Dead Bodies*. Tucson, Arizona: Galen Press, 1994.

Jellinek S. *Dying, Apparent-death and Resuscitation*. Baltimore: Williams and Wilkins Co., 1947.

Jude JR. Rediscovery of external heart compression in Dr. William Kouwenhoven's laboratory. Chapter in Safar P. (ed) *Advances in Cardiopulmonary Resuscitation*. New York: Springer-Verlag, 1970, pp. 286–291.

Jude JR, Kouwenhoven WB, Knickerbocker GG. Clinical and experimental application of a new treatment for cardiac arrest. *Surgical Forum* 1960;11:252–254.

Jude JR. Origins and development of cardiopulmonary resuscitation in Boulton TB, Atkinsons RS. *The History of Anesthesia*. New York: Parthenon, 2nd ed. 1989, pp. 452–464.

Kaye W and Bircher N (eds). *Cardiopulmonary Resuscitation*. New York: Livingstone, 1989.

Kowenhoven WB, Kay JH. A simple electrical apparatus for the clinical treatment of ventricular fibrillation. *Surgery* 1951;30:780–786.

Larsen MP, Eisenberg MS, Cummins RO, Hallstrom AP. Predicting survival from out-of-hospital cardiac arrest: A graphic model. *Annals of Emergency Medicine* 1993;22:1652–1658.

Lewis RP, Stang JM, Fulkerson PK, Sampson KL, Scoles A, Warren JV. Effectiveness of advanced paramedics in a mobile coronary care system. *Journal of the American Medical Association* 1979;241:1902–1904.

Lewis RP, Fulkerson PK, Stang JM, et al. The Colombus emergency medical service system. *Journal of the Ohio State Medical Association* 1979;75:391–394.

Lown B. Electrical reversion of cardiac arrhythmias. *British Heart Journal* 1967;29:469–488.

Lown B, Neuman J, Amarasingham B, Berkovits BV. Comparison of alternating current with direct current electroshock across the closed chest. *American Journal of Cardiology* 1962;223–233.

Lund I, Lind B, eds. Aspects of resuscitation, *Acta Anaesthesiologica Scandinavica* Supplement 29, 1968.

Meyer HW. *A History of Electricity and Magnetism*, Cambridge, Massachusetts: MIT Press, 1971.

Morgan JD. Attitudes toward death, in Reich WT (ed) *Encyclopedia of Bioethics*, New York: Simon & Schuster, 1995, pp. 523–529.

Nagel EL, Hirschman JC, Nussenfeld SR, Rankin D, Lundblad E. Telemetry-medical command in coronary and other mobile emergency care systems. *Journal of the American Medical Association* 1970;214:332–338.

Nagel EL, Hirshman JC, Mayer PW, Dennis F. Telemetry of physiologic data: An aid to fire-rescue in a metropolitan area. *Southern Medical Journal* 1968;61:598–601.

Nagel EL, Fine EG, Krischer JP, Davis JH. Complications of CPR. *Critical Care Medicine*,1981;9,424.

Negovski VA. Reanimatology—the science of resuscitation in Stephenson HE (ed) *Cardiac Arrest and Resuscitation*, St. Louis: C.V.Mosby, 1969, pp. 1–25.

Nielsen H. *The Holger Nielsen Method of Artificial Resuscitation*, London: Royal Life Saving Society, 1952.

Nuland SB. *How We Die*, New York: Alfred A. Knopf, Inc., 1994.

Pantridge JF, Adgey AAJ. Pre-hospital coronary care: The mobil coronary care unit. *American Journal of Cardiology* 1969;24:666–673.

Pantridge JF, Adgey AAJ. Prehospital management of acute myocardial infarction in Chung EK (ed) *Cardiac Emergency Care*, Philadelphia: Lea and Fegiger, 1974, pp. 52–65.

Pantridge JF, Adgey AAJ, Geddes JS, Webb SW. *The Acute Coronary Attack,* London: Grune & Stratton, 1975.

Paraskos J. Biblical accounts of resuscitation. *Journal of Medical History and Allied Sciences* 1992;47:310–320.

Payne JP. On the resuscitation of the apparently dead: An historical account. *Annals of Royal College of Surgery* (England)1969;45:98–107.

Perkins JF. Historical development of respiratory physiology. Chapter in Fenn WO, Rahn H, (eds). *Handbook of Physiology Volume I, Section 3: Respiration,* Washington, D.C.: American Physiological Society, 1964, pp. 1–64.

Price JL. The evolution of breathing machines. *Medical History* 1962;6:67–72.

Priestly J. *History and Present State of Electricity, with Original Experiments*, London, 1767.

Proceedings of the Symposium on Mouth-to-Mouth Resuscitation and External Cardiac Resuscitation (Stavanger, Norway, August 21–25, 1961) *Acta Anaesthesiologica Scandinavica*: Supplement 9, 1961.

Recent advances in emergency resuscitation. *Maryland State Medical Journal* 1961;August:398–411.

Recommendations of the symposium on emergency resuscitation, Stavanger, Norway. *Journal of the American Medical Association* 1961;178:748.

Redding JR, Commentary on the proceedings: Second Wolf Creek Conference on CPR. *Critical Care Medicine* 1981;9,432–435.

Resnekov L. Eighteenth century resuscitation. Chapter in *Advances in Cardiopulmonary Resuscitation* Safar P (ed), New York: Springer-Verlag, 1970, pp. 253–254.

Rose LB, Press E. Cardiac defibrillation by ambulance attendants. *Journal of the American Medical Association* 1972;219:63–68.

Rosen Z, Davidson JT. Respiratory resuscitation in ancient Hebrew sources. *Anesthesia and Analgesia* 1972;51:4:502–505.

Rosenthal RE. Cardiopulmonary resuscitation: Historical and future perspectives. *Postgraduate Medicine* 1987;81:90–103.

Rosner F. Artificial respiration in biblical times. *New York State Journal of Medicine* 1959 (April 15):1104–1105.

Roth N. Gaylord Wilshire's I-ON-A-CO. *Medical Instrumentation* 1978;12:1.

Roth N. Electroresuscitation and the occult. *Medical Instrumentation* 1980;14:120–121.

Roth N. Life-and-death decisions: Electrodiagnosis and premature burial. *Medical Instrumentation* 1980;14:322.

Roth N. The nineteenth century revival of electrotherapy. *Medical Instrumentation* 1977;11:236–237.

Roth N. Controversies and cures: the electrical medicine of J. G. Schaffer. *Medtronic News*, 1994,22:71–73

Ruben H. The immediate treatment of respiratory failure. *British Journal of Anesthesiolgy* 1964;36:542–549.

Safar P. Pathophysiology of dying and reanimation. Chapter in Schwartz R, Safar P,

Stone, Storey, Wagner (eds) *Principles and Practice of Emergency Medicine*, Philadelphia: W.B. Saunders, 1986, Vol. 1, pp. 2–41.

Safar P. History of cardiopulmonary resuscitation. *Acute Care* 1986;12:61–62.

Safar P. From back-pressure arm-lift to mouth-to-mouth, control of airway, and beyond. Chapter in Safar P (ed) *Advances in Cardiopulmonary Resuscitation*, New York: Springer-Verlag, 1970, pp. 266–275.

Safar P, Escarraga LA, Elam JO. A comparison of the mouth-to-mouth and mouth-to-airway methods of artificial respiration with the chest-pressure arm-lift methods. *New England Journal of Medicine* 1958;258:671–677.

Safar P, Escarraga LA, Chang F. Upper airway obstruction in the unconscious patient. *Journal of Applied Physiology* 1959;14:760–764.

Safar P, Brown TC, Holtey WJ, Wilder RJ. Ventilation and circulation with closed-chest cardiac massage in man. *Journal of the American Medical Association* 1961;176:574–576.

Safar P. Imitation of the closed-chest cardiopulmonary resuscitation in basic life support: A personal history. *Resuscitation* 1989;18:7–20.

Safar P, McMahon MC. *Resuscitation of the Unconscious Victim*, Springfield, Illinois: Charles C Thomas, 2nd ed, 1961.

Sanders AB, Meislin HW, Ewy GA. The physiology of cardiopulmonary resuscitation: An update. *Journal of the American Medical Association* 1984;252:3283–3286.

Schecter DC. Role of the Humane Societies in the history of resuscitation. *Surgical Gynecology and Obstetrics* 1969 (October):811–815.

Schecter DC. Application of electrotherapy to noncardiac thoratic disorders. *Bulletin of the New York Academy of Medicine* 1970;46:932–951.

Scherlis L. Poetical version of the rules of the Humane Society for recovering drowned persons. *Critical Care Medicine* 1981;9:430–431.

Scientific American. Our Abrams Investigation I-XI and Our Abrams Verdict. October 1923; September 1924.

Silvester HR. A new method of resuscitating still-born children, and of restoring persons apparently drowned or dead. *British Medical Journal* July 17, 1858.

Stephenson HE. Charles Claude Guthrie's contribution to cardiac resuscitation. *Critical Care Medicine* 1981;9:428–429.

Stephenson HE Jr, ed *Cardiac Arrest and Resuscitation*, 4th ed, St Louis: Mosby, 1974.

Stillings D. The Piscean origin of medical electricity. *Medical Instrumentation* 1973; 7:163.

Thangam S, Weil MH, Rackow EC. Cardiopulmonary resuscitation: A historical review. *Acute Care* 1986;12:63–94.

Wax PM. Elixirs, diluents, and the passage of the 1938 Federal Food, Drug and Cosmetic Act. *Annals of Internal Medicine*. 1955;122:456–461.

Wiggers CJ. The mechanism and nature of ventricular fibrillation. *American Heart Journal* 1940;20:399–411.

Wiggers CJ, Bell JR, Paine M, et al. Studies of ventricular fibrillation caused by electric shock. I. The revival of the heart from ventricular fibrillation by use of K and Ca. *American Journal of Physiology* 1930;92:223–239.

Wiggers CJ, Theisen H, Shaw HDB. Studies on ventricular fibrillation produced by electric shock. III. The action of antagonistic salts. *American Journal of Physiology* 1930;93:197–212.

Wilson LG. Erasistratus, Galen and the pneuma. *Bulletin of the History of Medicine* 1959;33:293–314.

Wilder RJ, Jude JR, Kouwenhoven WB, McMahon MC. Cardiopulmonary resuscitations by trained ambulance personnel. *Journal of the American Medical Association* 1964;190:531–534.

Wislicki L. A biblical case of hypothermia—resuscitation by rewarming (Elisha's method). *Clio Medica* 1974;9:213–214.

Wright-St. Claire RE. The development of resuscitation. *New Zealand Medical Journal* 1985;98:339–341.

Young JH. Device quackery in America. *Bulletin of the History of Medicine* 1965;39:154–162.

Zoll PM. Resuscitation of the heart in ventricular standstill by external electric stimulation. *New England Journal of Medicine* 1952;247:768–771.

Zoll PM. The First Successful External Cardiac Stimulation and A-C Defibrillation. Chapter in Safar P (ed) *Advances in Cardiopulmonary Resuscitation*, New York: Springer-Verlag, 1970, pp. 281–285.

Zoll PM, Linenthal AJ, Lucas JE. Resuscitation from cardiac arrest due to digitalis by external electric stimulation. *The American Journal of Medicine* 1957;23:832–837.

Zoll PM, Linenthal AJ, Norman LR, et al. Treatment of unexpected cardiac arrest by external electric stimulation of the heart. *New England Journal of Medicine* 1956;254:541–546.

INDEX

« »